REVISED
9TH EDITION

First Aid MANUAL

Written and authorised by the UK's leading first aid providers

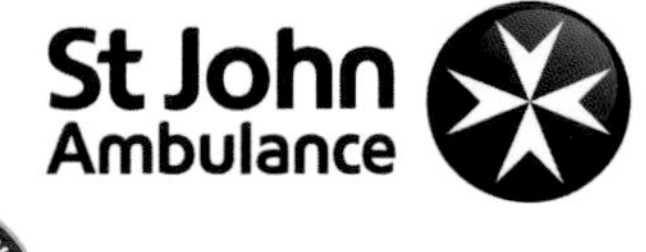

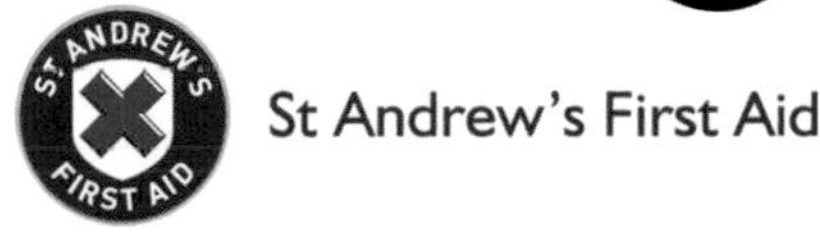

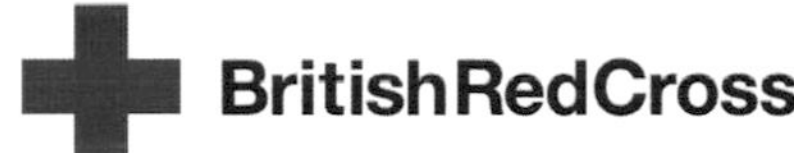

REVISED
9TH EDITION

First Aid MANUAL

The Authorised Manual of St John Ambulance, St Andrew's First Aid and the British Red Cross

ST JOHN AMBULANCE
Dr Margaret Austin LRCPI LRCSI LM
DEPUTY CHIEF MEDICAL OFFICER

ST ANDREW'S FIRST AID
Mr Rudy Crawford MBE BSc (Hons) MB ChB FRCS (Glasg) FCEM
CHAIRMAN OF THE BOARD

BRITISH RED CROSS
Dr Vivien J. Armstrong MBBS DRCOG FRCA PGCE (FE)
CHIEF MEDICAL ADVISER

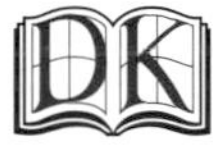

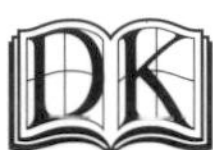

LONDON, NEW YORK, MUNICH, MELBOURNE, DELHI

St John Ambulance is a registered charity (No. 1077265/1); St Andrew's First Aid is the trading name of St Andrew's Ambulance Association, incorporated by Royal Charter 1899, is a charity registered in Scotland (No. SC006750); The British Red Cross Society, incorporated by Royal Charter 1908, is a charity registered in England and Wales (220949), and Scotland (SC037738). Each charity receives a royalty for every copy of the book sold by Dorling Kindersley. Details of the royalties payable can be obtained by writing to the publishers, Dorling Kindersley Limited, at 80 Strand, London WC2R 0RL. For the purposes of the Charities Acts no further seller of this book shall be deemed to be a commercial participator with these three Societies.

DORLING KINDERSLEY

Consultant editor Jemima Dunne
Project editor Janet Mohun, Nicola Hodgson
Production editor Jamie McNeill
Production controller Sophie Argyris
Managing editor Sarah Larter, Julie Oughton
Associate publisher Liz Wheeler
Publisher Jonathan Metcalf

Senior art editor Vicky Short
Designer Paul Drislane
Jacket designer Mark Cavanagh
Art direction for photography Bev Speight and Nigel Wright for XAB Design
Photographer Gerard Brown, Vanessa Davies
Managing art editor Michelle Baxter, Louise Dick
Art director Phil Ormerod, Bryn Walls

Text revised in line with the latest guidelines from the Resuscitation Council (UK).
Note: The masculine pronoun "he" is used when referring to the first aider or casualty, unless the individual shown in the photograph is female. This is for convenience and clarity and does not reflect a preference for either sex.

Ninth edition first published in Great Britain in 2009
This revised edition published 2011 by
Dorling Kindersley Limited, 80 Strand, London WC2R 0RL

A Penguin Company
2 4 6 8 10 9 7 5 3 1
001-179799-Apr/2011

All enquiries regarding any extracts or re-use of any material in this book should be addressed to the publishers, Dorling Kindersley Limited. A CIP catalogue record for this book is available from the British Library

ISBN: 978 1 4053 6214 6

Printed and bound in Slovakia by TBB

Discover more at
www.dk.com

THE FIRST AID SOCIETIES

Drawing on hundreds of years of combined experience, the First Aid Societies are the acknowledged experts in training and practising first aid. Each society offers distinct charitable, voluntary and training services, but all work together to raise standards in first aid. Our medical advisers have based the advice in this book on the most up-to-date research, and our training experts have presented it in a way that is both easy to learn and easy to recall.

ST JOHN AMBULANCE

As the nation's leading first aid charity, St John Ambulance believes that no one should die because they needed first aid and did not get it. This is why we teach people first aid (in schools, workplaces and the community), equipping them with the skills to be the difference between life and death. Some of the people we teach go on to become one of our 40,000 volunteers, providing first aid at events, acting as first responders to NHS emergency calls in the community, or supporting their local ambulance service.

You too can be the difference between a life lost and a life saved. To find out how, visit sja.org.uk, or call 08700 10 49 50

ST ANDREW'S FIRST AID

St Andrew's First Aid is Scotland's dedicated first aid charity and provider of first aid training, services and supplies. Our volunteers provide essential first aid services in communities across Scotland, including cover for events large and small, and teach life-saving skills to others. We also supply a full range of first aid products and training materials to first aid professionals, industry and the general public.

- Visit www.firstaid.org.uk
- Email info@firstaid.org.uk
- Call 0141 332 4031

BRITISH RED CROSS

The British Red Cross helps people in crisis worldwide. We are part of a global network of volunteers, responding to natural disasters, conflicts and individual emergencies.

The Red Cross is the world's leading first aid training provider. We train tens of thousands of people in the UK every year, building resilience within communities and preparing them to cope with all types of emergencies. We also provide first aid cover at public events and offer a wide range of first aid products.

For more information about the work of the Red Cross, training and products:

- Visit redcross.org.uk/firstaid
- Email firstaid@redcross.org.uk
- Call 0844 871 8000

CONTENTS

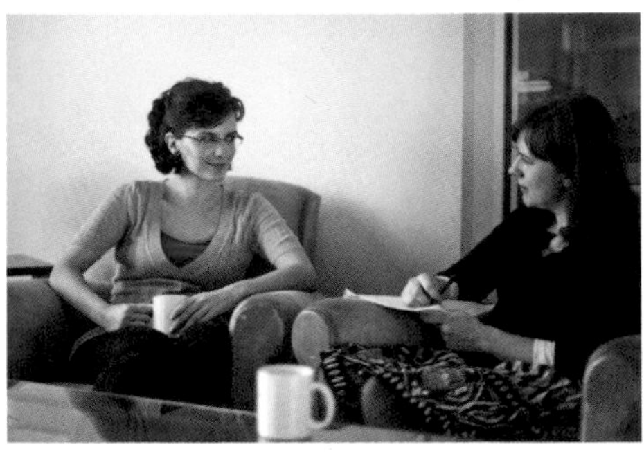

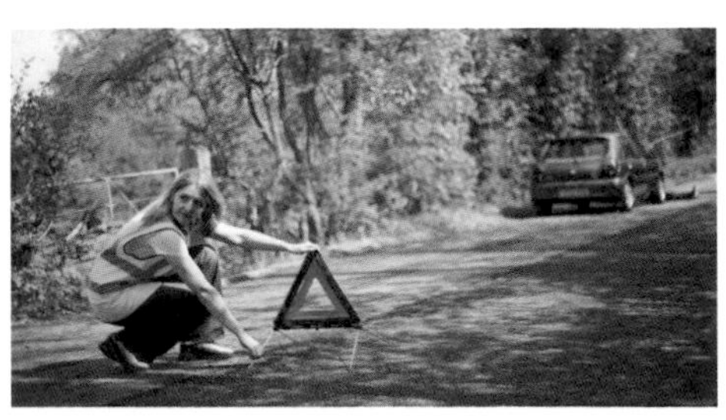

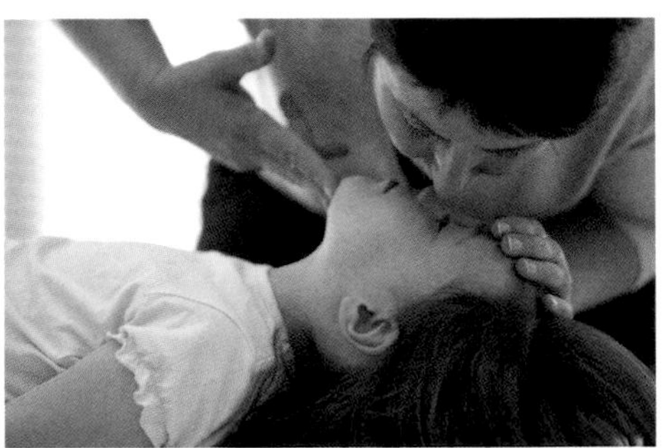

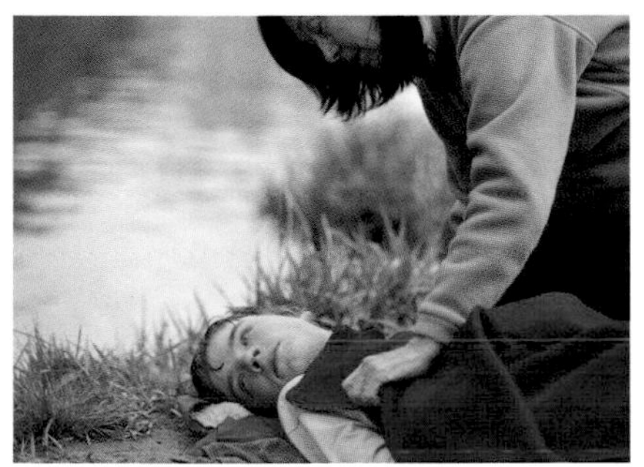

6 WOUNDS AND CIRCULATION 104

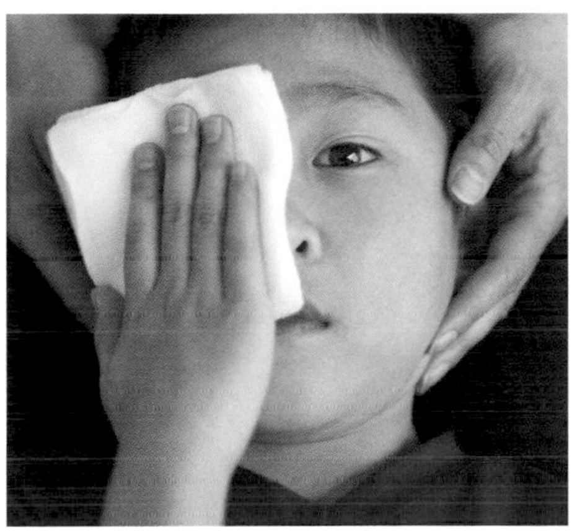

7 BONE, JOINT AND MUSCLE INJURIES 130

8 NERVOUS SYSTEM PROBLEMS 160

9 EFFECTS OF HEAT AND COLD 176

10 FOREIGN OBJECTS, POISONING, BITES & STINGS 198

INTRODUCTION

This publication, now in its revised 9th edition, is the authorised manual of the First Aid Societies – St John Ambulance, St Andrew's First Aid, and the British Red Cross. Together, they have endeavoured to ensure that this manual reflects the relevant guidance from informed authoritative sources, current at the time of publication. While the material contained here provides guidance on initial care and treatment, it must not be regarded as a substitute for medical advice.

The First Aid Societies do not accept responsibility for any claims arising from the use of this manual when the guidelines have not been followed. First aiders are advised to keep up-to-date with developments, to recognise the limits of their competence and to obtain first aid training from a qualified trainer.

The first three chapters provide background information to help you examine your role as a first aider, manage a situation safely and learn how to assess a sick or injured person effectively. Treatment for injuries and conditions is given in specific chapters that follow. Life-saving treatment for an unconscious casualty has an entire chapter. Other chapters are grouped by body system, for example *Breathing problems* or the type of injury, such as *Effects of heat and cold.*

HOW TO USE THIS BOOK

ANATOMY

The chapters are grouped by body system or cause of injury. Within the sections there are easy-to-understand anatomy features that explain the risks involved with particular injuries or conditions and how and why first aid can help.

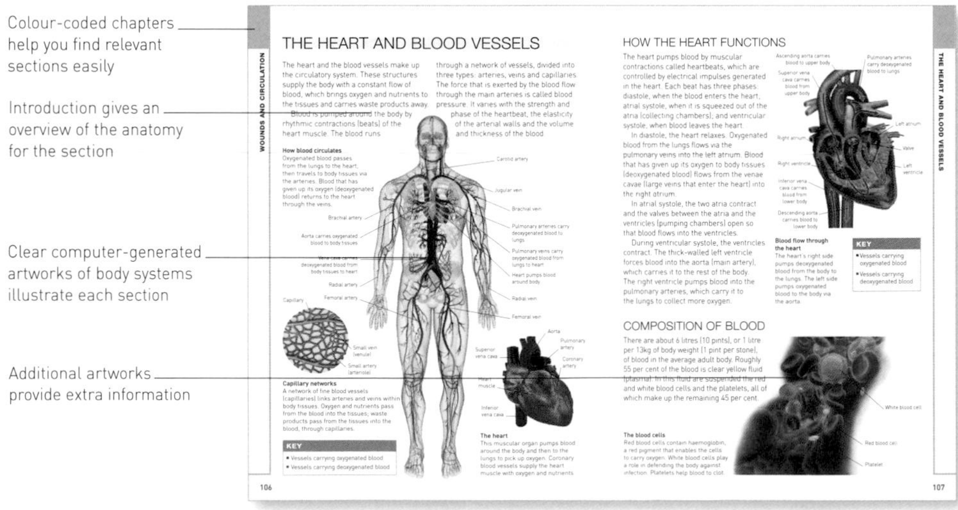

WOUNDS AND CIRCULATION

THE HEART AND BLOOD VESSELS

The heart and the blood vessels make up the circulatory system. These structures supply the body with a constant flow of blood, which brings oxygen and nutrients to the tissues and carries waste products away.

Blood is pumped around the body by rhythmic contractions (beats) of the heart muscle. The blood runs through a network of vessels, divided into three types: arteries, veins and capillaries. The force that is exerted by the blood flow through the main arteries is called blood pressure. It varies with the strength and phase of the heartbeat, the elasticity of the arterial walls and the volume and thickness of the blood.

How blood circulates
Oxygenated blood passes from the lungs to the heart, then travels to body tissues via the arteries. Blood that has given up its oxygen (deoxygenated blood) returns to the heart through the veins.

Carotid artery
Jugular vein
Brachial vein
Brachial artery
Pulmonary arteries carry deoxygenated blood to lungs
Aorta carries oxygenated blood to body tissues
Pulmonary veins carry oxygenated blood from lungs to heart
Vena cava carries deoxygenated blood from body tissues to heart
Heart pumps blood around body
Radial artery
Radial vein
Capillary
Femoral artery
Femoral vein
Small vein (venule)
Small artery (arteriole)
Aorta
Pulmonary artery
Superior vena cava
Coronary artery
Heart muscle
Inferior vena cava

Capillary networks
A network of fine blood vessels (capillaries) links arteries and veins within body tissues. Oxygen and nutrients pass from the blood into the tissues; waste products pass from the tissues into the blood, through capillaries.

KEY
- Vessels carrying oxygenated blood
- Vessels carrying deoxygenated blood

The heart
This muscular organ pumps blood around the body and then to the lungs to pick up oxygen. Coronary blood vessels supply the heart muscle with oxygen and nutrients.

106

HOW THE HEART FUNCTIONS

The heart pumps blood by muscular contractions called heartbeats, which are controlled by electrical impulses generated in the heart. Each beat has three phases: diastole, when the blood enters the heart; atrial systole, when it is squeezed out of the atria (collecting chambers); and ventricular systole, when blood leaves the heart.

In diastole, the heart relaxes. Oxygenated blood from the lungs flows via the pulmonary veins into the left atrium. Blood that has given up its oxygen to body tissues (deoxygenated blood) flows from the venae cavae (large veins that enter the heart) into the right atrium.

In atrial systole, the two atria contract and the valves between the atria and the ventricles (pumping chambers) open so that blood flows into the ventricles.

During ventricular systole, the ventricles contract. The thick-walled left ventricle forces blood into the aorta (main artery), which carries it to the rest of the body. The right ventricle pumps blood into the pulmonary arteries, which carry it to the lungs to collect more oxygen.

Ascending aorta carries blood to upper body
Pulmonary arteries carry deoxygenated blood to lungs
Superior vena cava carries blood from upper body
Left atrium
Right atrium
Valve
Right ventricle
Left ventricle
Inferior vena cava carries blood from lower body
Descending aorta carries blood to lower body

Blood flow through the heart
The heart's right side pumps deoxygenated blood from the body to the lungs. The left side pumps oxygenated blood to the body via the aorta.

KEY
- Vessels carrying oxygenated blood
- Vessels carrying deoxygenated blood

COMPOSITION OF BLOOD

There are about 6 litres (10 pints), or 1 litre per 13kg of body weight (1 pint per stone), of blood in the average adult body. Roughly 55 per cent of the blood is clear yellow fluid (plasma). In this fluid are suspended the red and white blood cells and the platelets, all of which make up the remaining 45 per cent.

White blood cell
Red blood cell
Platelet

The blood cells
Red blood cells contain haemoglobin, a red pigment that enables the cells to carry oxygen. White blood cells play a role in defending the body against infection. Platelets help blood to clot.

THE HEART AND BLOOD VESSELS

107

CONDITIONS AND INJURIES

The main part of the book features eight colour-coded chapters outlining first aid for over 110 conditions or injuries. For each one, an introduction describes the risks and likely cause, together with clear step-by-step instructions.

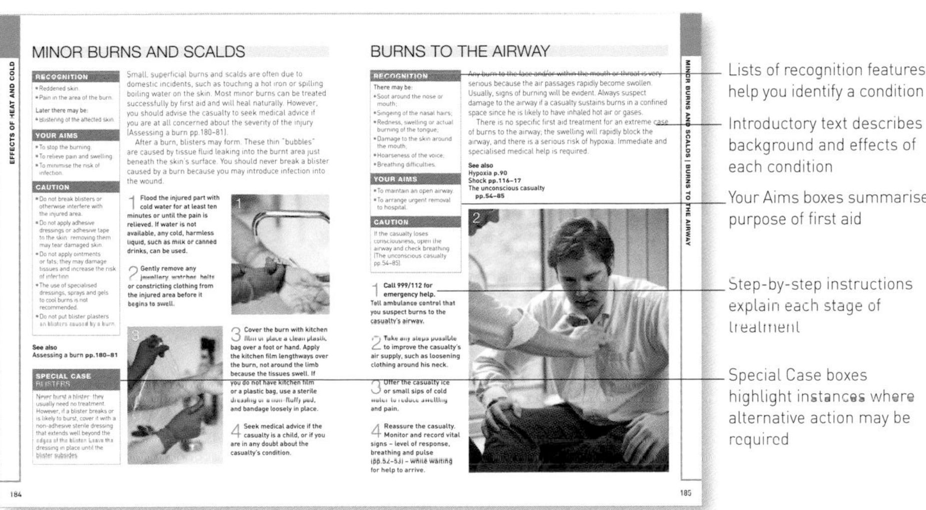

EFFECTS OF HEAT AND COLD

MINOR BURNS AND SCALDS

RECOGNITION

- Reddened skin.
- Pain in the area of the burn.

Later there may be:

- Blistering of the affected skin.

YOUR AIMS

- To stop the burning.
- To relieve pain and swelling.
- To minimise the risk of infection.

CAUTION

- Do not break blisters or otherwise interfere with the injured area.
- Do not apply adhesive dressings or adhesive tape to the skin: removing them may tear damaged skin.
- Do not apply ointments or fats; they may damage tissues and increase the risk of infection.
- The use of specialised dressings, sprays and gels to cool burns is not recommended.
- Do not put blister plasters on blisters caused by a burn.

See also
Assessing a burn pp.180–81

SPECIAL CASE
BLISTERS

Never burst a blister: they usually need no treatment. However, if a blister breaks or is likely to burst, cover it with a non-adhesive sterile dressing that extends well beyond the edges of the blister. Leave the dressing in place until the blister subsides.

Small, superficial burns and scalds are often due to domestic incidents, such as touching a hot iron or spilling boiling water on the skin. Most minor burns can be treated successfully by first aid and will heal naturally. However, you should advise the casualty to seek medical advice if you are at all concerned about the severity of the injury (Assessing a burn pp.180–81).

After a burn, blisters may form. These thin "bubbles" are caused by tissue fluid leaking into the burnt area just beneath the skin's surface. You should never break a blister caused by a burn because you may introduce infection into the wound.

1 **Flood the injured part with cold water for at least ten minutes or until the pain is relieved. If water is not available, any cold, harmless liquid, such as milk or canned drinks, can be used.**

2 **Gently remove any jewellery, watches, belts or constricting clothing from the injured area before it begins to swell.**

3 **Cover the burn with kitchen film or place a clean plastic bag over a foot or hand. Apply the kitchen film lengthways over the burn, not around the limb because the tissues swell. If you do not have kitchen film or a plastic bag, use a sterile dressing or a non-fluffy pad, and bandage loosely in place.**

4 **Seek medical advice if the casualty is a child, or if you are in any doubt about the casualty's condition.**

184

BURNS TO THE AIRWAY

RECOGNITION

There may be:

- Soot around the nose or mouth;
- Singeing of the nasal hairs;
- Redness, swelling or actual burning of the tongue;
- Damage to the skin around the mouth;
- Hoarseness of the voice;
- Breathing difficulties.

YOUR AIMS

- To maintain an open airway.
- To arrange urgent removal to hospital.

CAUTION

If the casualty loses consciousness, open the airway and check breathing (The unconscious casualty pp.54–85).

Any burn to the face and/or within the mouth or throat is very serious because the air passages rapidly become swollen. Usually, signs of burning will be evident. Always suspect damage to the airway if a casualty sustains burns in a confined space since he is likely to have inhaled hot air or gases.

There is no specific first aid treatment for an extreme case of burns to the airway; the swelling will rapidly block the airway, and there is a serious risk of hypoxia. Immediate and specialised medical help is required.

See also
Hypoxia p.90
Shock pp.116–17
The unconscious casualty pp.54–85

1 **Call 999/112 for emergency help. Tell ambulance control that you suspect burns to the casualty's airway.**

2 **Take any steps possible to improve the casualty's air supply, such as loosening clothing around his neck.**

3 **Offer the casualty ice or small sips of cold water to reduce swelling and pain.**

4 **Reassure the casualty. Monitor and record vital signs – level of response, breathing and pulse (pp.52–53) – while waiting for help to arrive.**

MINOR BURNS AND SCALDS | BURNS TO THE AIRWAY

185

Lists of recognition features help you identify a condition

Introductory text describes background and effects of each condition

Your Aims boxes summarise purpose of first aid

Step-by-step instructions explain each stage of treatment

Special Case boxes highlight instances where alternative action may be required

EMERGENCY ADVICE

At the back of the manual is a quick-reference emergency section that provides additional at-a-glance action plans for potentially life-threatening injuries and conditions from unconsciousness and bleeding to asthma and heart attack.

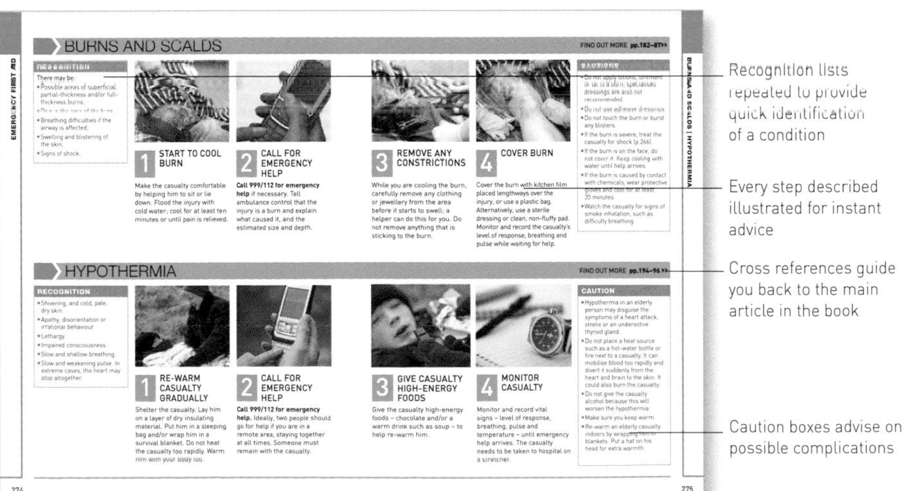

EMERGENCY FIRST AID

BURNS AND SCALDS

FIND OUT MORE pp.182–87>>

RECOGNITION

There may be:

- Possible areas of superficial, partial-thickness and/or full-thickness burns;
- Pain in the area of the burn;
- Breathing difficulties if the airway is affected;
- Swelling and blistering of the skin;
- Signs of shock.

1 START TO COOL BURN

Make the casualty comfortable by helping him to sit or lie down. Flood the injury with cold water; cool for at least ten minutes or until pain is relieved.

2 CALL FOR EMERGENCY HELP

Call 999/112 for emergency help if necessary. Tell ambulance control that the injury is a burn and explain what caused it, and the estimated size and depth.

3 REMOVE ANY CONSTRICTIONS

While you are cooling the burn, carefully remove any clothing or jewellery from the area before it starts to swell; a helper can do this for you. Do not remove anything that is sticking to the burn.

4 COVER BURN

Cover the burn with kitchen film placed lengthways over the injury, or use a plastic bag. Alternatively, use a sterile dressing or clean, non-fluffy pad. Monitor and record the casualty's level of response, breathing and pulse while waiting for help.

CAUTION

- Do not apply lotions, ointment or fat to a burn; specialised dressings are also not recommended.
- Do not use adhesive dressings.
- Do not touch the burn or burst any blisters.
- If the burn is severe, treat the casualty for shock (p.266).
- If the burn is on the face, do not cover it. Keep cooling with water until help arrives.
- If the burn is caused by contact with chemicals, wear protective gloves and cool for at least 20 minutes.
- Watch the casualty for signs of smoke inhalation, such as difficulty breathing.

HYPOTHERMIA

FIND OUT MORE pp.194–96>>

RECOGNITION

- Shivering, and cold, pale, dry skin.
- Apathy, disorientation or irrational behaviour.
- Lethargy.
- Impaired consciousness.
- Slow and shallow breathing.
- Slow and weakening pulse. In extreme cases, the heart may stop altogether.

1 RE-WARM CASUALTY GRADUALLY

Shelter the casualty. Lay him on a layer of dry insulating material. Put him in a sleeping bag and/or wrap him in a survival blanket. Do not heat the casualty too rapidly. Warm him with your body too.

2 CALL FOR EMERGENCY HELP

Call 999/112 for emergency help. Ideally, two people should go for help if you are in a remote area, staying together at all times. Someone must remain with the casualty.

3 GIVE CASUALTY HIGH-ENERGY FOODS

Give the casualty high-energy foods – chocolate and/or a warm drink such as soup – to help re-warm him.

4 MONITOR CASUALTY

Monitor and record vital signs – level of response, breathing, pulse and temperature – until emergency help arrives. The casualty needs to be taken to hospital on a stretcher.

CAUTION

- Hypothermia in an elderly person may disguise the symptoms of a heart attack, stroke or an underactive thyroid gland.
- Do not place a heat source such as a hot-water bottle or fire next to a casualty. It can mobilise blood too rapidly and divert it suddenly from the heart and brain to the skin. It could also burn the casualty.
- Do not give the casualty alcohol because this will worsen the hypothermia.
- Make sure you keep warm.
- Re-warm an elderly casualty indoors by wrapping him in blankets. Put a hat on his head for extra warmth.

274

BURNS AND SCALDS | HYPOTHERMIA

275

Recognition lists repeated to provide quick identification of a condition

Every step described illustrated for instant advice

Cross references guide you back to the main article in the book

Caution boxes advise on possible complications

1

First aid is the initial assistance or treatment given to a person who is injured or suddenly taken ill. The person who provides this help is a first aider. This chapter prepares you for being a first aider, psychologically and emotionally, as well as giving practical advice on what you should and should not do in an emergency situation.

The information provided throughout this book will help you to provide effective first aid to any casualty in any situation. However, to become a fully competent first aider, you should complete a recognised first aid course. Completing a course will also strengthen your skills and increase your confidence. St John Ambulance, St Andrew's First Aid, and the British Red Cross are all able to provide first aid education tailored to your needs.

AIMS AND OBJECTIVES

- To understand your own abilities and limitations.
- To stay safe and calm at all times.
- To assess a situation quickly and calmly and summon the appropriate help.
- To assist the casualty and provide the necessary treatment, with the help of those around where necessary.
- To pass on relevant information to the emergency services, or the person who takes responsibility for the casualty.
- To be aware of your own needs.

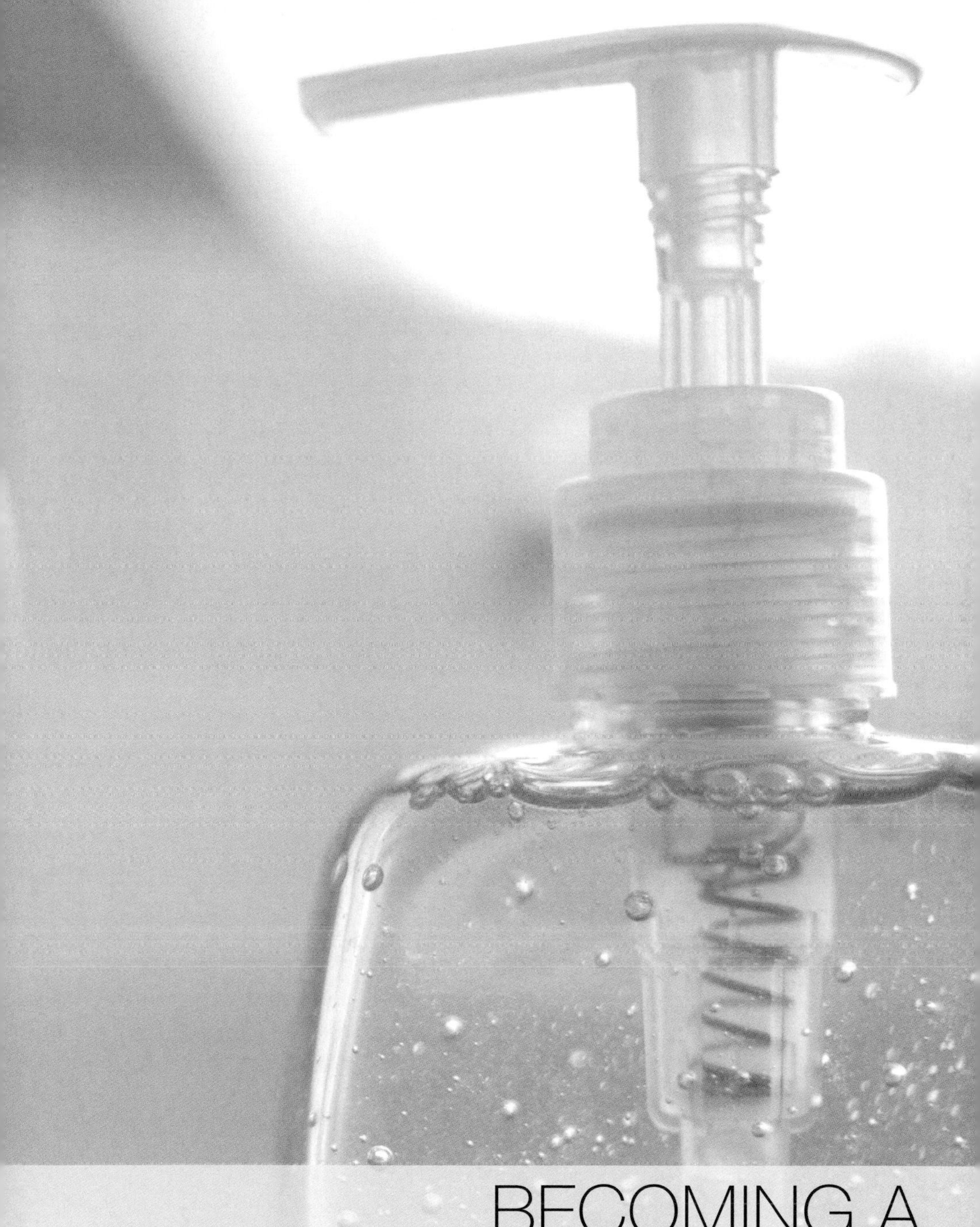

BECOMING A FIRST AIDER

WHAT IS A FIRST AIDER?

First aid refers to the actions taken in response to someone who is injured or suddenly taken ill. A first aider is a person who takes this action while taking care to keep everyone involved safe (p.28) and to cause no further harm while doing so.

Follow the actions that most benefit the casualty, taking into account your own skills, knowledge and experience, using the guidelines set out in this book.

This chapter prepares you for the role of first aider by providing guidance on responding to a first aid situation and assessing the priorities for the casualty. There is advice on the psychological aspect of giving first aid and practical guidance on how to protect yourself and a casualty. Chapter 2, Managing an Incident (pp.26–37), provides guidelines on dealing with events (traffic or water incidents or fires, for example). Chapter 3, Assessing a Casualty (pp.38–53), looks at the practical steps to take when assessing a sick or injured person's condition.

One of the primary rules of first aid is to ensure that an area is safe for you before you approach a casualty (p.28). Do not attempt heroic rescues in hazardous circumstances. If you put yourself at risk, you are unlikely to be able to help casualties and could become one yourself and cause harm to others. If it is not safe, do not approach the casualty, but call for emergency help.

FIRST AID PRIORITIES

- **Assess a situation** quickly and calmly.
- **Protect yourself** and any casualties from danger – never put yourself at risk (p.28).
- **Prevent cross infection** between yourself and the casualty as far as possible (p.16).
- **Comfort and reassure** casualties at all times.
- **Assess the casualty:** identify, as far as you can, the injury or nature of illness affecting a casualty (pp.38–53).
- **Give early treatment,** and treat the casualties with the most serious (life-threatening) conditions first.
- **Arrange for appropriate help:** call 999/112 for emergency help if you suspect serious injury or illness; take or send the casualty to hospital; transfer him into the care of a healthcare professional or to his home. Stay with a casualty until care is available.

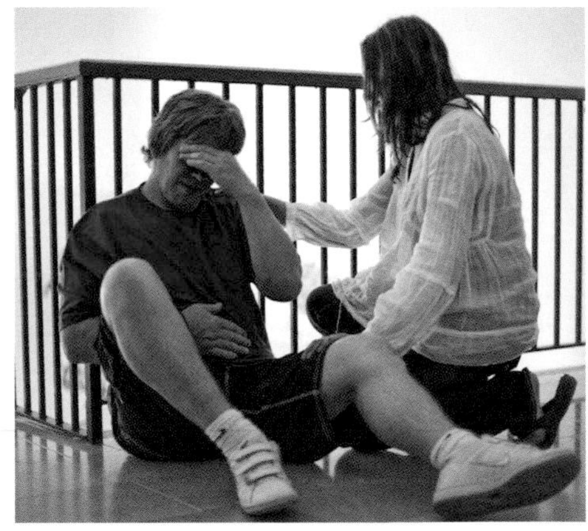

ASSESSING AN INCIDENT
When you come across an incident stay calm and support the casualty. Ask him what has happened. Try not to move the casualty; if possible, treat him in the position you find him.

HOW TO PREPARE YOURSELF

When responding to an emergency you should recognise both the emotional and physical needs of all involved, including your own. You should look after your own psychological health and be able to recognise stress if it develops (pp.24–25).

A calm, considerate response from you that facilitates trust and respect from those around you is fundamental to you being able to give or receive information from a casualty or witnesses effectively. This includes being aware of, and managing, your reactions, so that you can focus on the casualty and make an assessment. By talking to a casualty in a kind, considerate, gentle but firm manner, you will inspire confidence in your actions and this will generate trust between you and the casualty. Without this confidence he may not tell you about an important event, injury or symptom, and may remain in a highly distressed state.

The actions described in this chapter aim to help you facilitate this trust, minimise distress and provide support to promote the casualty's ability to cope and recover. The key steps to being an effective first aider are:

- **Be calm** in your approach;
- **Be aware of risks** (to yourself and others);
- **Build and maintain trust** (from the casualty and the bystanders);
- **Give early treatment,** treating the most serious (life-threatening) conditions first;
- **Call appropriate help;**
- **Remember your own needs.**

BE CALM

It is important to be calm in your approach. Consider what situations might challenge you, and how you would deal with them. In order to convey confidence to others and encourage them to trust you, you need to control your emotions and reactions.

People often fear the unknown. Becoming more familiar with first aid priorities and the key techniques in this book can help you feel more comfortable. By identifying your fears in advance, you can take steps to overcome them. Find out as much as you can, for example, by going on a first aid course, asking others how they dealt with similar situations or talking your fears through with a person you trust.

STAY IN CONTROL

In an emergency situation, the body responds by releasing hormones that may cause a "fight, flight or freeze" response. When this happens, your heart beats faster, your breathing quickens and you may sweat more. You may also feel more alert, want to run away or feel frozen to the spot.

If you feel overwhelmed and slightly panicky, you may feel pressured to do something before you are clear about what is needed. Pause and take a few slow breaths. Consider who else might help you feel calmer, and remind yourself of the first aid priorities (opposite). If you still feel overwhelmed, take another breath and say to yourself "be calmer" as a cue. When you are calm, you will be better able to think more clearly and plan your response.

The thoughts you have are linked to the way you behave and the way you feel. If you think that you cannot cope, you will have more trouble working out what to do and will feel more anxious: more ready to fight, flee or freeze. If you know how to calm yourself, you will be better able to deal with your anxiety and so help the casualty.

PROTECTION FROM INFECTION

When you give first aid, it is important to protect yourself (and the casualty) from infection as well as injury. Take steps to avoid cross infection – transmitting germs or infection to a casualty or contracting infection yourself from a casualty. Remember, infection is a risk even with relatively minor injuries. It is a particular concern if you are treating a wound, because blood-borne viruses, such as hepatitis B or C and Human Immunodeficiency Virus (HIV), may be transmitted by contact with body fluids. This risk increases if an infected person's blood makes contact with yours through a cut or graze.

Usually, taking measures such as washing your hands and wearing disposable gloves will provide sufficient protection for you and the casualty. There is no known evidence of these blood-borne viruses being transmitted during resuscitation. If a face shield or pocket mask is available, it should be used when you give rescue breaths (pp.68–69 and pp.76–77).

WHEN TO SEEK MEDICAL ADVICE

Take care not to prick yourself with any needle found on or near a casualty, or cut yourself on glass. If you accidentally prick or cut your skin, or splash your eye, wash the area thoroughly and seek medical help immediately. If you are providing first aid on a regular basis, it is advisable to seek guidance on additional personal protection, such as immunisation. If you think you have been exposed to an infection while giving first aid, seek medical advice as soon as possible.

MINIMISING THE RISK OF CROSS INFECTION

- **Do** wash your hands and wear latex-free disposable gloves. If gloves are not available, ask the casualty to dress his or her own wound, or enclose your hands in clean plastic bags.
- **Do** cover cuts and grazes on your hands with waterproof dressings.
- **Do** wear a plastic apron if dealing with large quantities of body fluids and wear plastic glasses to protect your eyes.
- **Do** dispose of all waste safely (p.18).
- **Do not** touch a wound with your bare hands and do not touch any part of a dressing that will come into contact with a wound.
- **Do not** breathe, cough or sneeze over a wound while you are treating a casualty.

CAUTION

To help protect yourself from infection you can carry protective equipment such as:

- Pocket mask or face shield;
- Latex-free disposable gloves;
- Alcohol gel to clean your hands.

THOROUGH HAND WASHING

If you can, wash your hands before you touch a casualty, but if this is not possible, wash them as soon as possible afterwards. For a thorough wash, pay attention to all parts of the hands – palms, wrists, fingers, thumbs and fingernails. Use soap and water if available, or rub your hands with alcohol gel.

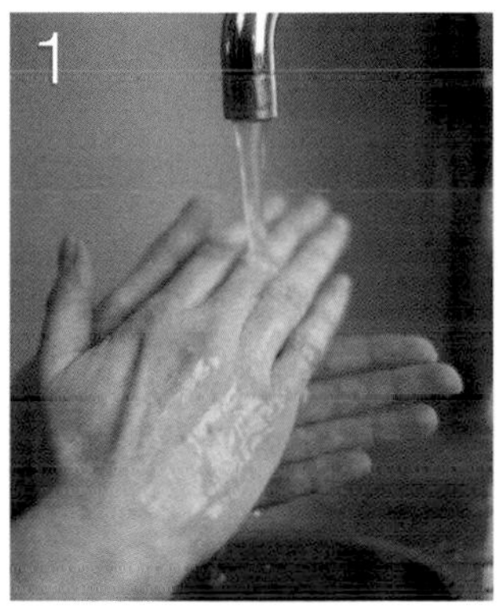

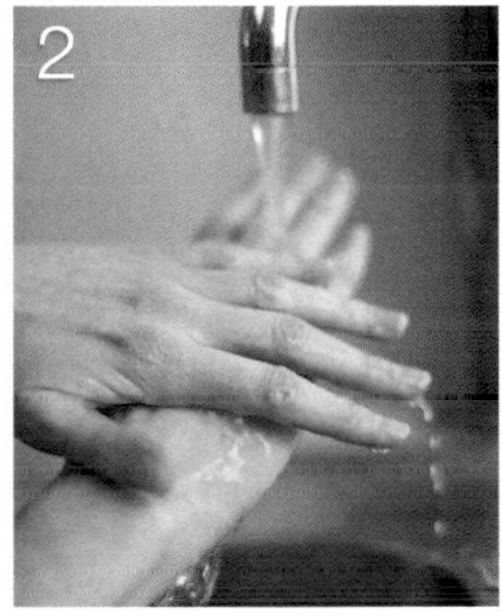

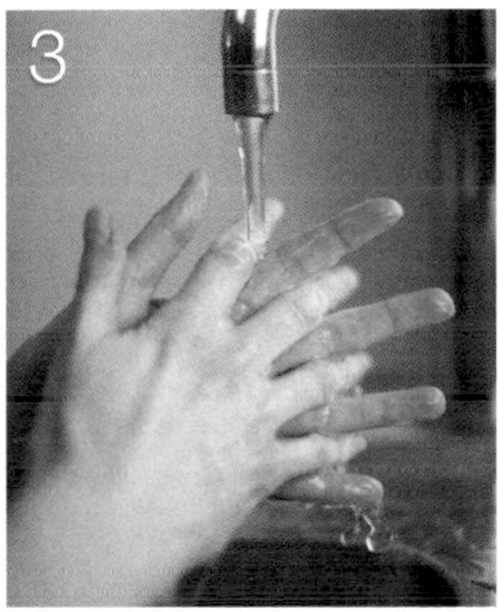

1 Wet your hands under running water. Put some soap into the palm of a cupped hand. Rub the palms of your hands together.

2 Rub the palm of your left hand against the back of your right hand, then rub the right palm on the back of your left hand.

3 Interlock the fingers of both hands and work the soap between them.

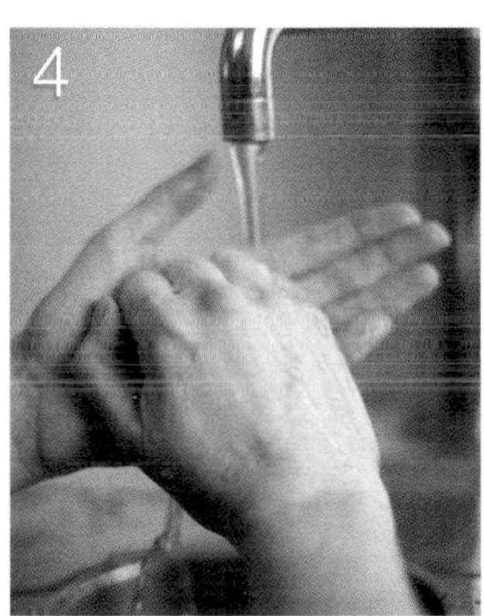

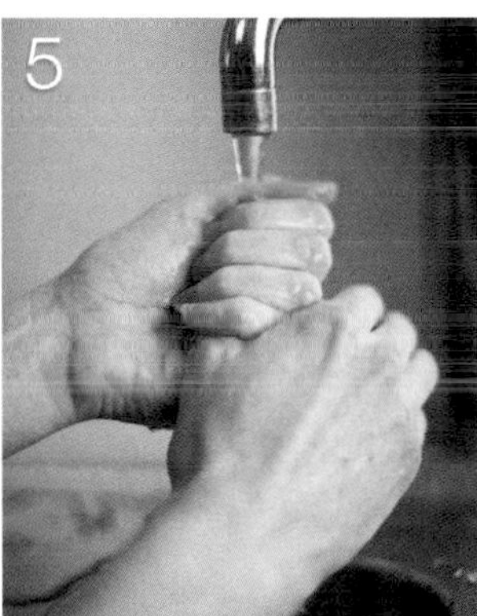

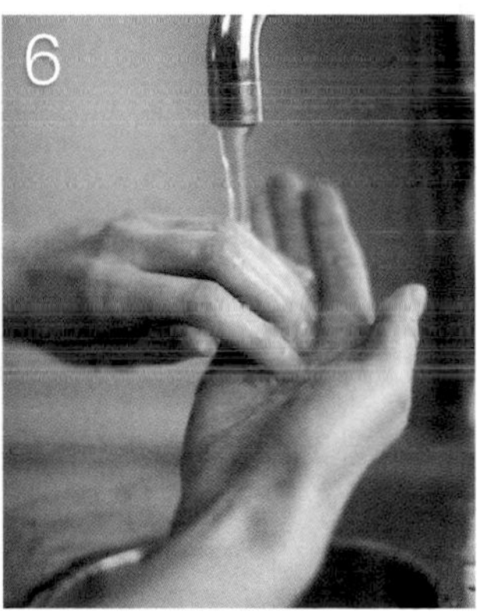

4 Rub the back of the fingers of your right hand against the palm of your left hand, then repeat with your left hand in your right palm.

5 Rub your right thumb in the palm of your left hand, then your left thumb in the right palm.

6 Rub the fingertips of your left hand in the palm of your right hand and vice versa. Rinse thoroughly, then pat dry with a disposable paper towel.

PROTECTION FROM INFECTION (continued)

USING PROTECTIVE GLOVES

In addition to hand washing, gloves give added protection against infection in a first aid situation. If possible, carry protective, disposable, latex-free gloves with you at all times. Wear them whenever there is a likelihood of contact with blood or other body fluids. If in doubt, wear them anyway.

Disposable gloves should only be used to treat one casualty. Put them on just before you approach a casualty and remove them as soon as the treatment is completed and before you do anything else.

When taking off the gloves, hold the top edge of one glove with your other gloved hand and peel it off so that it is inside out. Repeat with the other hand without touching the outside of the gloves. Dispose of them in a biohazard bag (below).

CAUTION

Always use latex-free gloves. Some people have a serious allergy to latex, and this may cause anaphylactic shock (p.221). Nitrile gloves (often blue or purple) are recommended.

PUTTING ON GLOVES

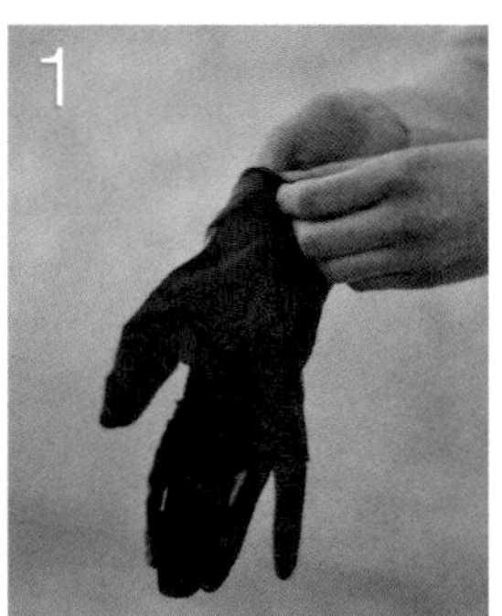

1 Ideally, wash your hands before putting on the gloves. Hold one glove by the top and pull it on. Do not touch the main part of the glove with your fingers.

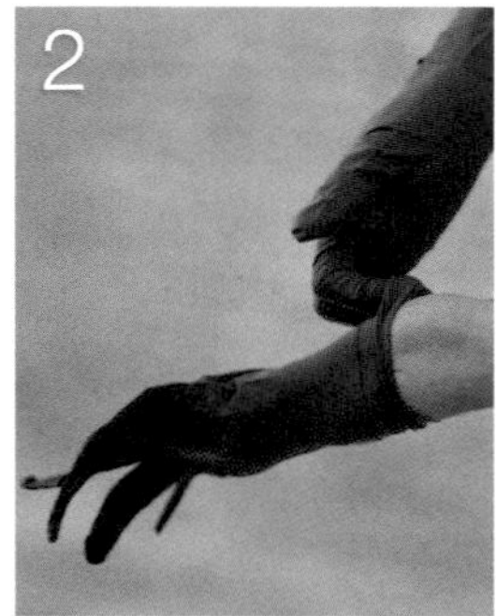

2 Pick up the second glove with the gloved hand. With your fingers under the top edge, pull it on to your hand. Your gloved fingers should not touch your skin.

DEALING WITH WASTE

Once you have treated a casualty, all soiled material must be disposed of carefully to prevent the spread of infection.

Place items such as dressings or gloves in a plastic bag – ideally a biohazard bag – and destroy it by burning (incineration), or ask the attending emergency service how to deal with this type of waste. Seal the bag tightly and label it to show that it contains clinical waste. Put sharp objects, such as needles, in a plastic container called a sharps container, which is usually yellow.

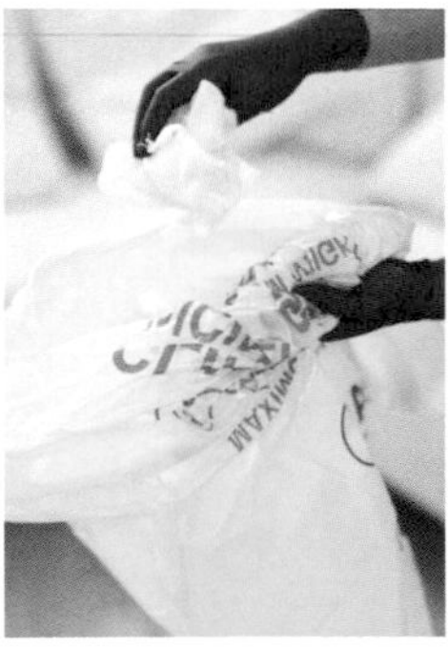

BIOHAZARD BAG

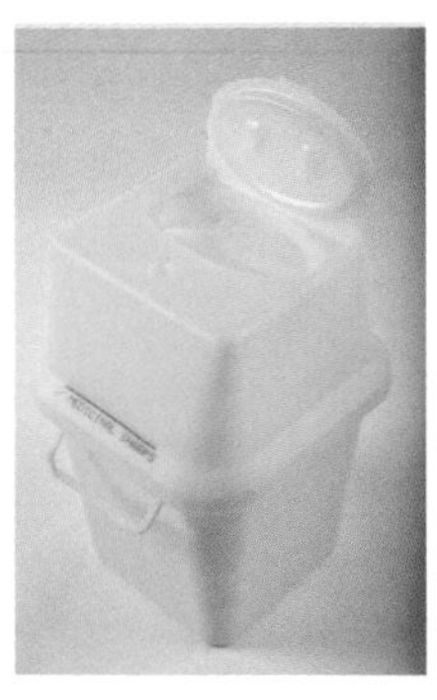

SHARPS CONTAINER

DEALING WITH A CASUALTY

Casualties are often frightened or become frightened because of what has just happened to them, their fears of what may happen next and of the pain and/or bleeding they are experiencing. Your role is to stay calm and take charge of the situation. However, be ready to stand back if someone better qualified is present to assist. If there is more than one casualty, assess each one using the primary survey (pp.44–45) and treat the most seriously injured casualty first.

BUILDING TRUST

Establish trust with your casualty by introducing yourself. Find out what the person likes to be called, and use his name each time you talk to him. Crouch or kneel down to the same height as the casualty. Explain what is happening and why. You will inspire trust if you say what you are doing before you do it. Treat the casualty with dignity and respect at all times. If possible, give him choices, for example, whether he would prefer to sit or lie down and/or who he would like to have with him.

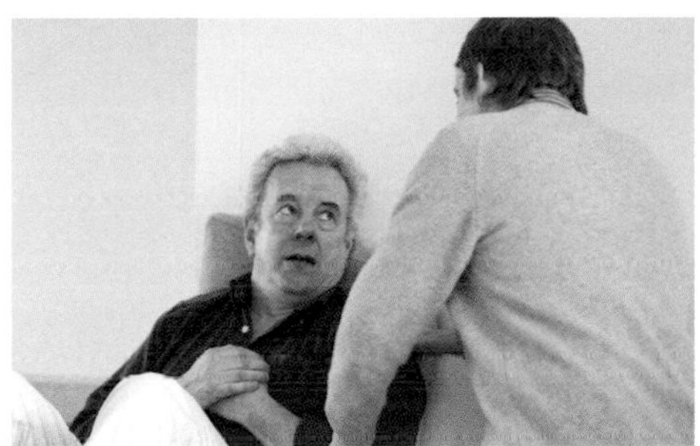

REASSURE THE CASUALTY
When treating a casualty, remain calm and do not do anything without explanation. Try to answer any questions he may have honestly.

DIVERSITY AND COMMUNICATION

Consider the age and appearance of your casualty when you talk to him, since different people need different responses. Respect people's wishes; accept that someone might want to be treated in a particular way. Communication can be difficult if a person speaks a different language or cannot hear you. Use simple language or signs or write questions down. Ask if anyone speaks the same language or knows the person or saw the incident and can describe what happened.

SPECIAL CASE TREATING CHILDREN

You will need to use simpler, shorter words when talking to children. If possible, make sure a child's parents or caregivers are with him, and keep them involved at all times. It is important to establish the carer's trust as well as the child's. Talk first to the parent/carer and get his or her permission to continue. Once the parent/carer trusts you, the child will also feel more confident.

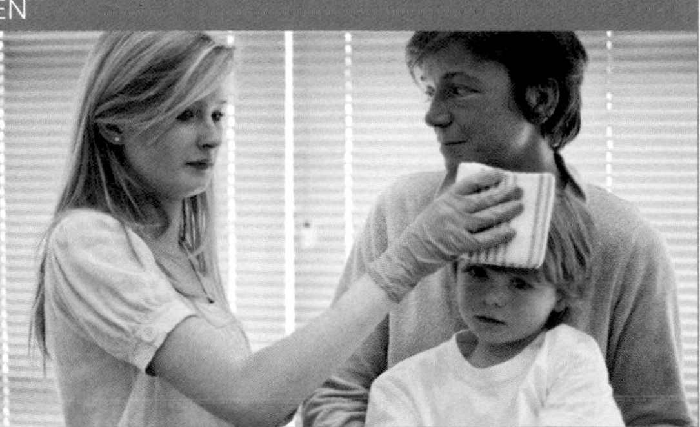

DEALING WITH A CASUALTY (continued)

LISTEN CAREFULLY

Use your eyes and ears to be aware of how a casualty responds. Listen by showing verbal and non-verbal listening skills.

- **Make eye contact,** but look away now and then so as not to stare.
- **Use a calm, confident voice** that is loud enough to be heard but do not shout.
- **Do not speak too quickly.**
- **Keep instructions simple:** use short sentences and simple words.
- **Use affirming nods** and "mmms" to show you are listening when the casualty speaks.
- **Check that the casualty understands** what you mean – ask to make sure.
- **Use simple hand gestures** and movements.
- **Do not interrupt the casualty,** but always acknowledge what you are told; for example, by summarising what a casualty has told you to show that you understand.

WHEN A CASUALTY RESISTS HELP

If someone is ill or injured he may be upset, confused, tearful, angry and/or keen to get away. Be sensitive to a casualty's feelings; let him know that his reactions are understandable. Also accept that you may not be able to help, or might even be seen as a threat. Stay at a safe distance until you have gained the person's permission to move closer, so that he does not feel crowded. Do not argue or disagree. A casualty may refuse help for example because he is suffering from a head injury or hypothermia. If you think a person needs something other than what he asks for, explain why. For example, you could say, "I think someone should look at where you're hurt before you move, in case moving makes it worse." If someone still refuses your help and you think they need urgent medical attention, call 999/112 for emergency help. A casualty has the right to refuse help, even if it causes further harm. Tell ambulance control that you have offered first aid and been refused. If you are worried that a person's condition is deteriorating, observe from a distance until help arrives.

TREATING THE CASUALTY

When treating a casualty, always relate to him calmly and thoughtfully to maintain trust. Think about how he might be feeling. Check that you have understood what the casualty said and consider the impact of your actions, for example, is the casualty becoming more (or less) upset, angry and tense? A change in emotional state can indicate that a condition is worsening.

Be prepared to change your manner, depending on what a person feels comfortable with; for example, ask fewer questions or talk about something else. Keep a casualty updated and give him options rather than telling him what to do. Ask the casualty about his next-of-kin or friends who can help, and help him to make contact with them. Ask if you can help to make arrangements so that any responsibilities the casualty may have can be taken care of.

Stay with the casualty. Do not leave someone who may be dying, seriously ill or badly injured alone except to go to call for emergency help. Talk to the casualty while touching his shoulder or arm, or holding a hand. Never allow a casualty to feel alone.

ENLISTING HELP FROM OTHERS

In an emergency situation you may be faced with several tasks at once: to maintain safety, to call for help and to start giving first aid. Some of the people at the scene may be able to help you do the following.

- **Make the area safe;** for example, control traffic and keep onlookers away.
- **Call 999/112 for emergency help** (p.23).
- **Fetch first aid equipment,** for example an automated external defibrillator (AED).
- **Control bleeding** with direct pressure, or support an injured limb.
- **Help maintain the casualty's privacy** by holding a blanket around the scene and encouraging onlookers to move away.
- **Transport the casualty** to a safe place if his life is in immediate danger, only if it is safer to move him than to leave him where he is, and you have the necessary help and equipment (p.234).

The reactions of bystanders may cause you concern or anger. They may have had no first aid training and feel helpless or frightened themselves. If they have seen or been involved in the incident, they too may be injured and distressed. Bear this in mind if you need to ask a bystander to help you. Talk to people in a firm but gentle manner. By staying calm yourself, you will gain their trust and help them remain calm too.

CARE OF PERSONAL BELONGINGS

Make sure the casualty's belongings are with them at all times. If you have to search belongings for identification or clues to a person's condition (medication, for example), do so in front of a reliable witness. If possible, ask the casualty's permission before you do this. Afterwards, ensure that all of the clothing and personal belongings accompany the casualty to hospital or are handed over to the police.

KEEPING NOTES

As you gather information about a casualty, write it down so that you can refer to it later. A written record of the timing of events is particularly valuable to medical personnel. Note, for example, the length of a period of unconsciousness, the duration of a seizure, the time of any changes in the casualty's condition, and the time of any intervention or treatment. Hand your notes to the emergency services when they arrive, or give them to the casualty. Useful information to provide includes:

- **Casualty's details,** including his name, age and contact details;
- **History** of the incident or illness;
- **Brief description** of any injuries;
- **Unusual behaviour,** or a change in behaviour;
- **Treatment** – where given, and when;
- **Vital signs** – level of response, breathing rate and pulse (pp.52–53);
- **Medical history;**
- **Medication** the casualty has taken, with details of the amounts taken and when;
- **Next-of-kin contact details;**
- **Your contact details** as well as the date, time and place of your involvement.

Remember that any information you gather is confidential. Never share it with anyone not involved in the casualty's care without his agreement. Let the casualty know why you are recording information and who you will give it to. When you are asking for such information, be sensitive to who is around and of the casualty's privacy and dignity.

REQUESTING HELP

Further help is available from a range of sources. If help is needed, you must decide both on the type of help and how to access it. First, carry out a primary survey (pp.44–45) to ascertain the severity of the casualty's condition. If it is not serious, explain the options and allow him to choose where to go. If a casualty's condition is serious, seek emergency help. Throughout the book there are guidelines for choosing appropriate level of help.

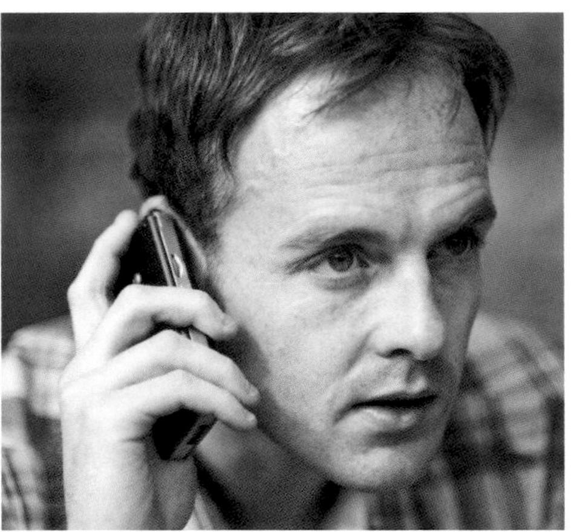

- **Call 999/112 for emergency help** if the casualty needs urgent medical attention and should be transported to hospital in an ambulance; for example, when you suspect a heart attack.
- **Take or send the casualty** to hospital. Choose this option when a casualty needs hospital treatment, but his condition is unlikely to worsen; for example, with a finger injury. You can take him yourself if you can arrange transport – either in your own car or in a taxi.
- **Seek medical advice.** Depending on what is available in his area, the casualty should be advised to call his own doctor's surgery, NHS walk-in centre or NHS advice line. He would do this, for example, when he has symptoms such as earache or diarrhoea.

CALLING FOR HELP
Use your mobile phone to call for help. Stay calm, be clear and concise, and give as much detail as possible.

TELEPHONING FOR HELP

You can telephone for help from:

- **Emergency services,** including police, fire and ambulance services; mine, mountain, cave and fell rescue; and HM Coastguard by calling 999 or 112;
- **Utilities,** including gas, electricity or water. The phone number will be in the telephone directory;
- **Health services,** including doctor, dentist, nurse, midwife or NHS helplines – this varies in different areas. The phone number will be in the telephone directory;

Calls to the emergency services are free from any phone, including mobiles. On motorways, emergency phones can be found every 1.5 km (1 mile); arrows on marker posts indicate the direction of (and distance to) the nearest phone. To summon help using these telephones, pick up the receiver and your call will be answered.

Keep time away from the casualty to a minimum. Ideally, tell someone else to make the call for you while you stay with the casualty. Ask the person to confirm that the call has been made and that help is on the way. If you have to leave a casualty to call for help, first take any necessary vital action (primary survey pp.44–45).

MAKING THE CALL

When you dial 999 or 112, you will be asked which service you require. If there are casualties, ask for the ambulance service; ambulance control will alert other services if required. Your call can be traced if you are unsure of your exact location. Always stay on the telephone until the ambulance control clears the line; you may be given important information about what to do for the casualty while you wait, and/or asked for further information as the situation develops. If someone else makes the call, ensure he is aware of the importance of his call and that he reports back to you.

TALKING TO THE EMERGENCY SERVICES

State your name clearly and say that you are acting in your capacity as a first aider. It is essential to provide the following:

- **Your telephone number** and/or the number you are calling from.
- **The exact location** of the incident; give a road name or number and postcode, if possible – some street signs include the postcode they are in. It can also be helpful to mention any junctions or other landmarks in the area. If you are on a motorway, say which direction the vehicles were travelling in.
- **The type and gravity** of the emergency. For example, "Traffic incident, two cars, road blocked, three people trapped."
- **Number, gender and age** of casualties. For example, "One man, early sixties, breathing difficulties, suspected heart attack."
- **Details of any hazards,** such as gas, toxic substances, power-line damage, or adverse weather conditions, such as fog or ice.

WHEN THE EMERGENCY SERVICES ARRIVE

Once the emergency services arrive, they will take over the care of the casualty. Tell them what has happened and any treatment given. Hand over any notes you made while attending the casualty. You may be asked to continue helping, for example, by assisting relatives or friends of the casualty while the paramedics provide emergency care.

You should also follow instructions given to you by the medical team. Remain until you are told you can go, since they may need to ask you more questions or the police may want to speak to you. Help maintain a clear and clean environment and to preserve the dignity and confidentiality of those involved.

You may be asked to contact a relative. Explain as simply and honestly as you can what has happenened and where the casualty has been taken. Do not be vague or exaggerate, since this may cause unnecessary alarm. It is better to admit ignorance than to give someone misleading information. However, the information you give may cause distress; if so, remain calm and be clear about what they need to do next.

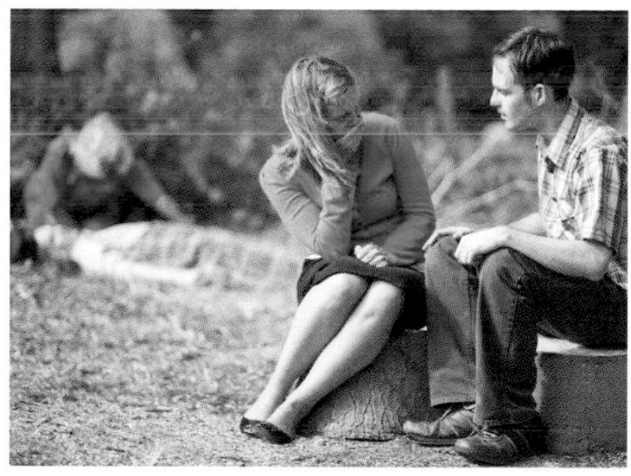

ASSISTING AT THE SCENE
Once the emergency services arrive, tell the team everything that you know. While they assess and treat the casualty, you may be asked to look after or reassure friends.

THE USE OF MEDICATION

In first aid, administering medication is largely confined to relieving general aches and pains. It usually involves helping a casualty to take his own painkillers.

A variety of medications can be bought without a doctor's prescription. However, you must not buy or borrow medication to administer to a casualty yourself.

If you administer, or advise taking, any medication other than that stipulated in this manual, the casualty may be put at risk, and you could face legal action as a consequence. Whenever a casualty takes medication, it is essential to make sure that:

- **It is appropriate** to the condition;
- **It is not out of date;**
- **It is taken as advised;**
- **Any precautions** are strictly followed;
- **The recommended dose** is not exceeded;
- **You keep a record** of the name and dose of the medication as well as the time and method of administration.

CAUTION

Aspirin should never be given to anyone under the age of 16 years as there is risk of a rare condition called Reye's syndrome.

REMEMBER YOUR OWN NEEDS

Most people who learn first aid gain significantly from doing so. As well as learning new skills and meeting new people, by learning first aid you can make a real difference to peoples' lives. Being able to help people who are ill or injured often results in a range of positive feelings. However, you may also feel stressed when you are called upon to administer first aid, and feel emotional once you have finished treating a casualty, whatever the outcome. Occasionally, that stress can interfere with your physical and mental well-being after an incident. Everyone responds to stressful situations in different ways, and some people are more susceptible to stress than others. It is important to learn how to deal with any stress in order to maintain your own health and effectiveness as a first aider. Gaining an understanding of your needs can help you be better prepared for future situations.

IMMEDIATELY AFTER AN INCIDENT

An emergency is an emotional experience. Many first aiders experience satisfaction, or even elation, and most cope well. However, after you have treated a casualty, depending on the type of incident and the outcome, you might experience a mixture of the following:

- **Satisfaction;**
- **Confusion, worry, doubt;**
- **Anger, sadness, fear.**

You may go through what has happened again and again in your mind, so it can be helpful to talk to someone you trust about how you feel and what you did. Consider talking to someone else who was there, or who you know has had a similar experience. Never reproach yourself or hide your feelings. This is especially important if the outcome was not as you had hoped. Even with appropriate treatment, and however hard you try, a casualty may not recover.

LATER REACTIONS

Delivering first aid can lead to positive feelings as you notice new things about yourself, such as, for example, your ability to deal with a crisis. However, occasionally, the effect of an incident on you will depend on your first aid experience as well as on the nature of the actual incident.

The majority of the incidents you will deal with will be of a minor nature and they will probably involve people you know. If you have witnessed an incident that involved a threat to life or you have experienced a feeling of helplessness, you may find yourself suffering from feelings of stress after the incident. In most cases, these feelings should disappear over time.

WHEN TO SEEK HELP

If, however, you experience persistent or distressing symptoms associated with a stressful incident, such as nightmares and flashbacks, seek further help from someone you trust and feel you can confide in.

See your doctor if you feel overwhelmed by your symptoms. Your doctor will talk through them with you and together you can decide what is best for you. Seeking help is nothing to be embarrassed about, and it is important to be able to overcome these feelings. This will not only help you deal with your current reactions, but it will also help you learn how to respond to situations in the future.

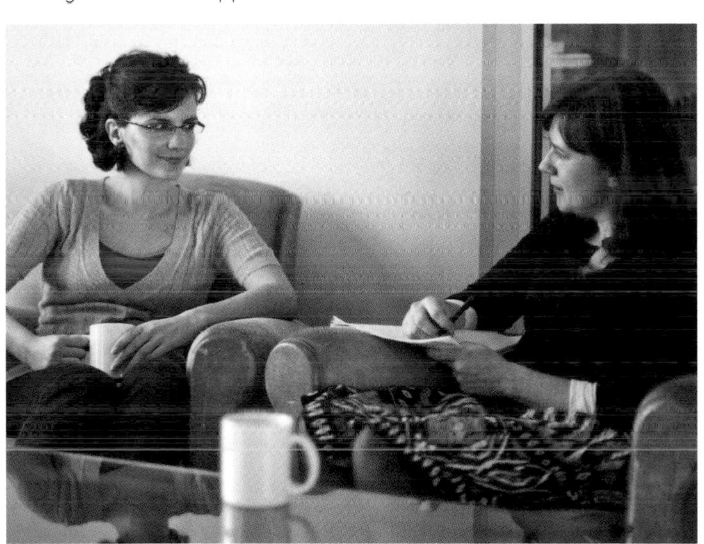

TALKING THINGS OVER
Confiding in a friend or relative is often useful. Ideally, talk to someone who also attended the incident; she may have the same feelings about it as you. If you are unable to deal with the effects of the event you were part of or witnessed, seek help from your doctor.

2

The scene of any incident can present many potential dangers, whether someone has suddenly become ill or has been injured, whether in the home or outside at the scene of an incident. Before any first aid can be provided you must make sure that approaching the scene of the incident does not present unacceptable danger to you, the casualty or anyone else who is helping.

This chapter provides advice for first aiders on how to ensure safety in an emergency situation. There are specific guidelines for emergencies that pose a particular risk. These include fires, traffic incidents and incidents involving electricity and drowning.

The procedures used by the emergency services for major incidents, where particular precautions are necessary and where first aiders may be called on to help, are also described here.

AIMS AND OBJECTIVES

- To protect yourself from danger and make the area safe.
- To assess the situation quickly and calmly and summon help if necessary.
- To assist any casualties and provide necessary treatment with the help of bystanders.
- To call 999/112 for emergency help if you suspect serious injury or illness.
- To be aware of your own needs.

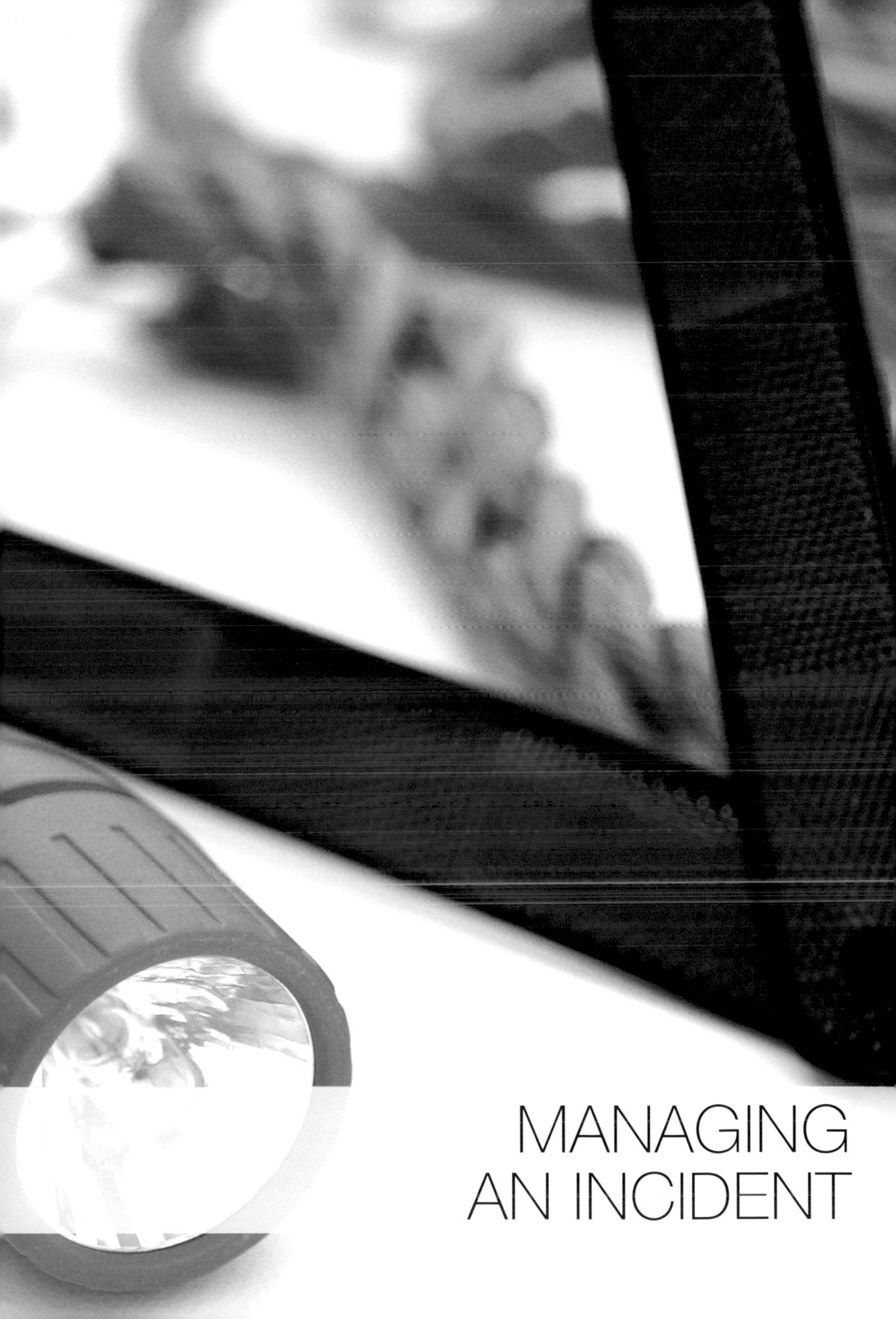

MANAGING AN INCIDENT

ACTION AT AN EMERGENCY

In any emergency you must follow a clear plan of action. This will enable you to prioritise the demands that may be made upon you, and help you decide on your response. The principle steps are: to assess the situation, to make the area safe (if possible) and to give emergency aid. Assess any casualties by carrying out a primary survey (pp.44–45) to identify the most seriously injured.

ASSESSING THE SITUATION

Evaluating the scene accurately is one of the most important factors in the management of an incident. You should stay calm. State that you have first aid training and, if there are no medical personnel in attendance, calmly take charge.

Identify any safety risks and assess the resources available. Action for key dangers you may face, such as fire, are dealt with in this chapter, but be aware, too, of trip hazards, sharp objects, chemical spills and falling masonry.

All incidents should be managed in a similar manner. Consider the following:

- **Safety** What are the dangers and do they still exist? Are you wearing protective equipment? Is it safe for you to approach?
- **Scene** What factors are involved at the incident? What are the mechanisms of the injuries (pp.42–43)? How many casualties are there? What are the potential injuries?
- **Situation** What happened? How many people are involved and what age are they? Are any of them children or elderly?

MAKING AN AREA SAFE

The conditions that give rise to an incident may still present a danger and must be eliminated if possible. It may be that a simple measure, such as turning off the ignition of a car to reduce the risk of fire, is sufficient. As a last resort, move the casualty to safety. Usually specialist help and equipment is required for this.

When approaching a casualty make sure you protect yourself: wear high-visibility clothing, gloves and head protection if you have them. Remember, too, that a casualty faces the risk of injury from the same hazards that you face. If extrication from the scene is delayed, try to protect the casualty from any additional hazards.

If you cannot make an area safe, then call 999/112 for emergency help. Stand clear of the incident until the emergency services have secured the scene.

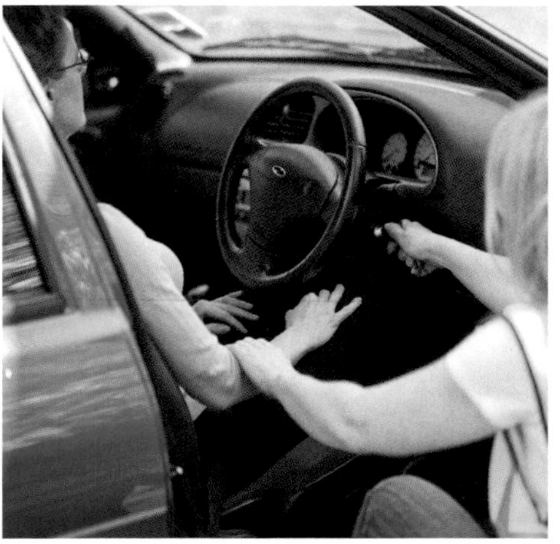

MAKING A VEHICLE SAFE
Wear a high-visibility jacket if you have one to alert others of your presence. Switch off the ignition (even if the engine is no longer running); this reduces the risk of a spark causing a fire.

GIVING EMERGENCY HELP

Once an area has been made safe, use the primary survey (pp.44–45) to quickly carry out an initial assessment of the casualty or casualties to establish treatment priorities. If there is more than one casualty, attend to those with life-threatening conditions first. If possible, treat casualties in the position in which you find them; move them only if they are in immediate danger or if it is necessary to provide life-saving treatment.

Enlist help from others if possible. Ask bystanders to call for the emergency services (p.23). They can also help to protect a casualty's privacy, put out warning triangles in the event of a vehicle incident (p.30) or fetch equipment while you begin first aid.

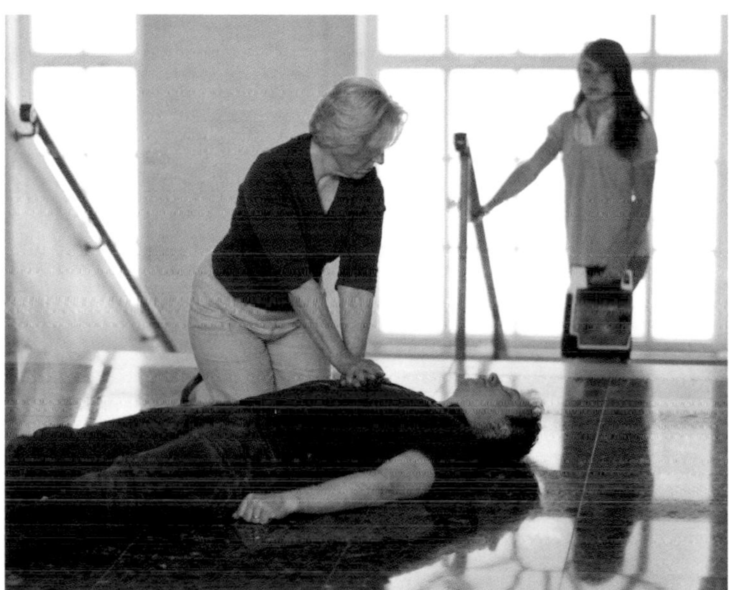

BEGIN TREATMENT
Start life-saving first aid as soon as possible. Ask others to call for help and fetch equipment such as an automated external defibrillator (AED).

ASSISTING THE EMERGENCY SERVICES

Hand over any notes you have made to the emergency services when they arrive (p.21). Answer any questions they may have and follow any instructions. As a first aider you may be asked to help, for example, to move a casualty using specialist equipment. If so, you should always follow their instructions.

HELICOPTER RESCUE

Occasionally, helicopter rescue is required. If a casualty is being rescued in this way, there are a number of safety rules to follow. The emergency services may already be in attendance, in which case you should keep clear unless they give you specific instructions. If the emergency services are not in attendance, it is important to keep bystanders clear. Make sure everyone is at least 50m (55yd) away, and that no-one is smoking. Kneel down as the helicopter approaches, keeping well away from the rotor blades. Once it has landed do not approach it. Keep bystanders back and wait for a member of the crew to approach you.

TRAFFIC INCIDENTS

The severity of traffic incidents can range from a fall from a bicycle to a major vehicle crash involving many casualties. Often, the incident site will present serious risks to safety, largely because of passing traffic.

It is essential to make the incident area safe before attending any casualties (p.28); this protects you, the casualties and other road users. Once the area is safe, quickly assess the casualties and prioritise treatment. Give first aid to those with life-threatening injuries before treating anyone else. Call 999/112 for emergency help, giving as much detail as you can about the incident, indicating number and age of the casualties, and types of injury.

MAKING THE INCIDENT AREA SAFE

Do not put yourself or others in further danger. Take the following precautions.

- **Park safely,** well clear of the incident site, set your hazard lights flashing and put on a high-visibility jacket/vest if you have one.
- **Set up warning triangles** (or another vehicle with hazard lights) at least 45m (49yd) from the incident in each direction; bystanders can do this while you attend to the casualty. If possible, send helpers to warn other drivers to slow down.
- **Make vehicles safe.** For example, switch off the ignition of any damaged vehicle and, if you can, disconnect the battery. Pull the supply cut-off on large diesel vehicles; this is normally found on the outside of the vehicle and will be marked.
- **Stabilise vehicles.** If a vehicle is upright, apply the handbrake, put it in gear and/or place blocks in front of the wheels. If it is on its side, do not attempt to right it, but try to prevent it from rolling over further.
- **Watch out for physical dangers,** such as traffic. Make sure that no-one smokes anywhere near the incident.
- **Alert the emergency services** to damaged power lines, spilt fuel or any vehicles with Hazchem signs (opposite).

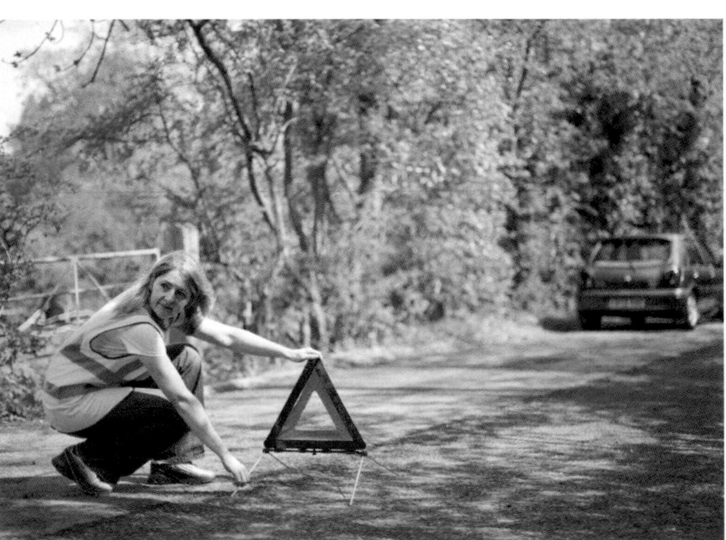

WARN OTHER ROAD USERS
Ask a bystander to set up warning triangles in both directions. Advise the person to watch for other vehicles while she is doing this.

SPECIAL CASE HAZARDOUS SUBSTANCES

Traffic incidents may be complicated by spillages of substances or toxic vapours. Keep bystanders away from the scene and stand upwind of the vehicle. Hazchem signs on the back of the vehicle indicate that it may be carrying a potentially dangerous substance. Give all the details to the emergency services so they can assess the risks involved. If in doubt about your safety or the meaning of a symbol, keep your distance. If the top left panel of a sign contains the letter "E", the substance is a public safety hazard.

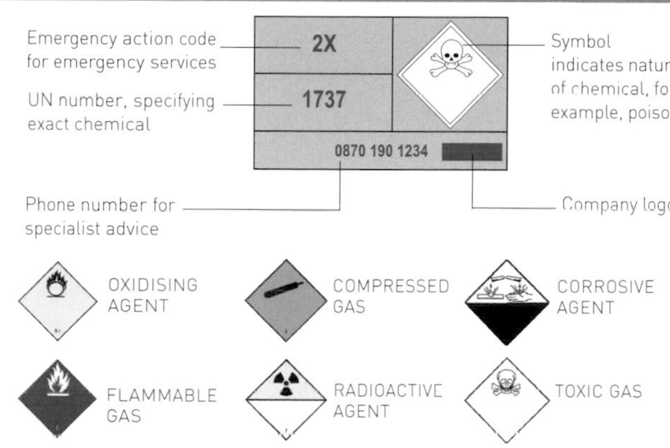

ASSESSING THE CASUALTIES

Quickly assess any casualties by carrying out a primary survey (pp.44–45). Deal first with those who have life-threatening injuries. Assume that any casualty who has been involved in a road-traffic incident may have a neck or spinal injury (pp.171–73). If possible, treat casualties in the position in which you find them, supporting the head and neck at all times, and wait for the emergency services.

Search the area around the incident thoroughly to make sure you do not overlook any casualty who may have been thrown clear, or who has wandered away from the site. Bystanders can help. If a person is trapped inside or under a vehicle, she will need to be released by the fire service. Monitor and record the casualty's vital signs – level of response, breathing and pulse (pp.52–53) – while you are waiting.

CAUTION

- Do not cross a motorway to attend to an incident or casualty.
- At night, wear or carry something light or reflective, such as a high-visibility jacket, and use a torch.
- Do not move the casualty unless it is absolutely necessary. If you do have to move her, the method will depend on the casualty's condition and available help.
- Be aware that road surfaces may be slippery because of fuel, oil or even ice.
- Watch out for undeployed air bags and unactivated seat-belt tensioners.
- Find out as much as you can about the incident and relay this information to the emergency services when they arrive.

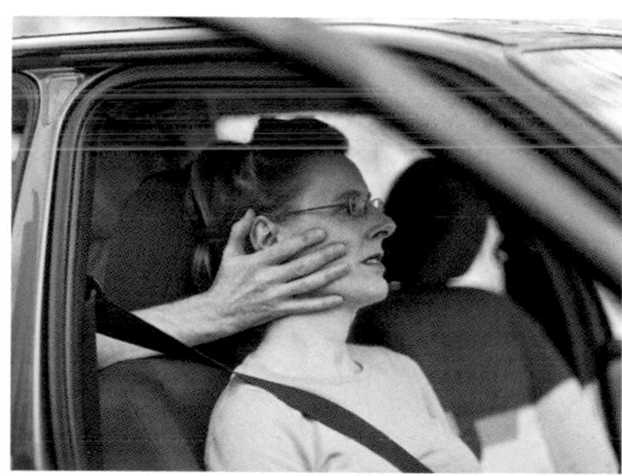

CASUALTY IN A VEHICLE
Assume that any injured casualty in a vehicle has a neck injury. Support the head while you await help. Reassure her and keep her ears uncovered so that she can hear you.

FIRES

Fire spreads very quickly, so your first priority is to warn any people at risk. If in a building, activate the nearest fire alarm, call 999/112 for emergency help, then leave the building. However, if doing this delays your escape, make the call when you are out of the building. As a first aider, try to keep everyone calm. Encourage and assist people to evacuate the area.

When arriving at an incident involving fire, stop, observe, think: do not enter the area. A minor fire can escalate in minutes to a serious blaze. Call 999/112 for emergency help and wait for it to arrive.

THE ELEMENTS OF FIRE

A fire needs three components to start and maintain it: ignition (a spark or flame); a source of fuel (petrol, wood or fabric); and oxygen (air). Removing one of these elements can break this "triangle of fire".

- **Remove combustible materials,** such as paper or cardboard, from the path of a fire, as they can fuel the flames.
- **Cut off a fire's oxygen** supply by shutting a door on a fire or smothering the flames with a fire blanket. This will cause the fire to suffocate and go out.
- **Switch off a car's ignition,** or pull the fuel cut-off on a large diesel vehicle, normally marked on the outside of the vehicle, or switch off the gas supply.

LEAVING A BURNING BUILDING

If you see or suspect a fire in a building, activate the first fire alarm you see. Try to help people out of the building without putting yourself at risk. Close doors behind you to help prevent the fire from spreading. If you are in a public building, use the fire exits and look for assembly points outside.

You should already know the evacuation procedure at your workplace. If, however, you are visiting other premises you are not familiar with, follow the signs for escape routes and obey any instructions given by their fire marshals.

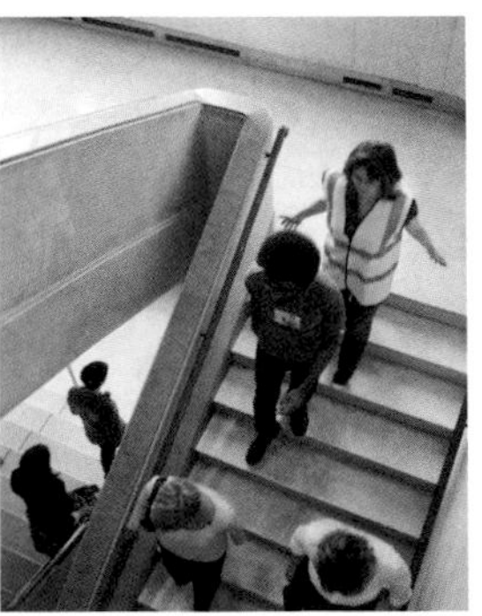

EVACUATING OTHER PEOPLE Encourage people to leave the building calmly but quickly by the nearest exit. If they have to use the stairs, make sure they do not rush and risk falling down.

CAUTION

When escaping from a fire:

- Do not re-enter a burning building to collect personal possessions;
- Do not use lifts;
- Do not go back to a building until cleared to do so by a fire officer.

Fire precautions:

- Do not move anything that is on fire;
- Do not smother flames with flammable materials;
- Do not fight a fire if it puts your own safety at risk;
- If your clothes catch fire and help is not available, extinguish the flames by wrapping yourself up tightly in suitable material and rolling along the ground;
- Do not put water on an electrical fire: pull the plug out or switch the power off at the mains;
- Smother a hot fat fire with a fire blanket; never use water.

CLOTHING ON FIRE

Always follow this procedure: Stop, Drop and Roll.

- **Stop** the casualty panicking, running around or going outside; any movement or breeze will fan the flames.
- **Drop** the casualty to the ground. If possible, wrap him tightly in a fire blanket, or heavy fabric such as a coat, curtain, blanket (not a nylon or cellular type) or rug.
- **Roll** the casualty along the ground until the flames have been smothered. Treat any burns (pp.182–88): help the casualty to lie down with the burned side uppermost and cool the burn.

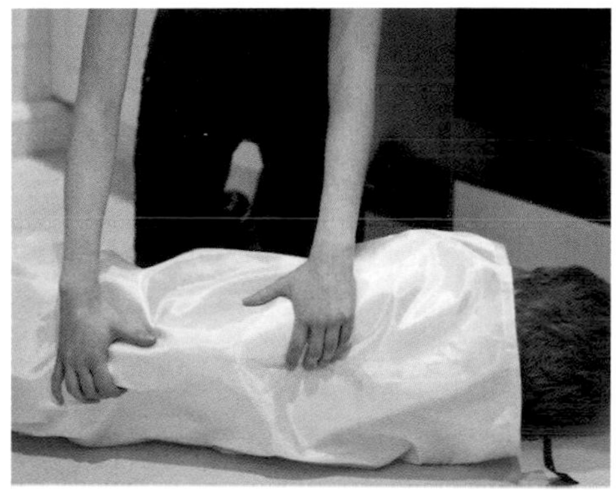

PUTTING OUT FLAMES
Help the casualty on to the ground to stop flames rising to his face. Wrap him in a fire blanket to starve flames of oxygen, and roll him on the ground until the flames are extinguished.

SMOKE AND FUMES

Any fire in a confined space creates a highly dangerous atmosphere that is low in oxygen and may also be polluted by carbon monoxide and other toxic fumes. Never enter a smoke- or fume-filled building or open a door leading to a fire. Let the emergency services do this.

- **If you are trapped** in a burning building, if possible go into a room at the front of the building with a window and shut the door. Block gaps under the door by placing a rug or similar heavy fabric across the bottom of the door to minimise smoke. Open the window and shout for help.
- **Stay low** if you have to cross a smoke-filled room: air is clearest at floor level.
- **If escaping** through a high window, climb out backwards feet first; lower yourself to the full length of your arms before dropping down.

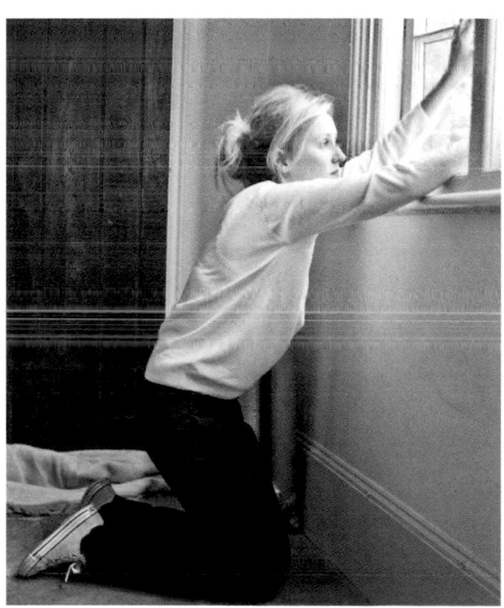

AVOIDING SMOKE AND FUMES
Shut the door of the room you are in and put a rug or blanket against the door to keep smoke out. Open the window and shout for help. Keep as low as possible to avoid fumes in the room.

ELECTRICAL INCIDENTS

When a person is electrocuted, the passage of electrical current through the body may stun him, causing his breathing and heartbeat to stop. The electrical current can also cause burns both where it enters and where it exits the body to go to "earth". An electrical burn may appear very small or not be visible on the skin, but the damage can extend deep into the tissues (p.186).

Factors that affect the severity of the injury are: the voltage; the type of current; and the path of the current. A low voltage of 240 volts is found in a home or workplace, a high voltage of 440–1,000 volts is found in industry and voltage of more than 1,000 volts is found in power lines. The type of current will either be alternating (AC) or direct (DC), and the path of the current can be hand-to-hand, hand-to-foot or foot-to-foot.

Most low-voltage and high-tension currents are AC, which causes muscular spasms (tetany) and the "locked-on" phenomenon – the casualty's grasp is "locked" on to the object preventing him from letting go, so he may remain electrically charged ("live"). In contrast, DC tends to produce a single large muscular contraction that often throws the person away from the source. Be aware that the jolt may cause the casualty to be thrown or to fall, resulting in injuries such as spinal injuries and fractures.

CAUTION

- Do not touch the casualty if he is in contact with the electrical current.
- Do not use anything metallic to break the electrical contact.
- Do not approach high-voltage wires until the power is turned off.
- Do not move a person with an electrical injury unless he is in immediate danger and is no longer in contact with the electricity.
- If the casualty is unconscious, and it is safe to touch him, open the airway and check breathing (The unconscious casualty pp.54–85).

HIGH-VOLTAGE CURRENT

Contact with a high-voltage current, found in power lines and overhead cables, is usually immediately fatal. Anyone who survives will have severe burns, since the temperature of the electricity may reach up to 5,000°C (9,032°F). Furthermore, the shock produces a muscular spasm that propels the casualty some distance, causing additional injuries.

High-voltage electricity may jump ("arc") up to 18m (20yd). The power must be cut off and isolated before anyone approaches the casualty. A casualty who has suffered this type of shock is likely to be unconscious. Once you have been officially informed that it is safe to approach, assess the casualty, open the airway and check breathing (The unconscious casualty pp.54–85).

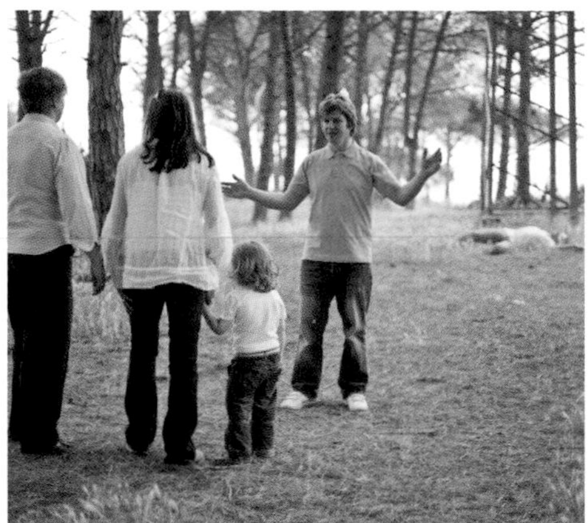

PROTECT BYSTANDERS
Keep everyone away from the incident. Bystanders should stay at least 18m (20yd) from the damaged cable and/or casualty.

LOW-VOLTAGE CURRENT

Domestic current, as used in homes and workplaces, can cause serious injury or even death. Incidents are usually due to faulty switches, frayed flexes or defective appliances. Young children are at risk since they are naturally curious, and may put fingers or other objects into electrical wall sockets. Water is also a very efficient conductor of electricity, so presents additional risks. Handling an otherwise safe electrical appliance with wet hands, or when you are standing on a wet floor, greatly increases the risk of an electric shock.

BREAKING CONTACT WITH THE ELECTRICITY

1 **Before beginning any treatment, look first, do not touch. If the casualty is still in contact with the electrical source, she will be "live" and you risk electrocution.**

2 **Turn off the source of electricity, if possible, to break the contact between the casualty and the electrical supply. Switch off the current at the mains or meter point if possible. Otherwise remove the plug or wrench the cable free.**

3 **Alternatively, move the source away from both you and the casualty. Stand on some dry insulating material, such as a wooden box, plastic mat or telephone directory. Using a wooden pole or broom, push the casualty's limb away from the electrical source or push the source away from her.**

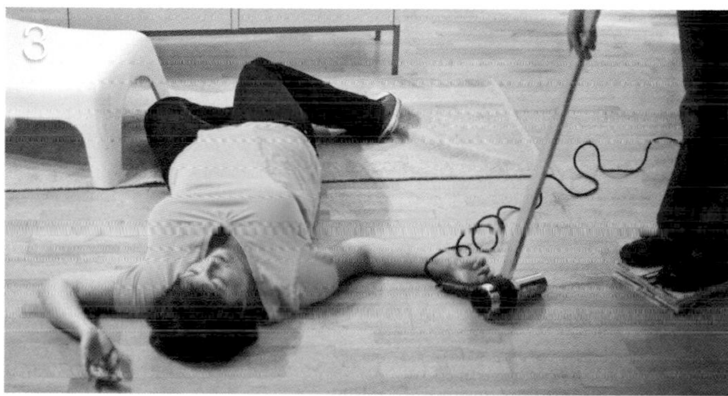

4 **If it is not possible to break the contact using a wooden object, loop a length of rope around the casualty's ankles or under the arms, taking great care not to touch her, and pull her away from the source of the electrical current.**

5 **Once you are sure that the contact between the casualty and the electricity has been broken, perform a primary survey (pp.44–45) and treat any condition found. Call 999/112 for emergency help.**

LIGHTNING

A natural burst of electricity discharged from the atmosphere, lightning forms an intense trail of light and heat. Lightning seeks contact with the ground through the nearest tall feature in the landscape and, sometimes, through anyone standing nearby. However, the short duration of a lightning strike usually precludes serious thermal injury. It may, however, set clothing on fire, knock the casualty down or cause the heart and breathing to stop (cardiac arrest). If cardiopulmonary resuscitation/ CPR (pp.66–67) is started promptly, many victims survive. Always clear everyone from the site of a lightning strike since it can strike again in the same place.

WATER INCIDENTS

Incidents around water may involve people of any age. However, drowning is one of the most common causes of accidental death among young people under the age of 16. Young children can drown in fish ponds, paddling pools, baths and even in the toilet if they fall in head first as well as in swimming pools, in the sea and in open water. Many cases of drowning involve people who have been swimming in strong currents or very cold water, or who have been swimming or boating after drinking alcohol.

There are particular dangers connected with incidents involving swimmers in cold water. Open water around Great Britain and Ireland is cold, even in summer. Sea temperatures range from 5°C (41°F) to 15°C (59°F); inland waters may be colder.

The sudden immersion in cold water can result in an overstimulation of nerves, causing the heart to stop (cardiac arrest). Cold water may cause hypothermia (p.194) and exacerbate shock (pp.116–17). Spasm in the throat and inhalation of water can block the airway (Hypoxia p.90). Inhaled or swallowed water may be absorbed into the circulatory system, causing water overload to the brain, heart or lungs. The exertion of swimming can also strain the heart.

CAUTION

- If the casualty is unconscious, lift him clear of the water, support his head and neck, and carry him with his head lower than his chest. This stops him inhaling water and protects the airway if he vomits.
- When you reach land, open the airway and check breathing (The unconscious casualty pp.54–85).

WATER RESCUE

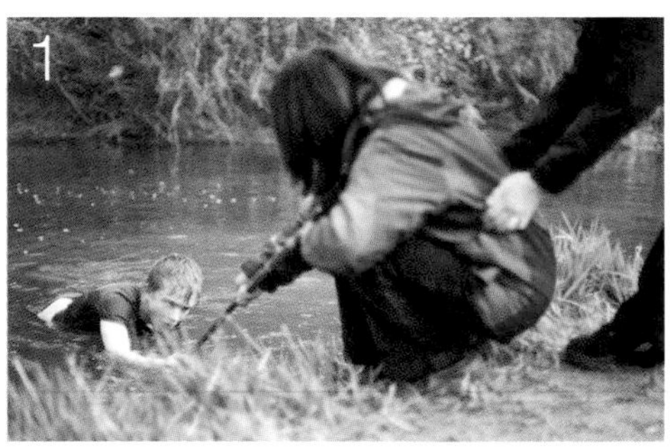

1 Your first priority is to get the casualty on to dry land with the minimum of danger to yourself. Stay on dry land, hold out a stick, a branch or a rope for him to grab, then pull him from the water. Alternatively, throw him a float.

2 If you are a trained life-saver, there is no danger to yourself and the casualty is unconscious, wade or swim to the casualty and tow him ashore. If you cannot do this safely, **call 999/112 for emergency help.**

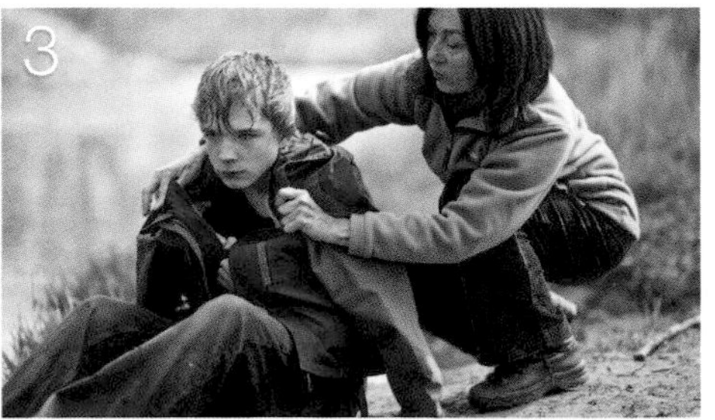

3 Once the casualty is out of the water, shield him from the wind, if possible. Treat him for drowning (p.98) and the effects of severe cold (pp.195–96). If possible, replace any wet clothing with dry clothing.

4 Arrange to take or send the casualty to hospital, even if he seems to have recovered completely. If you are at all concerned, **call 999/112 for emergency help.**

MAJOR INCIDENTS

A major incident is one that presents a serious threat to the safety of a community, or may cause so many casualties that it requires special arrangements from the emergency services. Events of this kind can overwhelm the resources of the emergency services in the area because there may be more casualties to treat than there are personnel available.

It is the responsibility of the emergency services to declare a situation to be a major incident, and certain procedures will be activated by them if necessary. The area around the incident will be sealed off and hospitals and specialist medical teams will be notified. It is not a first aider's responsibility to organise this, but you may be asked to help.

If you are the first person on the scene of what may be a major incident, do not approach it. Call 999/112 for emergency help immediately (pp.22–23). The ambulance control will need to know the type of incident that has occurred (for example, a fire, a traffic incident or an explosion), the location, the access, any particular hazards and the approximate number of casualties that may be involved.

EMERGENCY SERVICE SCENE ORGANISATION

First, the area immediately around the incident will be cordoned off – the inner cordon. Around this an outer cordon, the minimum safe area for emergency personnel (fire, ambulance and police), will be established. No one without the correct identification and safety equipment will be allowed inside the area. A casualty clearing station, where treatment takes place, a survivor reception centre, where the uninjured assemble, and ambulance parking and loading areas will be established inside the cordons.

TRIAGE

The emergency services initially use a system called a triage sieve to assess casualties. All casualties undergo a primary survey (pp.44–45) at the scene to establish treatment priorities. This will be followed by a secondary survey (pp.46–48) in the casualty clearing station. This check will be repeated and any change monitored until a casualty recovers or is transferred into the care of a medical team.

- **Casualties who cannot walk** will undergo further assessment. Depending on the findings, casualties will be assigned to Red Priority One (immediate) or Yellow Priority Two (urgent) areas for treatment and will be transferred to hospital by ambulance as soon as possible.
- **Walking casualties** with minor injuries will be assigned to the Green Priority Three area for treatment and will be transferred to hospital if necessary.
- **Uninjured people** will be taken to the survivor reception centre.

FIRST AIDER'S ROLE

You will not be allowed to enter the cordoned area without adequate personal safety equipment. You may be asked to assist the emergency services at an incident by, for example, helping to identify those casualties with minor injuries, supporting injured limbs or making a note of casualties' names and/or helping to contact their relatives.

3

When a person is suddenly taken ill or has been injured, it is important to find out what is wrong as quickly as possible. However, your first priority is to make sure that you are not endangering yourself by approaching a casualty.

Once you are sure that an incident area is safe, you need to begin your assessment of the casualty or casualties. This chapter explains how to approach each casualty and plan your assessment using a methodical two-stage system, first to check and treat life-threatening conditions (primary survey), then to carry out a detailed assessment (secondary survey). There is advice on deciding treatment priorities, managing more than one casualty and arranging aftercare. A casualty's condition may improve or deteriorate while in your care, so there is guidance on how to monitor changes in his condition.

AIMS AND OBJECTIVES

- To assess a situation quickly and calmly, while first protecting yourself and the casualty from any danger.
- To assess each casualty and treat life-threatening injuries first.
- To carry out a more detailed assessment of each casualty.
- To seek appropriate help. Call 999/112 for emergency help if you suspect serious injury or illness.
- To be aware of your own needs.

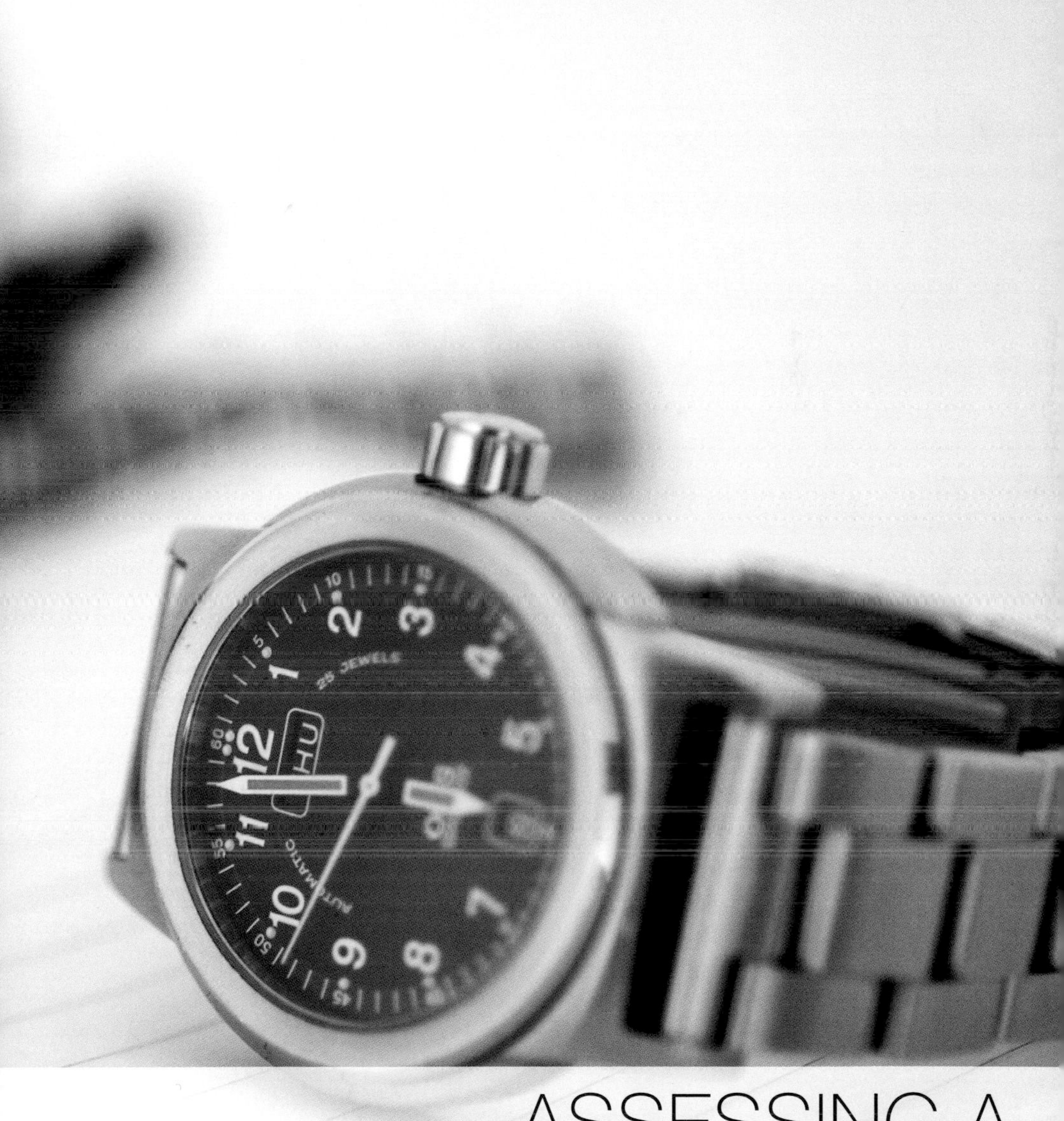

ASSESSING A CASUALTY

ASSESSING THE SICK OR INJURED

From the previous chapters you will now know that to ensure the best possible outcome for anyone who is injured or suddenly becomes ill you need to take responsibility for making assessments. Tell those at the scene that you are a trained first aider and calmly take charge. However, as indicated in Chapter 2 (pp.26–37), resist the temptation to begin dealing with any casualty until you have the assessed the overall situation, ensured that everyone involved is safe and, if appropriate, taken steps to organise the necessary help. As you read this chapter, look back at Chapter 1 (pp.12–25) and remember the following:

- **Be calm;**
- **Be aware of risks;**
- **Build and maintain** the casualty's trust;
- **Call appropriate help;**
- **Remember your own needs.**

MANAGING THE INJURED OR SICK

There are three aspects to this:

- **First,** find out what is wrong with the casualty;
- **Second,** treat conditions found in order of severity – life-threatening conditions first;
- **Third,** arrange for the next step of a casualty's care. You will need to decide what type of care a casualty needs. You may need to call for emergency help, suggest the casualty seeks medical advice or allow him to go home, accompanied if necessary.

Other people at the incident can help you with this. Ask one of them to call 999/112 for emergency help while you attend a casualty. Alternatively, they may be able to look after less seriously injured casualties, or fetch first aid equipment.

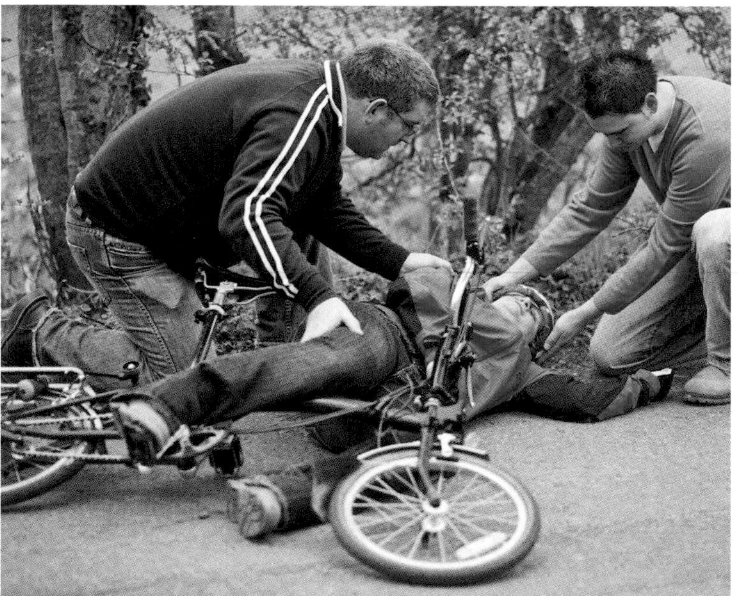

FIRST ACTIONS
Support the casualty; a bystander may be able to help. Ask the casualty what happened, and try to identify the most serious injury.

METHODS OF ASSESSMENT

When you assess a casualty you first need to identify and deal with any life-threatening conditions or injuries – primary survey. Deal with each life-threatening condition as you find it, working in the following order – airway, breathing, then circulation – before you progress to the next stage. Depending on your findings you may not move on to the next stage of the assessment. If the life-threatening injuries are successfully managed, or there are none, you carry on the assessment and perform a secondary survey.

THE PRIMARY SURVEY

This is an initial rapid assessment of a casualty to establish and treat conditions that are an immediate threat to life (pp.44–45).

If a casualty is conscious, suffering from minor injuries and is talking to you, then this survey will be completed very quickly. If, however, a casualty is more seriously injured (for example, unconscious), this assessment will take longer.

Follow the ABC principle: Airway, Breathing and Circulation.

- **Airway** Is the airway open and clear? If not, open and clear it. An obstructed airway will prevent breathing, causing hypoxia (p.93) and ultimately death. If the casualty is talking to you, the airway is open and clear.
- **Breathing** Is the casualty breathing normally? If he is breathing, you need to check for and treat any breathing difficulty (for example, asthma). If he is not breathing, call 999/112 for emergency help, then start chest compressions with rescue breaths (cardiopulmonary resuscitation/CPR). If this happens, you are unlikely to move on to the next stage.
- **Circulation** Is the casualty bleeding severely? This must be treated since it can lead to a life-threatening condition known as shock (pp.116–17).

SPECIAL CASE SEVERAL CASUALTIES

If there is more than one casualty, you will need to prioritise those that must be treated first according to the severity of their injuries. Use the primary survey ABC principles (above) to do this. Remember that unresponsive casualties are at greatest risk.

THE SECONDARY SURVEY

This is a detailed examination of a casualty to look for other injuries or conditions that may not be apparent (pp.46–48). To do this, carry out a head-to-toe examination (pp.49–51). Your aim is to find out:

- **History** What actually happened and any relevant medical history.
- **Symptoms** Injuries or abnormalities that the casualty tells you about.
- **Signs** Injuries or abnormalities that you can see.

By checking the recognition features of the different injuries and conditions explained in the chapters of this book you can identify what may be wrong. Record your findings and pass on any relevant information to the medical team.

LEVEL OF RESPONSE

You will initially have noted whether or not a casualty is conscious. He may have spoken to you or made eye contact or some other gesture (p.44). Or perhaps there has been no response to your questions such as "Are you all right?" or "What happened?" Now you need to establish the level of response using the AVPU scale (p.52). This is important since some illnesses and injuries cause a deterioration in a casualty's level of response, so it is vital to assess the level, then monitor him for any change.

MECHANISMS OF INJURY

The type of injury that a person sustains is directly related to how the injury is caused. In addition, whether a casualty sustains a single or multiple injury is also determined by the mechanisms that caused it. This is the reason why a history of the incident is important. In many situations, this vital information can only be obtained by those people who deal with the casualty at the scene – often first aiders. Look, too, at the circumstances in which an injury was sustained and the forces involved.

The information is useful since it also helps the emergency services and medical team predict the type and severity of injury, as well as the treatment. This therefore helps the diagnosis, treatment and likely outcome for the casualty.

CIRCUMSTANCES OF INJURY

The extent and type of injuries sustained due to impact – for example, a fall from a height or the impact of a car crash – can be predicted if you know exactly how the incident happened. For example, a car occupant is more likely to sustain serious injuries in a side-impact collision than in a frontal collision at the same speed. This is because the side of the car provides less protection and cannot absorb as much energy as the front of the vehicle. For a driver wearing a seatbelt whose vehicle is struck either head-on or from behind, a specific pattern of injuries can be suspected. The driver's body will be suddenly propelled one way, but the driver's head will lag behind briefly before moving. This results in a "whiplashing" movement of the neck (below). The casualty may also have injuries caused by the seatbelt restraint; for example, fracture of the breastbone and possibly bruising of the heart or lungs. There may be injuries to the face due to contact with the steering wheel or an inflated airbag.

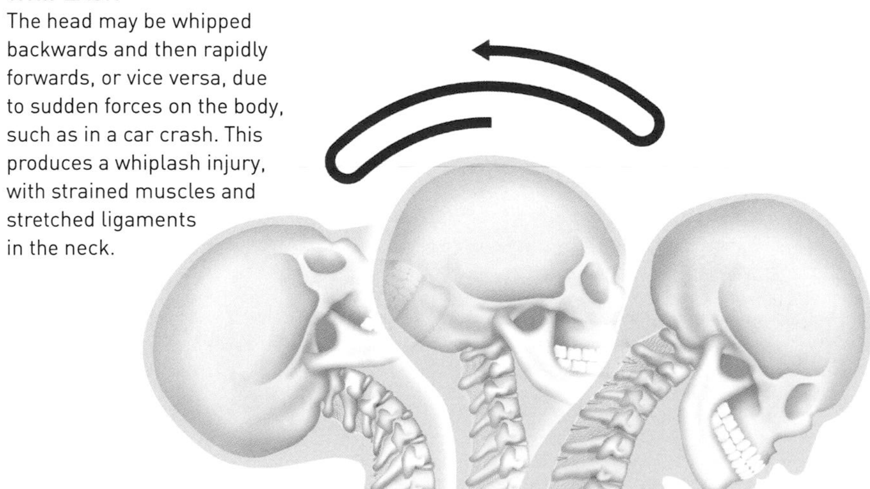

WHIPLASH
The head may be whipped backwards and then rapidly forwards, or vice versa, due to sudden forces on the body, such as in a car crash. This produces a whiplash injury, with strained muscles and stretched ligaments in the neck.

FORCES EXERTED ON THE BODY

The energy forces exerted during an impact are another important indicator of the type or severity of any injury. For example, if a man falls from a height of 1m (3ft 3in) or less on to hard ground, he will probably suffer bruising but no serious injury. A fall from a height of more than 2m (6ft 6in), however, is likely to produce more serious injuries, such as a pelvic fracture and internal bleeding. An apparently less serious fall can mask a more dangerous injury. If a person falls down the stairs, for example, she may tell you that she injured her ankle. If she has fallen awkwardly onto a hard surface, however, she may have sustained a spine and/or head injury.

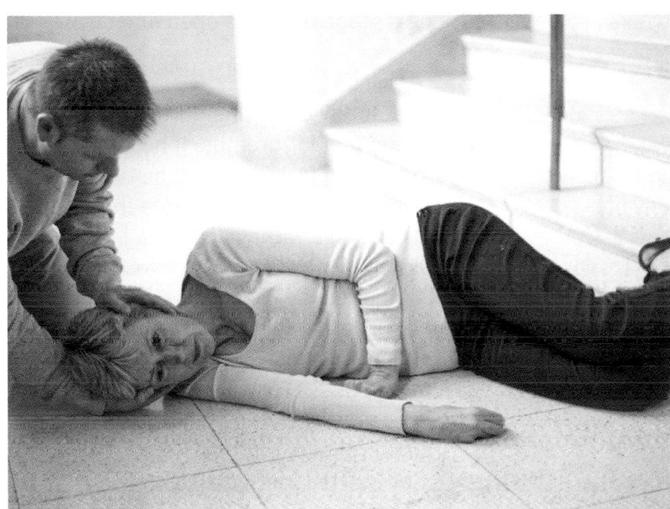

MOST SERIOUS INJURY MAY BE HIDDEN
A first aider should keep the casualty still, ask someone to support her head and **call 999/112 for emergency help**.

QUESTIONS TO ASK AT THE SCENE

When you are attending a casualty, ask the casualty, or any witnesses, questions to try to find out the mechanism of the injury. Witnesses are especially important if the casualty is unable to talk to you. Possible questions include:

- Was the casualty ejected from a vehicle?
- Was the casualty wearing a correctly adjusted seat-belt?
- Did the vehicle roll over?
- Was the casualty wearing a helmet?
- How far did the casualty fall?
- What type of surface did he land on?
- Is there evidence of body contact with a solid object, such as the floor or a vehicle's windscreen or dashboard?
- How did he fall? (For example, twisting falls can stretch or tear the ligaments or tissues around a joint such as the knee or ankle.)

Pass on all the information that you have gathered to the emergency services (p.21).

SECONDARY SURVEY

Once you have completed the primary survey and dealt with any life-threatening conditions, start the methodical process of checking for other injuries or illnesses by performing a head-to-toe examination. This is called the secondary survey. Question the casualty and the people around him. Make a note of your findings if you can, and pass all the details to the emergency services or hospital, or whoever takes responsibility for the casualty (p.29).

Ideally, the casualty should remain in the position found, at least until you are satisfied that it is safe to move him into a more comfortable position appropriate for his injury or illness.

This survey includes two further checks beyond the ABC (pp.44–45).

- **Disability** is the casualty's level of response (p.52).
- **Examine the casualty.** You may need to remove or cut away clothing to examine and/or treat the injuries.

By conducting this survey you are aiming to discover the following:

- **History** What happened leading up to the injury or sudden illness and any relevant medical history.
- **Symptoms** Information that the casualty gives you about his condition.
- **Signs** you find on examination of the casualty.

HISTORY

There are two important aspects to the history: what happened and any previous medical history.

EVENT HISTORY

The first consideration is to find out what happened. Your initial questions should help you to discover the immediate events leading up to the incident. The casualty can usually tell you this, but sometimes you have to rely on information from people nearby so it is important to verify that they are telling you facts and not just their opinions. There may also be clues, such as the impact on a vehicle, which can indicate the likely nature of the casualty's injury. This is often referred to as the mechanism of injury (pp.42–43).

PREVIOUS MEDICAL HISTORY

The second aspect to consider is a person's medical history. While this may have nothing to do with the present condition, it could be a clue to the cause. Clues to the existence of such a condition may include a medical bracelet or medication in the casualty's possessions (p.48).

TAKING A HISTORY

- **Ask what happened;** for example, establish whether the incident is due to illness or an accident.
- **Ask about medication** the casualty is taking currently.
- **Ask about medical history.** Find out if there are ongoing and previous conditions.
- **Find out** if a person has any allergies.
- **Check when** the person last had something to eat or drink.
- **Note the presence** of a medical warning bracelet – this may indicate an ongoing medical condition, such as epilepsy, diabetes or anaphylaxis.

SYMPTOMS

These are the sensations that the casualty feels and describes to you. When you talk to the casualty, ask him to give you as much detail as possible. For example, if he complains of pain, ask where it is. Ask him to describe the pain (is it constant or intermittent, sharp or dull). Ask him what makes the pain better (or worse), whether it is affected by movement or breathing and, if it did not result from an injury, where and how it began. The casualty may describe other symptoms, too, such as nausea, giddiness, heat, cold or thirst. Listen very carefully to his answers (p.20) and do not interrupt him while he is speaking.

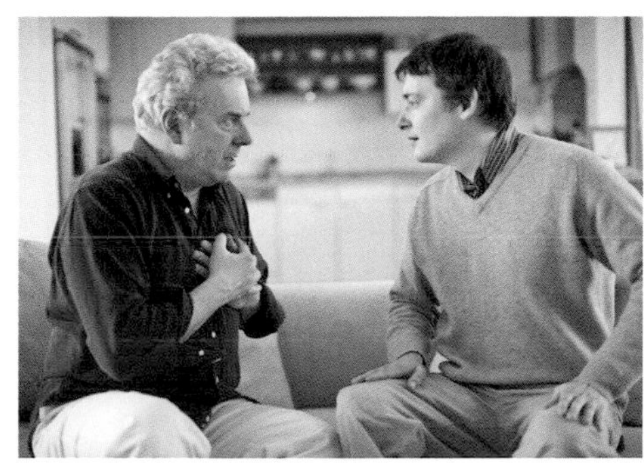

LISTEN TO THE CASUALTY
Make eye contact with the casualty as you talk to him. Keep your questions simple, and listen carefully to the symptoms he describes.

SIGNS

These are features such as swelling, bleeding, discoloration, deformity and smells that you can detect by observing and feeling the casualty. Use all of your senses – look, listen, feel and smell. Always compare the injured and uninjured sides of the body. You may also notice that the person is unable to perform normal functions, such as moving his limbs or standing. Make a note of any obvious superficial injuries, going back to treat them only when you have completed your examination.

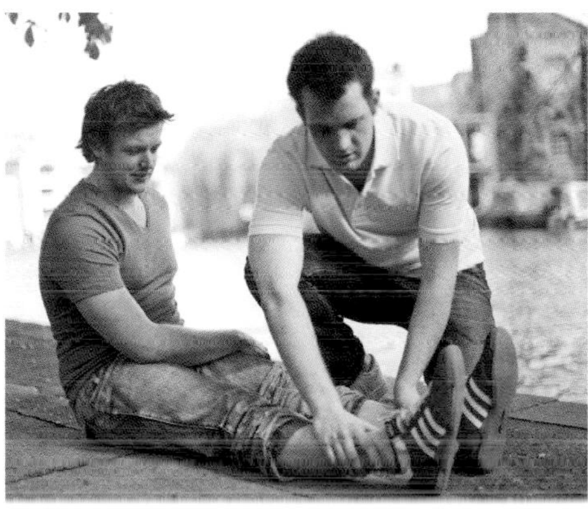

COMPARE BOTH SIDES OF THE BODY
Always compare the injured part of the body with the uninjured side. Check for swelling, deformity and/or discoloration.

QUICK REMINDER

Use the mnemonic **A M P L E** as a reminder when assessing a casualty to ensure that you have covered all aspects of the examination. When the emergency services arrive, they may ask:

A – Allergy – does the person have any allergies?
M – Medications – is the person on any medication?
P – Previous medical history.
L – Last meal – when did the person last eat?
E – Event history – what happened?

SECONDARY SURVEY (continued)

LOOK FOR EXTERNAL CLUES

As part of your assessment, look for external clues to a casualty's condition. If you suspect drug abuse, take care as he may be carrying needles and syringes. You may find an appointment card for a hospital or clinic, or a card indicating a history of allergy, diabetes or epilepsy. Horse-riders or cyclists may carry such a card inside their riding hat or helmet. Food or medication may also give valuable clues about the casualty's condition; for example, people with diabetes may carry sugar lumps or glucose gel. A person with a known disorder may also have medical warning information on a special locket, bracelet, medallion or key ring (such as a "MedicAlert" or "SOS Talisman"). Keep any such item with the casualty or give it to the emergency services.

If you need to search a casualty's belongings, always try to ask first and perform the search in front of a reliable witness (p.21).

MEDICAL CLUES	
	MEDICATION A casualty may be carrying tablets such as phenytoin for epilepsy, or a glyceryl trinitrate spray for angina.
	MEDICAL BRACELET This may be inscribed with information about a casualty's medical history (e.g., epilepsy, diabetes or anaphylaxis), or there may be a number to call.
	"PUFFER" INHALER The presence of an inhaler usually indicates that the casualty has asthma; reliever inhalers are generally blue and preventive inhalers are usually brown or white.
	INSULIN PEN This may indicate that a person has diabetes. The casualty may also have a glucose testing kit.
	AUTO-INJECTOR This contains adrenaline (epinephrine), for people at risk of anaphylactic shock.

HEAD-TO-TOE EXAMINATION

Once you have taken the casualty's history (p.46) and asked about any symptoms she has (p.47), you should carry out a detailed examination. Use all your senses when you examine a casualty: look, listen, feel and smell. Always start at the head and work down; this "head-to-toe" routine is both easily remembered and thorough. You may have to sensitively loosen, open, cut away or remove clothing where necessary to examine the casualty (p.232). Always be sensitive to a casualty's privacy and dignity, and ask her permission before doing this.

Protect yourself and the casualty by wearing disposable gloves. Make sure that you do not move the casualty more than is strictly necessary. If possible, examine a conscious casualty in the position found, or one that best suits her condition, unless her life is in immediate danger. If an unconscious breathing casualty has been placed in the recovery position, leave her in this position while you carry out the head-to-toe examination.

Check the casualty's breathing and pulse rates (pp.52–53), then work from her head downwards. Initially, note minor injuries but continue your examination to make sure that you do not miss any concealed potentially serious conditions; return to them only when you have completed your examination.

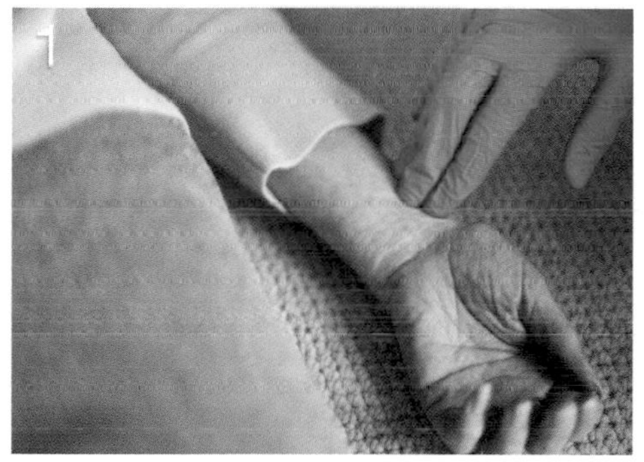

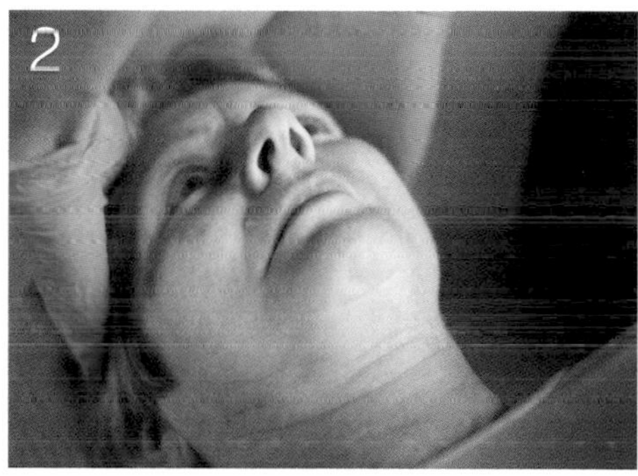

1 **Assess breathing (p.52). Check the rate (fast or slow), depth (shallow or deep) and nature (is it easy or difficult, noisy or quiet). Check the pulse (p.53). Assess the rate (fast or slow), rhythm (regular or irregular) and strength (strong or weak).**

2 **Start the physical examination at the casualty's head. Run your hands carefully over the scalp to feel for bleeding, swelling or depression, which may indicate a fracture. Be careful not to move the casualty if you suspect that she may have injured her neck.**

3 **Speak clearly to the casualty in both ears to find out if she responds or if she can hear. Look for clear fluid or watery blood coming from either ear. These discharges may be signs of a serious head injury (pp.165–67).**

4 **Examine both eyes. Note whether they are open. Check the size of the pupils (the black area). If the pupils are not the same size it may indicate head injury. Look for any foreign object, blood or bruising in the whites of the eyes.**

HEAD-TO-TOE EXAMINATION (continued)

5 Check the nose for discharges as you did for the ears. Look for clear fluid or watery blood (or a mixture of both) coming from either nostril. Any of these discharges might indicate serious head injury.

6 Look in the mouth for anything that might obstruct the airway. If the casualty has dentures that are intact and fit firmly, leave them. Look for mouth wounds or burns and check for irregularity in the line of the teeth.

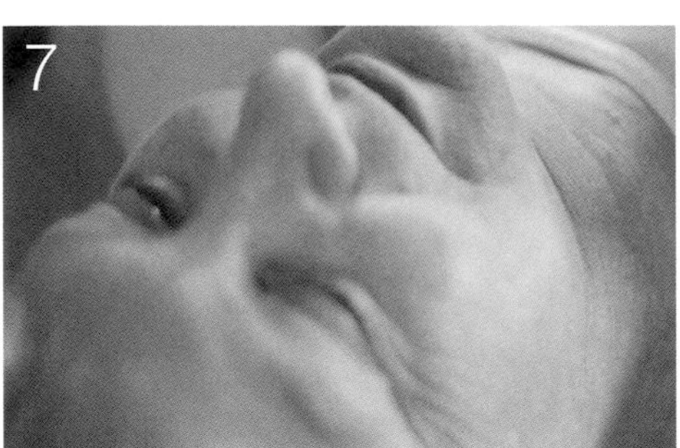

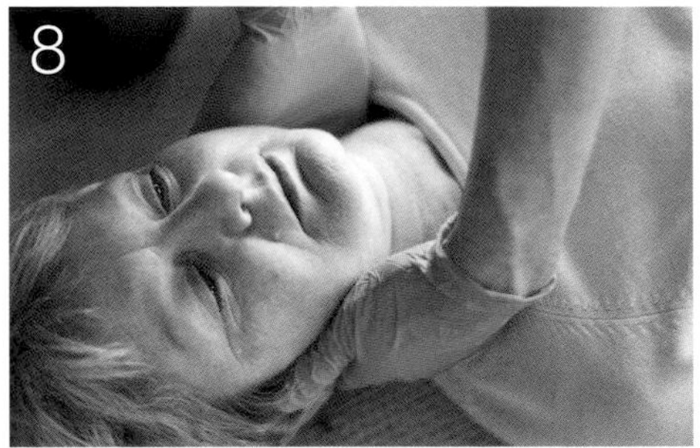

7 Look at the skin. Note the colour and temperature: is it pale, flushed or grey-blue (cyanosis); is it hot or cold, dry or damp? Pale, cold, sweaty (clammy) skin suggests shock; a flushed, hot face suggests fever or heatstroke. A blue tinge indicates lack of oxygen; look for this in the lips, ears and face.

8 Loosen clothing around the neck, and look for signs such as a medical warning medallion (p.48) or a hole (stoma) in the windpipe. Run your fingers gently along the spine from the base of the skull down as far as possible without moving the casualty; check for irregularity, swelling, tenderness or deformity.

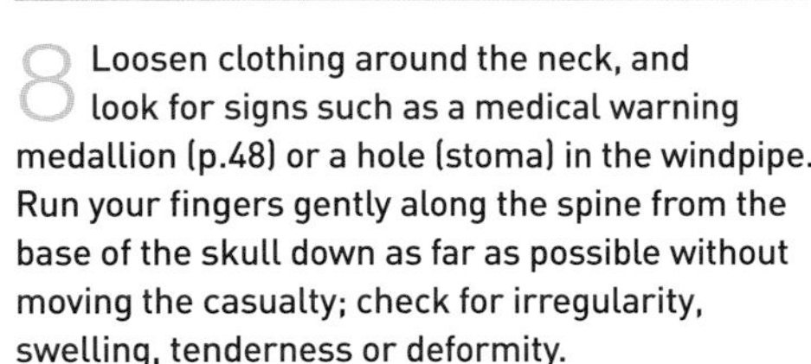

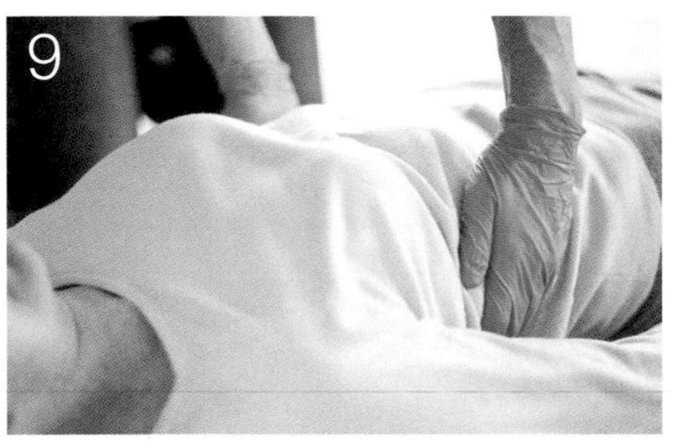

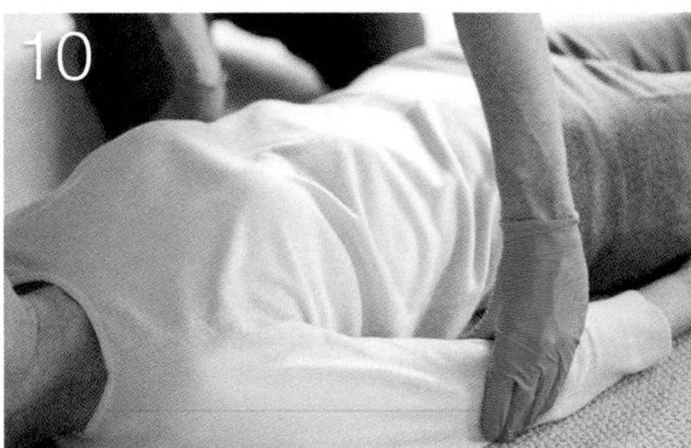

9 Look at the chest. Ask the casualty to breathe deeply, and note whether the chest expands evenly, easily and equally on both sides. Feel the ribcage to check for deformity, irregularity or tenderness. Ask the casualty if she is aware of grating sensations when breathing, and listen for unusual sounds. Note whether breathing causes any pain. Look for any external injuries, such as bleeding or stab wounds.

10 Feel along the collar bones, shoulders, upper arms, elbows, hands and fingers for any swelling, tenderness or deformity. Check the movements of the elbows, wrists and fingers by asking the casualty to bend and straighten each joint. Check that the casualty has no abnormal sensations in the arms or fingers. If the fingertips are pale or grey-blue there may be a problem with blood circulation. Look out for needle marks on the forearms, or a medical warning bracelet (p.48).

11 If there is any impairment in movement or loss of sensation in the limbs, do not move the casualty to examine the spine, since these signs suggest spinal injury. Otherwise, gently pass your hand under the hollow of the back and check for swelling and tenderness.

12 Gently feel the casualty's abdomen to detect any evidence of bleeding, and to identify any rigidity or tenderness of the abdomen's muscular wall, which could be a sign of internal bleeding. Compare one side of the the abdomen with the other.

13 Feel both sides of the hips, and examine the pelvis for signs of fracture. Check clothing for any evidence of incontinence, which suggests spinal or bladder injury, or bleeding from orifices, which suggests pelvic fracture.

14 Check the legs. Look and feel for bleeding, swelling, deformity or tenderness. Ask the casualty to raise each leg in turn, and to move her ankles and knees.

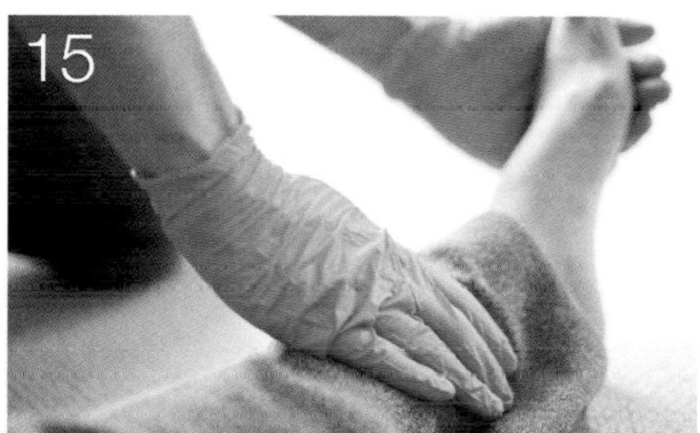
15

15 Check the movement and feeling in the toes. Check that the casualty has no abnormal sensations in her feet or toes. Compare both feet. Look at the skin colour: grey-blue skin may indicate a circulatory disorder or an injury due to cold.

POSSIBLE FINDINGS ON EXAMINATION

METHOD OF IDENTIFICATION	SYMPTOMS OR SIGNS
The casualty may tell you of these symptoms	■ Pain ■ Anxiety ■ Heat ■ Cold ■ Loss of sensation ■ Abnormal sensation ■ Thirst ■ Nausea ■ Tingling ■ Pain on touch or pressure ■ Faintness ■ Stiffness ■ Momentary unconsciousness ■ Weakness ■ Memory loss ■ Dizziness ■ Sensation of broken bone ■ Sense of impending doom
You may see these signs	■ Anxiety and painful expression ■ Unusual chest movement ■ Burns ■ Sweating ■ Wounds ■ Bleeding from orifices ■ Response to touch ■ Response to speech ■ Bruising ■ Abnormal skin colour ■ Muscle spasm ■ Swelling ■ Deformity ■ Foreign bodies ■ Needle marks ■ Vomit ■ Incontinence ■ Loss of normal movement ■ Containers and other circumstantial evidence
You may feel these signs	■ Dampness ■ Abnormal body temperature ■ Swelling ■ Deformity ■ Irregularity ■ Grating bone ends
You may hear these signs	■ Noisy or distressed breathing ■ Groaning ■ Sucking sounds from a penetrating chest injury ■ Response to touch ■ Response to speech ■ Grating bone (crepitus)
You may smell these signs	■ Acetone ■ Alcohol ■ Burning ■ Gas or fumes ■ Solvents or glue ■ Urine ■ Faeces ■ Cannabis

MONITORING VITAL SIGNS

When treating a casualty, you may need to assess and monitor his level of response, breathing and pulse. This information can help you to identify problems and indicate changes in a casualty's condition. Monitoring should be repeated regularly, and your findings recorded and handed over to the medical assistance taking over (p.21). In addition, if a casualty has a condition that affects his body temperature, such as fever, heat stroke or hypothermia, you will also need to monitor his temperature.

LEVEL OF RESPONSE

You need to monitor a casualty's level of response to assess her level of consciousness and any change in her condition. Any injury or illness that affects the brain may affect consciousness, and any deterioration is potentially serious. Assess the level of response using the AVPU scale (right) and make a note of any deterioration or improvement.

- **A** – Is the casualty Alert? Are her eyes open and does she respond to questions?
- **V** – Does the casualty respond to Voice? Can she answer questions and obey commands?
- **P** – Does the casualty respond to Pain? Does she open her eyes or move if pinched?
- **U** – Is the casualty Unresponsive to any stimulus (i.e. unconscious)?

BREATHING

When assessing a casualty's breathing, check the rate of breathing and listen for any breathing difficulties or unusual noises.

An adult's normal breathing rate is 12–16 breaths per minute; in babies and young children, it is 20–30 breaths per minute. When checking breathing, listen for breaths and watch the casualty's chest movements. For a baby or young child, it might be easier to place your hand on the chest and feel for movement of breathing.

Record the following information.

- **Rate** – count the number of breaths per minute.
- **Depth** – are the breaths deep or shallow?
- **Ease** – are the breaths easy, difficult or painful?
- **Noise** – is the breathing quiet or noisy, and if noisy, what are the types of noise?

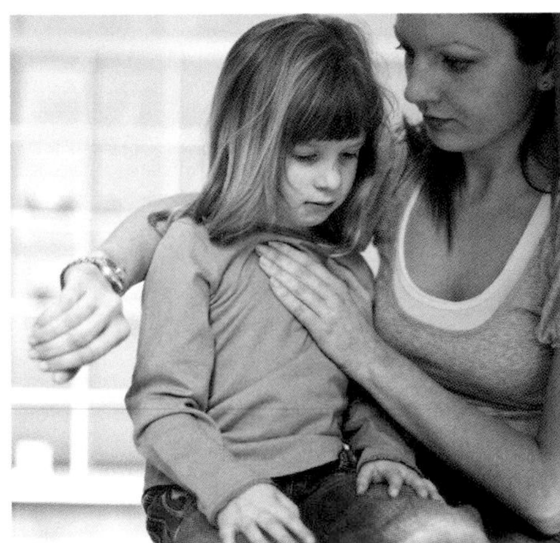

CHECKING A CASUALTY'S BREATHING RATE
Observe the chest movements and count the number of breaths per minute. Use a watch to time breaths. For a baby or young child, place your hand on the chest and feel for movement.

PULSE

Each heartbeat creates a wave of pressure as blood is pumped along the arteries (pp.106–07). Where arteries lie close to the skin surface, such as on the inside of the wrist and at the neck, this pressure wave can be felt as a pulse. The normal pulse rate in adults is 60–80 beats per minute. The rate is faster in children and may be slower in very fit adults. An abnormally fast or slow pulse may be a sign of illness.

The pulse may be felt at the wrist (radial pulse), or if this is not possible, the neck (carotid pulse). In babies, the pulse in the upper arm (brachial pulse) is easier to find.

When checking a pulse, use your fingers (not your thumb) and press lightly against the skin. Record the following points.

- **Rate** (number of beats per minute).
- **Strength** (strong or weak).
- **Rhythm** (regular or irregular).

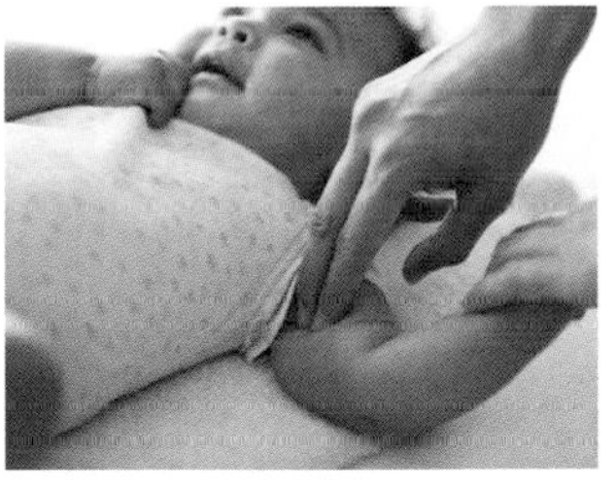

BRACHIAL PULSE
Place the pads of two fingers on the inner side of an infant's upper arm.

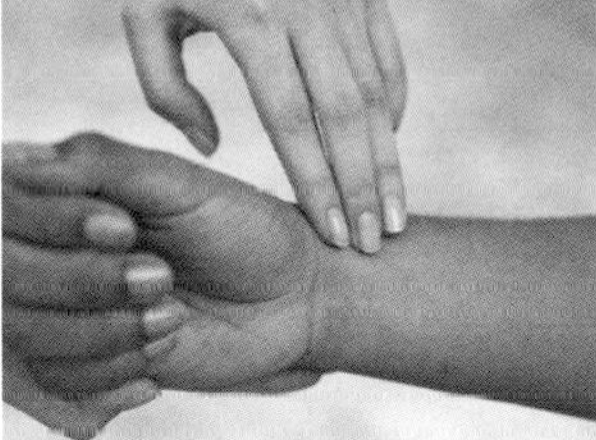

RADIAL PULSE
Place the pads of three fingers just below the wrist creases at the base of the thumb.

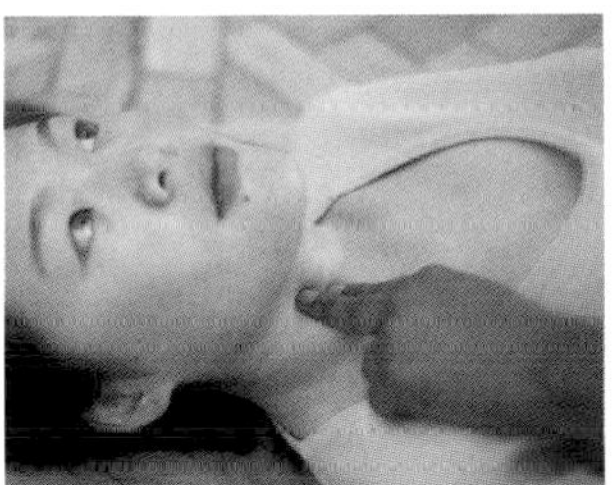

CAROTID PULSE
Place the pads of two fingers in the hollow between the large neck muscle and the windpipe.

BODY TEMPERATURE

Although not a vital sign, you may need to record temperature to assess body temperature. You can feel exposed skin but use a thermometer to obtain an accurate reading. Normal body temperature is 37°C (98.6°F). A temperature above this (fever) is usually caused by infection, but can be the result of heat exhaustion or heatstroke (pp.192–93). A lower body temperature may result from exposure to cold and/or wet conditions – hypothermia (p.194). There are several types of thermometer.

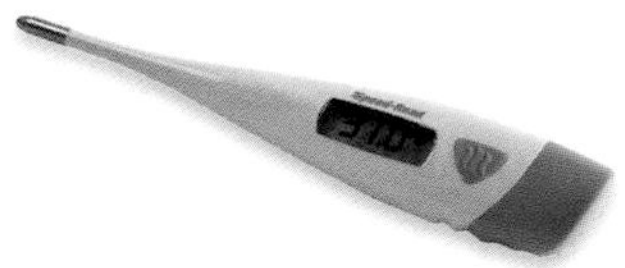

DIGITAL THERMOMETER
Used to measure temperature under the tongue or armpit. Leave it in place until it makes a beeping sound (about 30 seconds), then read the display.

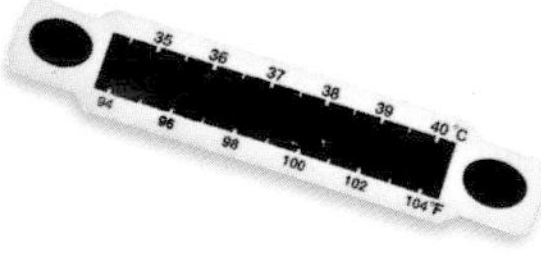

FOREHEAD THERMOMETER
A heat-sensitive strip for use on a small child. Hold against the child's forehead for about 30 seconds. The colour on the strip indicates temperature.

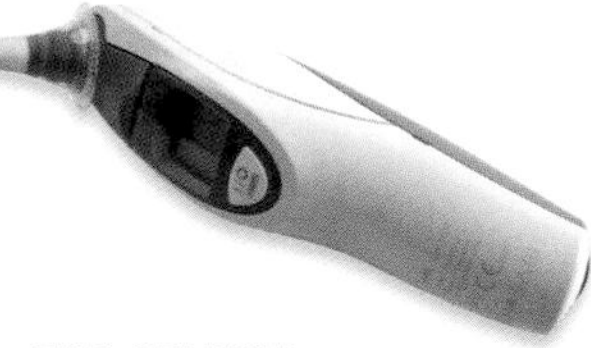

EAR SENSOR
Place the tip inside the ear for a reading within one second. The sensor is easy to use and is ideal for a sick child. It can be used while a person is asleep.

4

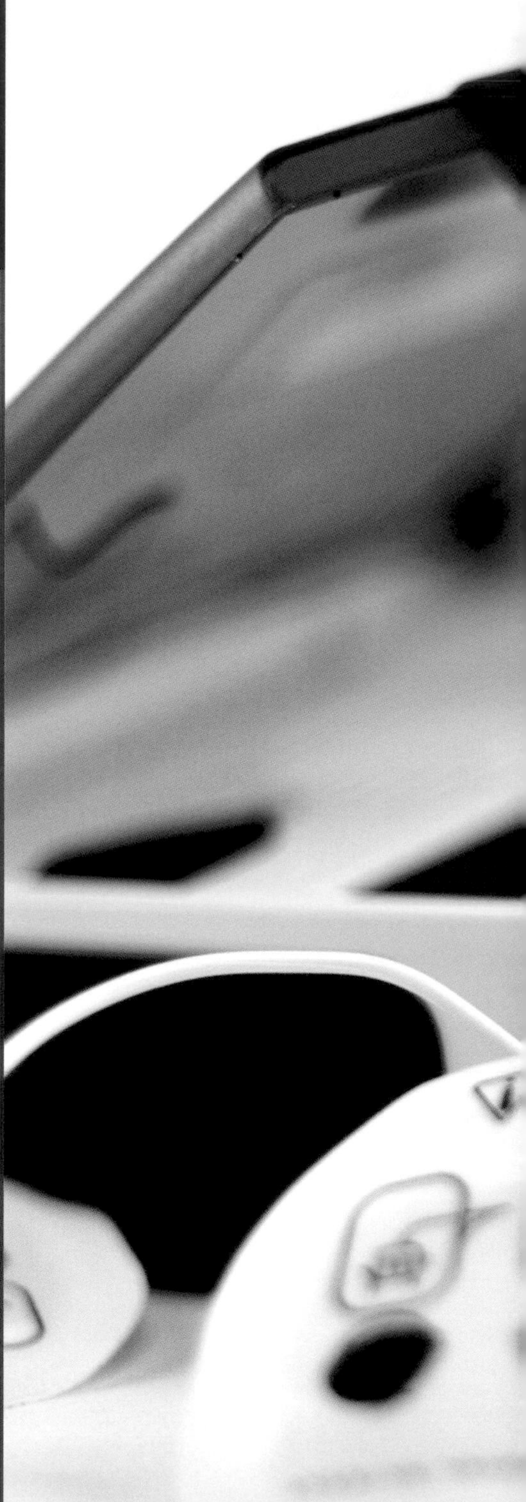

To stay alive we need an adequate supply of oxygen to enter the lungs and be transferred to all cells in the body by the circulating blood. If a person is deprived of oxygen for any length of time, the brain will begin to fail. As a result, the casualty will eventually lose consciousness, breathing will cease, the heart will stop and death results.

The airway must be kept open so that breathing can occur, allowing oxygen to enter the lungs and be circulated in the body.

Therefore, the priority of a first aider when treating any collapsed casualty is to establish an open airway and maintain breathing and circulation. An automated external defibrillator (AED) may be used to "shock" the heart back into a normal rhythm. This chapter outlines the priorities to remember when dealing with an unconscious adult, child, or infant.

There are important differences in the treatment for unconscious children and adults; this chapter gives separate step-by-step instructions for dealing with each of these groups.

AIMS AND OBJECTIVES

- To maintain an open airway, to check breathing and resuscitate if required.
- To call 999/112 for emergency help.

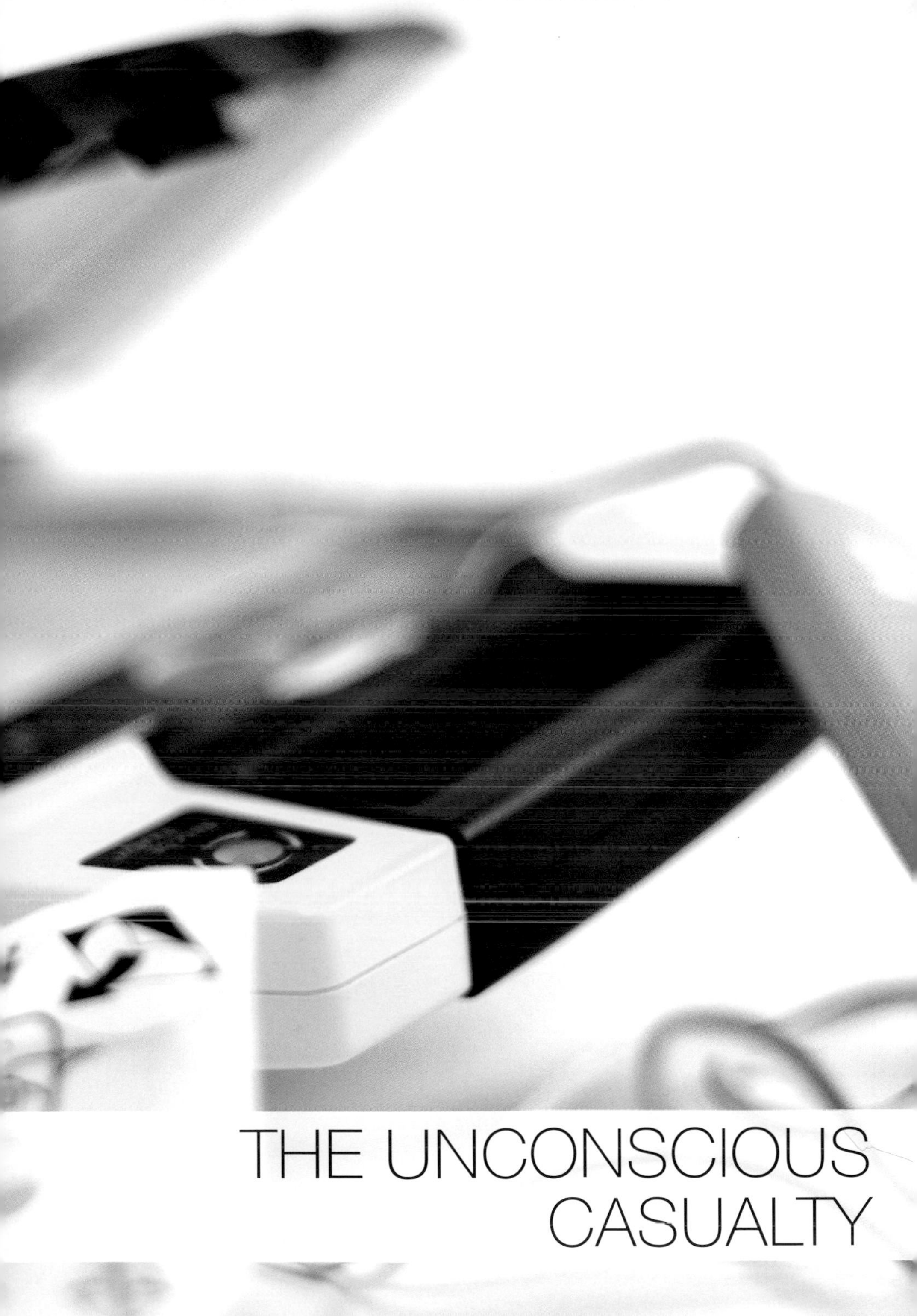

THE UNCONSCIOUS CASUALTY

BREATHING AND CIRCULATION

Oxygen is essential to support life. Without it, cells in the body die – those in the brain survive only a few minutes without oxygen. Oxygen is taken in when we breathe in (pp.88–89), and it is then circulated to all the body tissues via the circulatory system (p.106). It is vital to maintain breathing and circulation in order to sustain life.

The process of breathing enables air, which contains oxygen, to be taken into the air sacs (alveoli) in the lungs. Here, the oxygen is transferred across blood vessel walls into the blood, where it combines with blood cells. At the same time, the waste product of breathing, carbon dioxide, is released and exhaled in the breath.

When oxygen has been transferred to the blood cells it is carried from the lungs to the heart through the pulmonary veins. The heart pumps the oxygenated blood to the rest of the body via blood vessels called arteries. Deoxygenated blood is brought back to the heart by blood vessels called veins (p.89). The heart pumps this blood to the lungs via the pulmonary arteries, where the carbon dioxide is released and the blood is reoxygenated before circulating around the body again.

See also
How breathing works p.89
The heart and blood vessels pp.106–07
The respiratory system pp.88–89

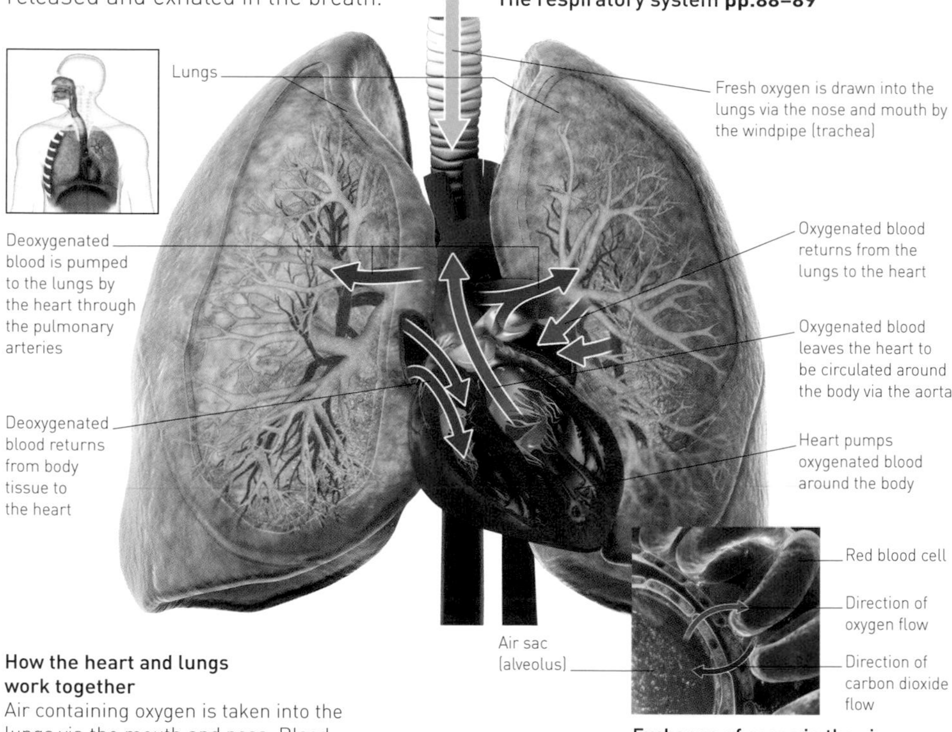

How the heart and lungs work together
Air containing oxygen is taken into the lungs via the mouth and nose. Blood is pumped from the heart to the lungs, where it absorbs oxygen. Oxygenated blood is returned to the heart before being pumped around the body.

Exchange of gases in the air sacs
Carbon dioxide passes out of blood cells into air sacs (alveoli). Oxygen crosses the walls of alveoli into blood cells.

LIFE-SAVING PRIORITIES

The procedures set out in this chapter can maintain a casualty's circulation and breathing.

With an unconscious casualty your priorities are to maintain an open airway, to maintain blood circulation (to get oxygenated blood to the tissues), and to breathe for the casualty (to get oxygen into the body). In an adult during the first minutes after the heart stops (cardiac arrest), the blood oxygen level remains constant, so chest compressions are more important than rescue breaths in the initial phase of resuscitation. After about two to four minutes, the blood oxygen level falls and rescue breathing becomes more important. The combination of chest compressions and rescue breaths is called cardiopulmonary resuscitation, or CPR.

In addition to CPR, a machine called an automated external defibrillator (AED) can be used to deliver an electric shock that may restore a normal heartbeat (pp.82–85).

In children and infants, a problem with breathing is the most likely reason for the heart to stop. They are therefore given FIVE initial rescue breaths before chest compressions are started.

CHEST COMPRESSION-ONLY CPR

Give chest compressions only if you have not had formal training in CPR or you are unwilling or unable to give rescue breaths. The ambulance dispatcher will give instructions for chest compression-only CPR.

KEY ELEMENTS FOR SURVIVAL

If all of the following elements are complete, the casualty's chances of survival are as good as they can possibly be:

- **Emergency help** is called quickly;
- **CPR** is used to provide circulation and oxygen to the body tissues;
- **AED** is used promptly;
- **Specialised treatment** and advanced care arrive quickly.

CHAIN OF SURVIVAL

EARLY HELP

Call 999/112 for emergency help so that an AED and expert help can be brought to the casualty.

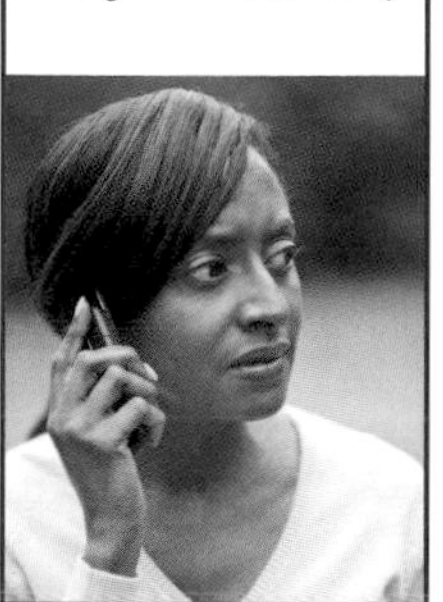

EARLY CPR

Chest compressions and rescue breaths are used to "buy time" until expert help arrives.

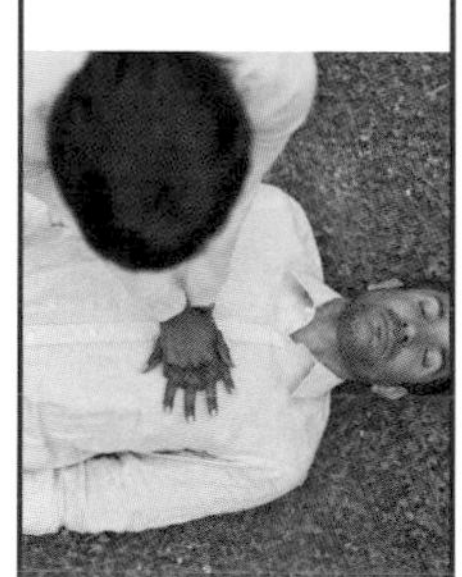

EARLY DEFIBRILLATION

A controlled electric shock from an AED is given. This can "shock" the heart into a normal rhythm.

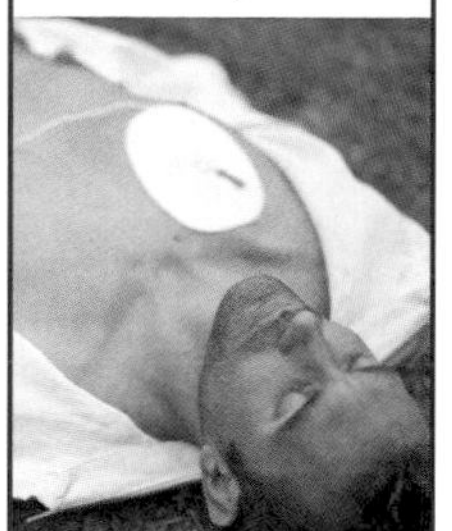

EARLY ADVANCED CARE

Specialised treatment by paramedics and in hospital stabilises the casualty's condition.

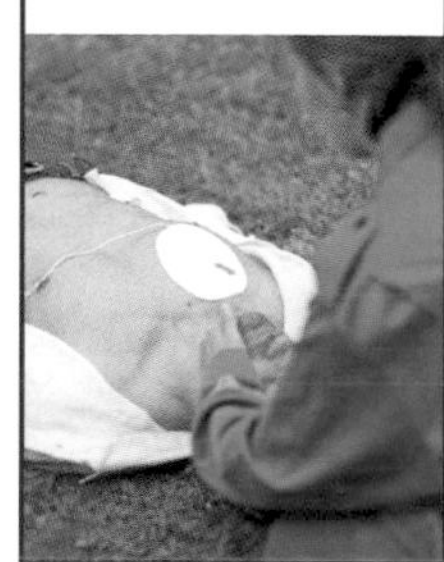

LIFE-SAVING PRIORITIES (continued)

IMPORTANCE OF MAINTAINING CIRCULATION

If the heart stops beating, blood does not circulate through the body. As a result, vital organs – most importantly the brain – become starved of oxygen. Brain cells are unable to survive for more than a few minutes without a supply of oxygen.

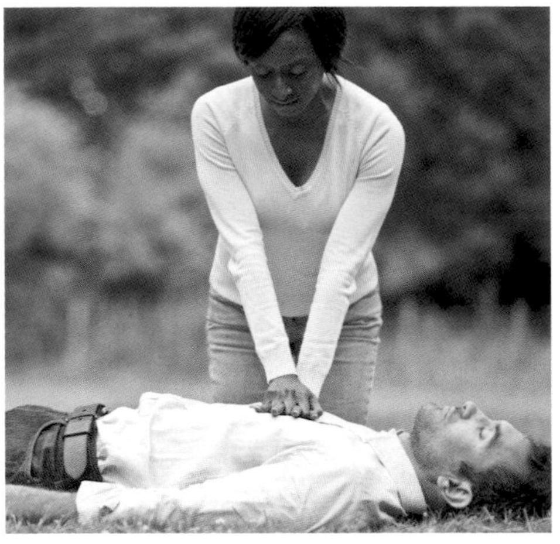

GIVING CHEST COMPRESSIONS

Some circulation can be maintained artificially by chest compressions (p.66). These act as a mechanical aid to the heart in order to get blood flowing around the body. Pushing vertically down on the centre of the chest increases the pressure in the chest cavity, expelling blood from the heart and forcing it into the tissues. As pressure on the chest is released, the chest recoils, or comes back up, and more blood is "sucked" into the heart; this blood is then forced out of the heart by the next compression. It is possible to find the hand position for chest compressions without removing clothing.

To ensure that the blood is supplied with enough oxygen, chest compressions should be combined with rescue breathing (opposite).

RESTORING HEART RHYTHM

A machine called an automated external defibrillator (AED) will be used to attempt to restart the heart when it has stopped (pp.82–85). The earlier the AED is used, the greater the chance of the casualty surviving. With each minute's delay, the chances of survival fall. AEDs can be used safely and effectively without any prior training in their use.

AEDs are found in many public places, such as railway stations, shopping centres, airports, coach stations and ferry ports. They are generally housed in cabinets, often marked with a recognised symbol, and placed where they can be easily accessed, on station platforms for example. The cabinets are not locked, but most are fitted with an alarm that is activated when the door is opened.

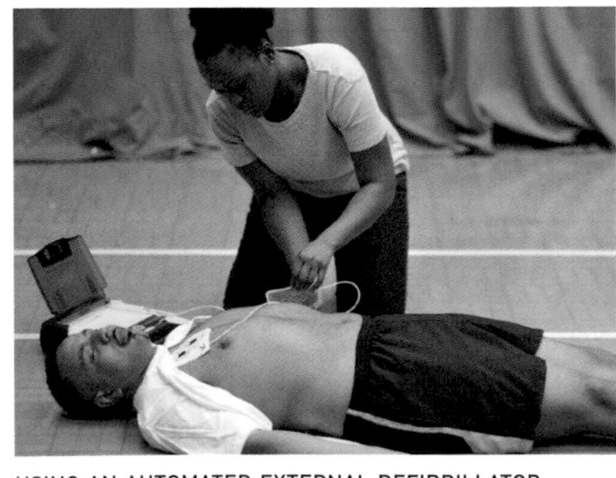

USING AN AUTOMATED EXTERNAL DEFIBRILLATOR

AN OPEN AIRWAY

An unconscious casualty's airway can become narrowed or blocked. This may be due to muscular control being lost, which allows the tongue to fall back and block the airway. When this happens, the casualty's breathing becomes difficult and noisy and may stop. Lifting the chin and tilting the head back lifts the tongue away from the entrance to the air passage, allowing the casualty to breathe.

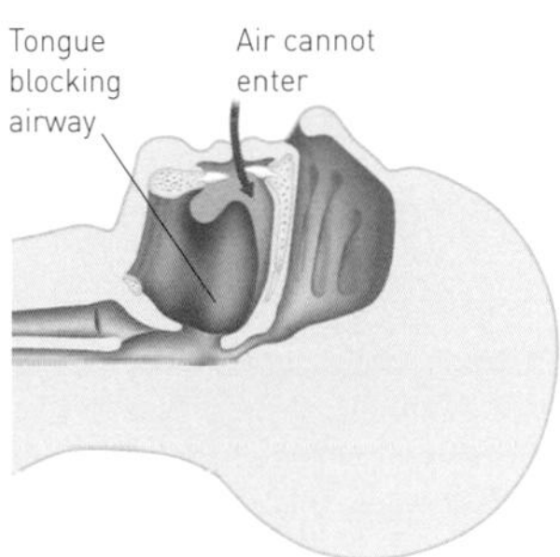

Blocked airway
In an unconscious casualty, the tongue falls back, blocking the throat and airway.

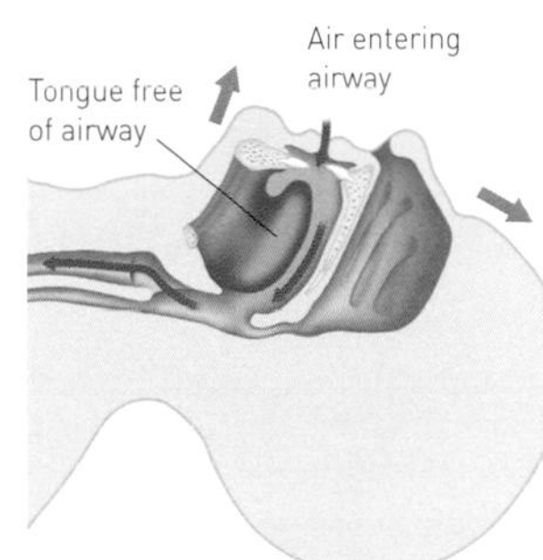

Open airway
In the head tilt, chin lift position, the tongue is lifted from the back of the throat and the trachea is open, so the airway will be clear.

BREATHING FOR A CASUALTY

Exhaled air contains about 16 per cent oxygen (only five per cent less than inhaled air) and a small amount of carbon dioxide. Your exhaled breath therefore contains enough oxygen to supply another person with oxygen – and potentially keep him alive – when it is forced into his lungs during rescue breathing.

By giving a casualty rescue breaths (p.67), you force air into his air passages. This reaches the air sacs (alveoli) in the lungs, and oxygen is then transferred to the blood vessels in the lungs.

When you take your mouth away from the casualty's, his chest falls, and air containing waste products is pushed out, or exhaled, from his lungs. This process, performed together with chest compressions (pp.66–67), can supply the tissues with oxygen until help arrives.

CAUTION

AGONAL BREATHING

This type of breathing usually takes the form of short, irregular gasps for breath. It is common in the first few minutes after a cardiac arrest. It should not be mistaken for normal breathing and, if it is present, chest compressions and rescue breaths (cardiopulmonary resuscitation/CPR) should be started without hesitation.

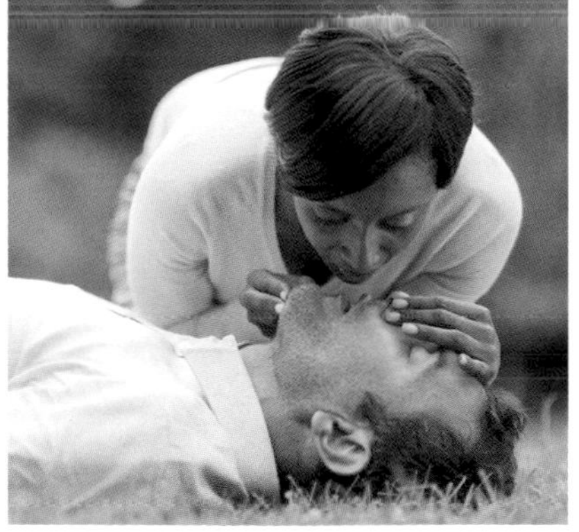

GIVING RESCUE BREATHS

LIFE-SAVING PRIORITIES (continued)

ADULT RESUSCITATION

This action plan is a summary of the techniques to use when attending a collapsed adult – more detailed instructions are given on the following pages. The plan assumes that neither you nor the casualty is in immediate danger.

CHECK CASUALTY'S RESPONSE

- Try to get a response by asking questions and gently shaking his shoulders (p.62).

Is there a response?

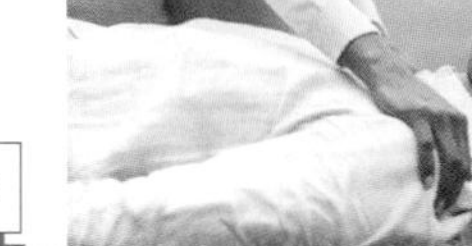

YES → Leave the casualty in the position found, check and treat life-threatening injuries and summon help, if needed following the ABC check (p.45).

NO ↓

OPEN THE AIRWAY; CHECK FOR BREATHING

- Tilt the head back and lift the chin to open the airway (p.63).
- Check for breathing (p.63).

Is he breathing normally?

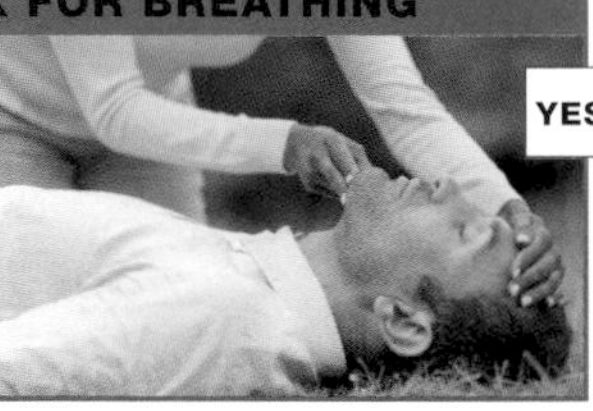

YES → If possible, leave the casualty in the position found. Check and treat life-threatening injuries. Place the casualty in the recovery position (pp.64–65). **Call 999/112 for emergency help.**

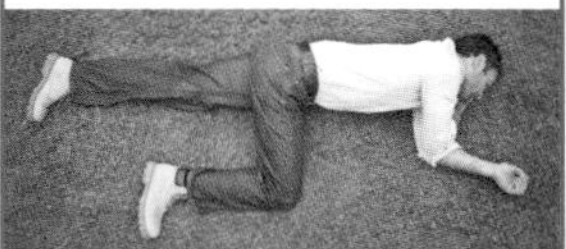

NO ↓

Ask a helper to **call 999/112 for emergency help and ask for an AED.**

- If you are on your own make the call yourself.

↓

BEGIN CPR

- Give 30 chest compressions (p.66).
- Give TWO rescue breaths (p.67)
- Alternate 30 chest compressions with TWO rescue breaths until help arrives, the casualty shows signs of regaining consciousness, such as coughing, opening his eyes, speaking, or moving purposefully, AND starts to breathe normally, or you are too exhausted to continue.

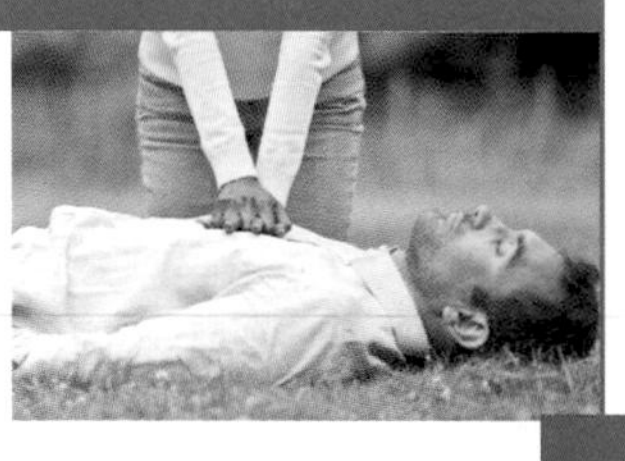

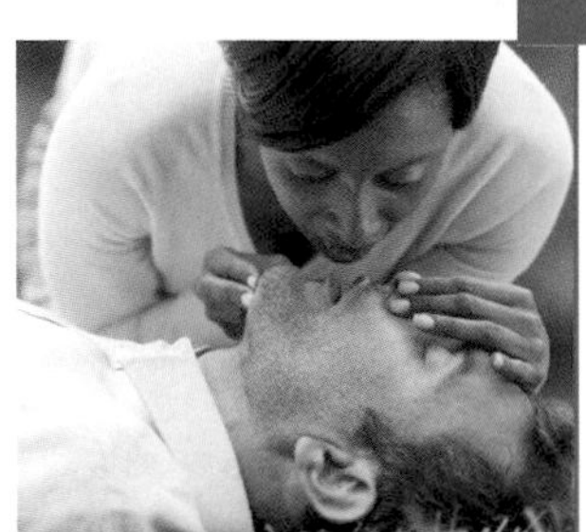

→
- Give chest compressions only if you have not had formal training in CPR or you are unwilling or unable to give rescue breaths. The ambulance dispatcher will give instructions for chest compression only CPR.
- If the casualty starts breathing normally, but remains unconscious, place him in the recovery position (pp.64–65).

CHILD/INFANT RESUSCITATION

This action plan shows the order for the techniques to use when attending a child between the ages of one and puberty or an infant under one year.

CHECK CHILD'S RESPONSE

- Try to get a response by asking questions and gently tapping the child's shoulder or an infant's foot.

Is there a response?

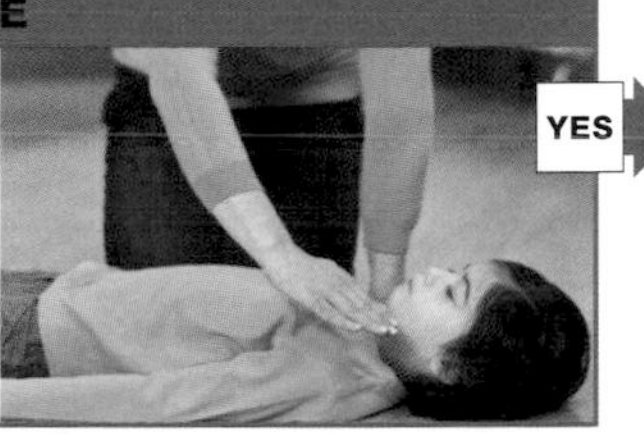

YES → Leave the child in the position found, check and treat life-threatening injuries and summon help if needed following the ABC check (p.45).

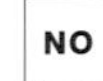

NO ↓

OPEN THE AIRWAY; CHECK FOR BREATHING

- Tilt the head back and lift the chin to open the airway (child p.71 or infant p.78).
- Check for breathing (child p.71 or infant p.79).

Is she breathing normally?

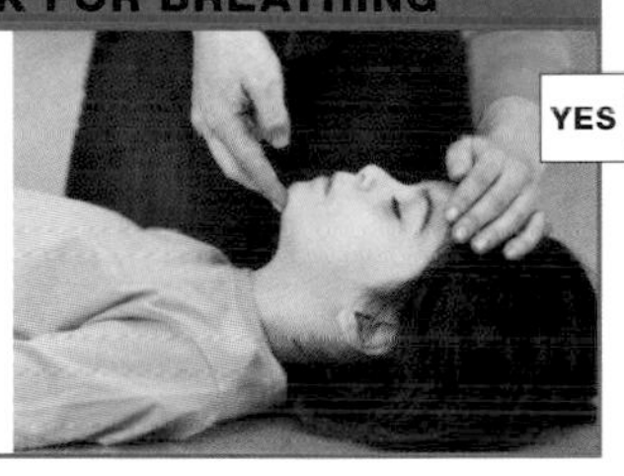

YES → If possible, leave the casualty in the position found. Check and treat life-threatening injuries. Place the child in the recovery position (pp.72–73), or hold infant (p.79). **Call 999/112 for emergency help.**

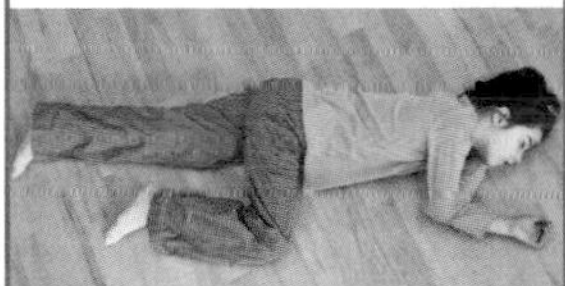

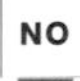

NO ↓

Ask a helper to **call 999/112 for emergency help and, for a child, ask for an AED** ideally with paediatric pads.

- Do not use an AED on an infant.

GIVE INITIAL RESCUE BREATHS

- Carefully remove any visible obstruction from the mouth.
- Give FIVE initial rescue breaths (child p.74 or infant p.80).

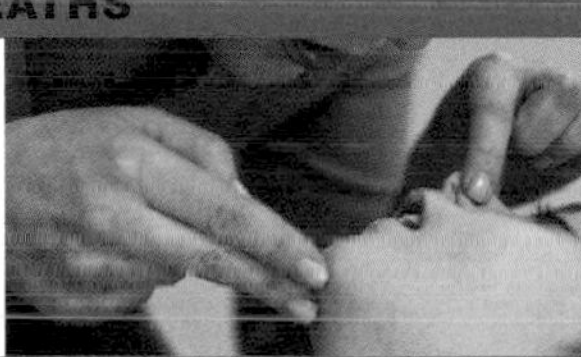

BEGIN CPR

- Give 30 chest compressions (child p.75 or infant p.81).
- Follow with TWO rescue breaths.
- Alternate 30 chest compressions with TWO rescue breaths until emergency help arrives, she shows signs of regaining consciousness, such as coughing, opening her eyes, speaking, or moving purposefully, AND starts to breathe normally, or you are too exhausted to continue.

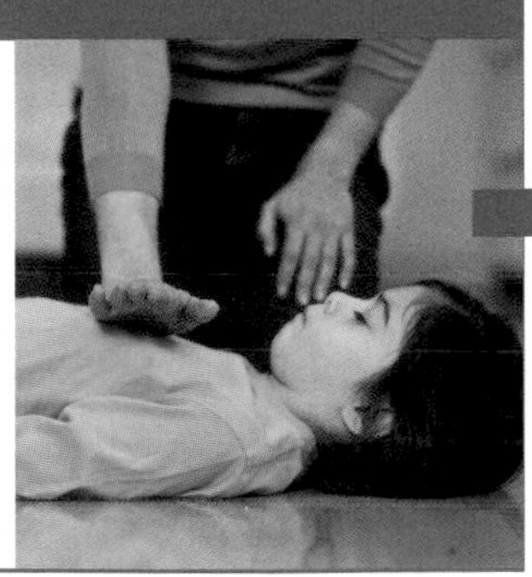

- Give chest compressions only if you have not had formal training in CPR or you are unwilling or unable to give rescue breaths. The ambulance dispatcher will give instructions for chest compression-only CPR.
- If you are alone, carry out CPR for one minute before calling for emergency help.
- If the child starts breathing normally, but remains unconscious, place her in the recovery position (pp.72–73).

UNCONSCIOUS ADULT

The following pages describe techniques for the management of an unconscious adult who may require resuscitation. Always approach and treat the casualty from the side, kneeling down next to his head or chest. You will then be in the correct position to perform all the stages of resuscitation: opening the airway; checking breathing; and giving chest compressions and rescue breaths (together called cardiopulmonary resuscitation, or CPR).

At each stage in the process you will have decisions to make – for example, is the casualty breathing? The steps given here tell you what to do next.

The first priority is to open the casualty's airway so that he can breathe or you can give rescue breaths. If normal breathing returns at any stage, you should place the casualty in the recovery position.

If the casualty is not breathing, the early use of an AED may increase his chance of survival.

HOW TO CHECK RESPONSE

CAUTION

Always assume that there is a neck injury and shake the shoulders very gently.

On discovering a collapsed casualty, you should first make sure the scene is safe and then establish whether he is conscious or unconscious. Do this by gently shaking the casualty's shoulders. Ask "What has happened?" or give a command such as, "Open your eyes". Always speak loudly and clearly to the casualty.

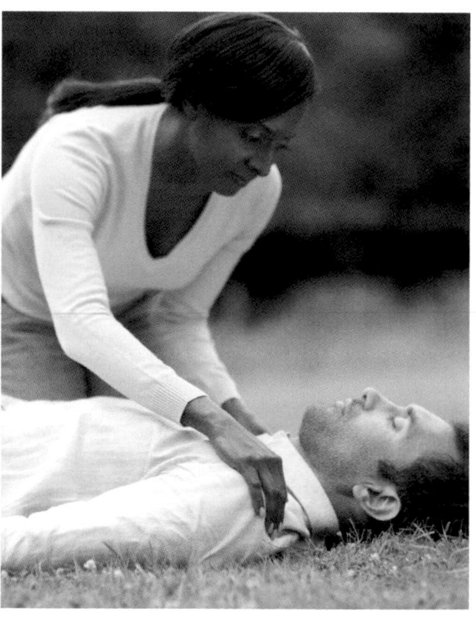

IF THERE IS A RESPONSE

1 **If there is no further danger, leave the casualty in the position in which he was found, check for life-threatening injuries and summon help if needed.**

2 **Treat any condition found and monitor and record vital signs – level of response, breathing and pulse (pp.52–53) – until emergency help arrives or the casualty recovers.**

IF THERE IS NO RESPONSE

1 **Shout for help. Leave the casualty in the position in which he was found and open the airway.**

2 **If you are unable to open the airway in the position in which he was found, roll him on to his back and open the airway. Go to *How to open the airway* (opposite).**

HOW TO OPEN THE AIRWAY

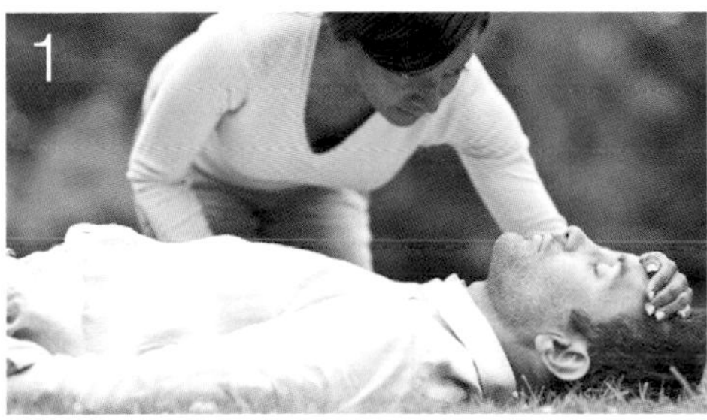

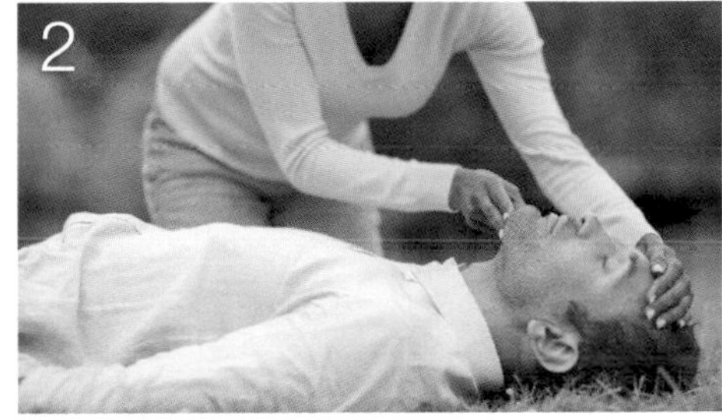

1 Place one hand on his forehead. Gently tilt his head back. As you do this, the mouth will fall open slightly.

2 Place the fingertips of your other hand on the point of the casualty's chin and lift the chin. Check the casualty's breathing. Go to *How to check breathing*, below.

HOW TO CHECK BREATHING

Keeping the airway open, look, listen and feel for normal breathing: look for chest movement; listen for sounds of breathing; and feel for breaths on your cheek. Do this for no more than ten seconds before deciding whether the casualty is breathing normally. Breathing may be agonal (p.59). If there is any doubt, act as if it is not normal

IF THE CASUALTY IS BREATHING

1 Check the casualty for any life-threatening injuries, such as severe bleeding, and treat as necessary.

2 Place the casualty in the recovery position (p.64) and **call 999/112 for emergency help.**

3 Monitor and record vital signs – level of response, breathing and pulse (pp.52–53) – while waiting for help to arrive. Go to *How to place casualty in recovery position* (pp.64–65).

IF THE CASUALTY IS NOT BREATHING

1 Ask a helper to **call 999/112 for emergency help.** Ask the person to bring an AED if one is available. If you are alone, make the call yourself.

2 Begin CPR with chest compressions. Go to *How to give CPR* (pp.66–67).

UNCONSCIOUS ADULT (continued)

HOW TO PLACE CASUALTY IN RECOVERY POSITION

If the casualty is found lying on his side or front, rather than his back, not all the following steps will be necessary to place him in the recovery position. If the mechanisms of injury suggest a spinal injury, treat as on pp.171–73.

1 Kneel beside the casualty. Remove his spectacles and any bulky objects, such as mobile phones or large bunches of keys, from his pockets. Do not search his pockets for small items.

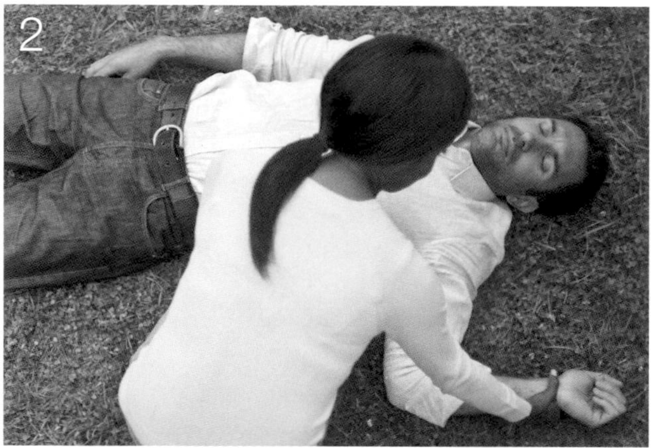

2 Make sure that both of the casualty's legs are straight. Place the arm that is nearest to you at right angles to the casualty's body, with the elbow bent and the palm facing upwards.

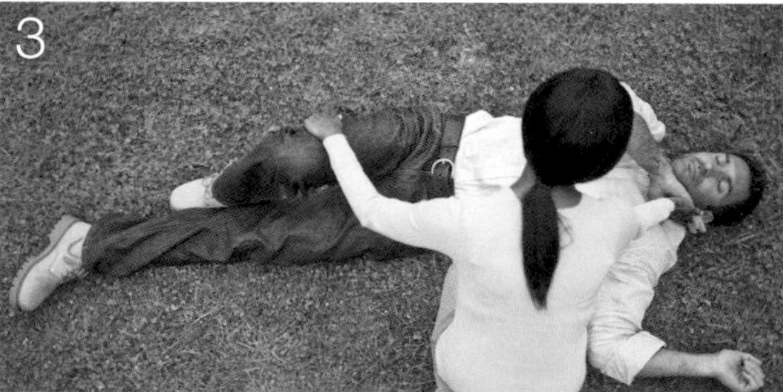

3 Bring the arm that is farthest from you across the casualty's chest, and hold the back of his hand against the cheek nearest to you. With your other hand, grasp the far leg just above the knee and pull it up, keeping the foot flat on the ground.

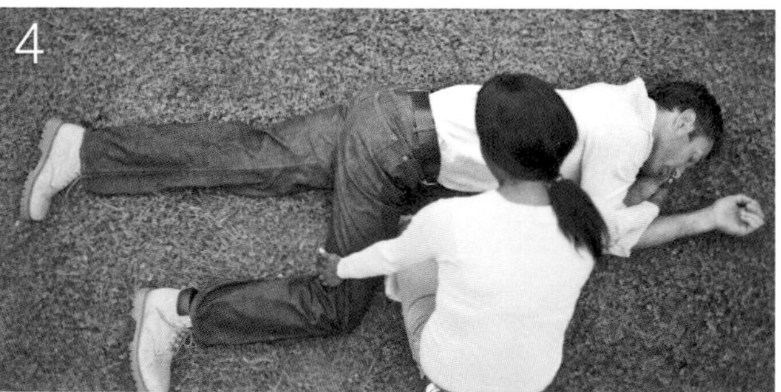

4 Keeping the casualty's hand pressed against his cheek, pull on the far leg and roll the casualty towards you and on to his side.

5 Adjust the upper leg so that both the hip and the knee are bent at right angles.

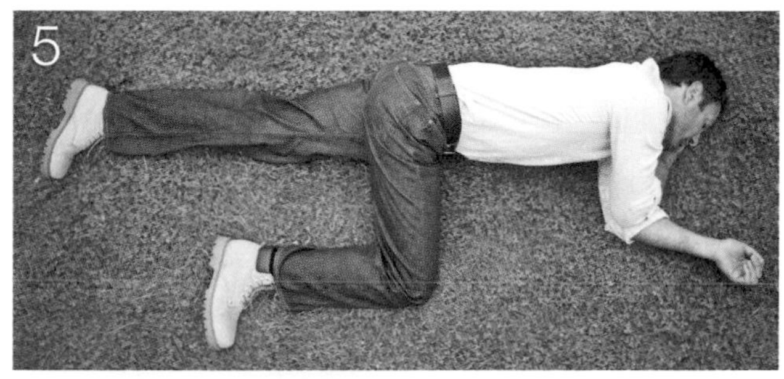

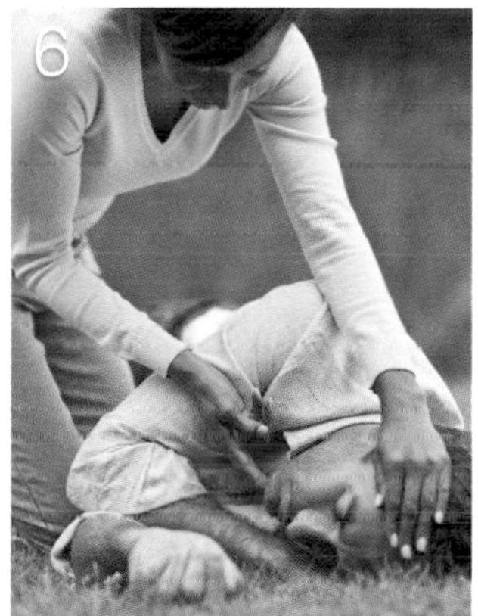

6 Tilt the casualty's head back and tilt his chin so that the airway remains open (p.63).

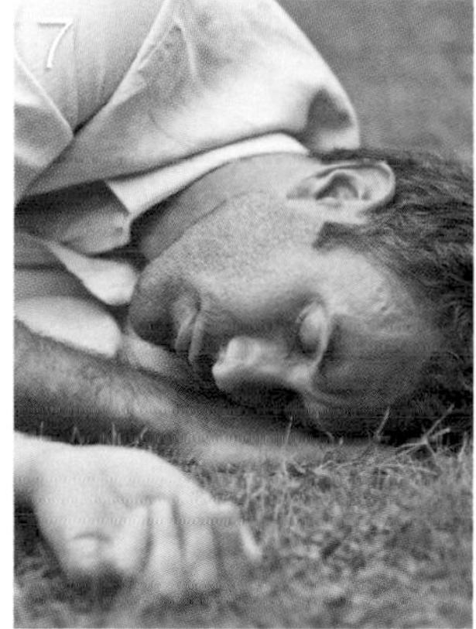

7 If necessary, adjust the hand under the cheek to keep the airway open.

8 If it has not already been done, **call 999/112 for emergency help.** Monitor and record vital signs – level of response, breathing and pulse (pp.52–53) – while waiting for help to arrive.

9 If the casualty has to be left in the recovery position for longer than 30 minutes, roll him on to his back, and then roll him on to the opposite side – unless other injuries prevent you from doing this.

SPECIAL CASE RECOVERY POSITION FOR SUSPECTED SPINAL INJURY

If you suspect a spinal injury (p.171) and need to place the casualty in the recovery position because you can't maintain an open airway, try to keep the spine straight using the following guidelines.

- If you are alone, use the technique shown opposite and above.
- If you have a helper, one of you should steady the head while the other turns the casualty (right).
- With three people, one person should steady the head while another turns the casualty. The third person should keep the casualty's back straight during the manoeuvre.
- If there are four or more people in total, use the log-roll technique (p.173).

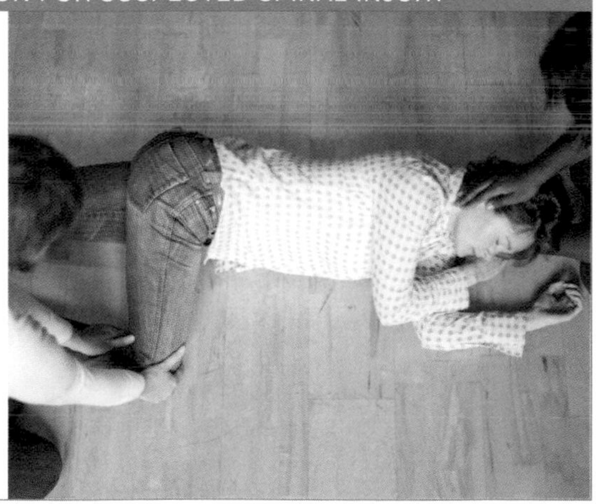

UNCONSCIOUS ADULT (continued)

HOW TO GIVE CPR

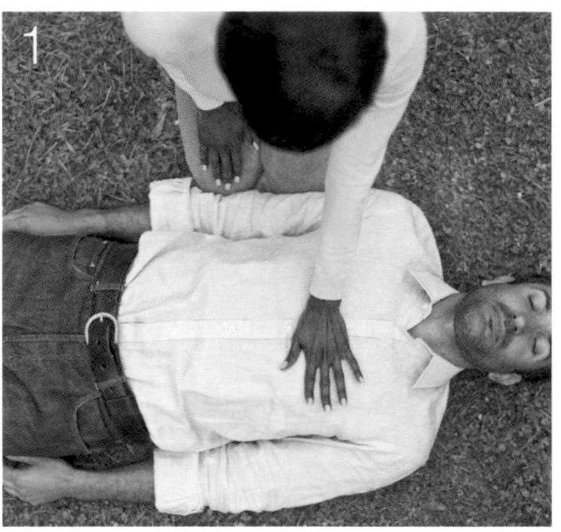

1 Kneel beside the casualty level with his chest. Place the heel of one hand on the centre of the casualty's chest. You can identify the correct hand position for chest compressions through a casualty's clothing.

HAND POSITION

Place your hand on the casualty's breastbone as indicated here. Make sure that you do not press on the casualty's ribs, the lower tip of the breastbone or the upper abdomen.

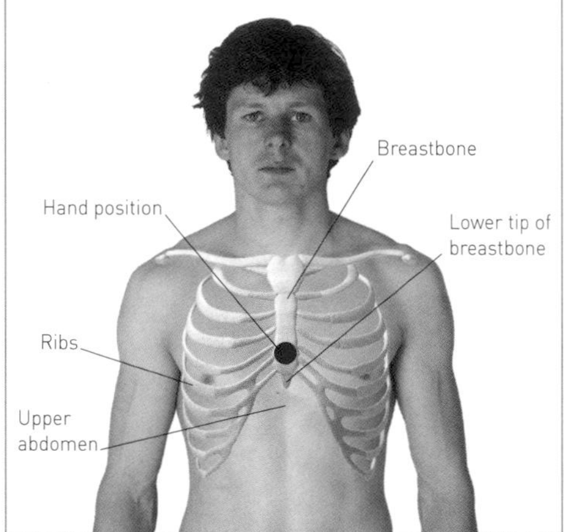

2 Place the heel of your other hand on top of the first hand, and interlock your fingers, making sure the fingers are kept off the ribs.

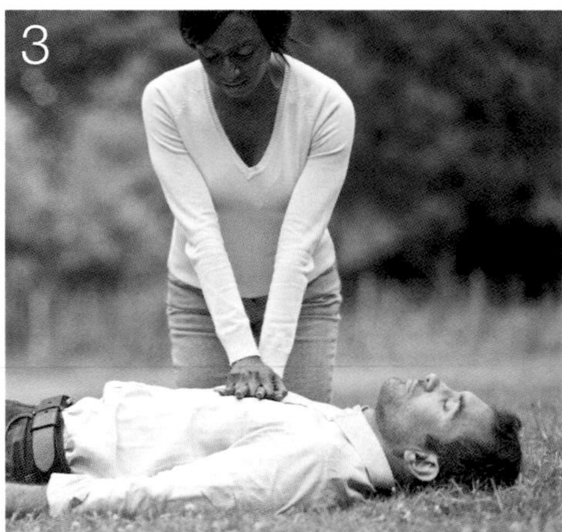

3 Leaning over the casualty, with your arms straight, press down vertically on the breastbone and depress the chest by 5–6cm (2–2½in). Release the pressure without removing your hands from his chest. Allow the chest to come back up fully (recoil) before giving the next compression.

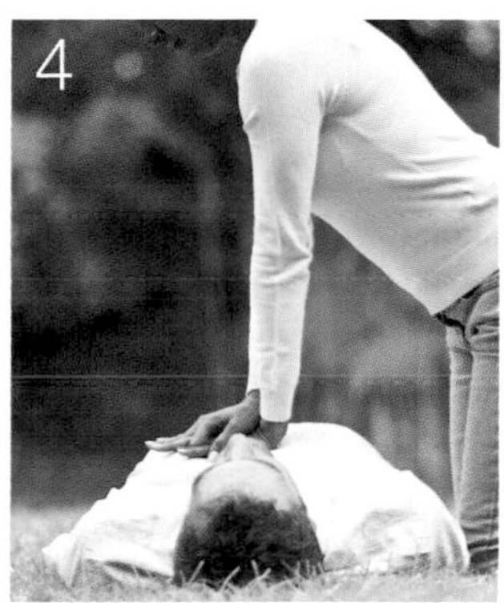

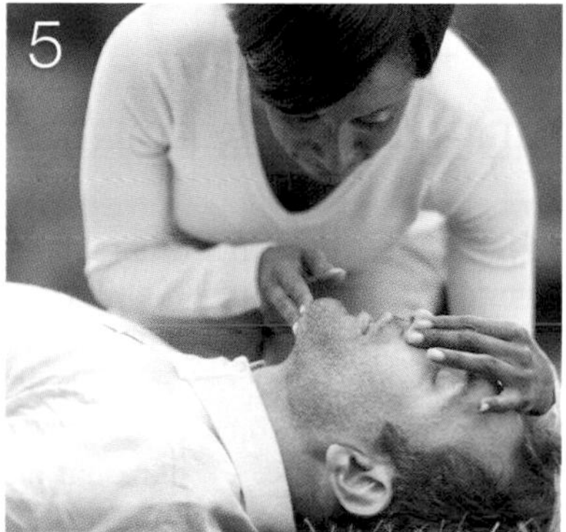

CAUTION

If there is more than one rescuer, change over every 1–2 minutes, with minimal interruption to chest compressions.

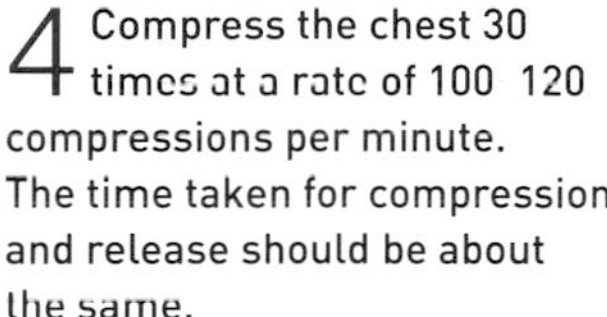

4 Compress the chest 30 times at a rate of 100–120 compressions per minute. The time taken for compression and release should be about the same.

5 Move to the casualty's head and make sure that the airway is still open. Put one hand on his forehead and two fingers of the other hand under the tip of his chin. Move the hand that was on the forehead down to pinch the soft part of the nose with the finger and thumb. Allow the casualty's mouth to fall open.

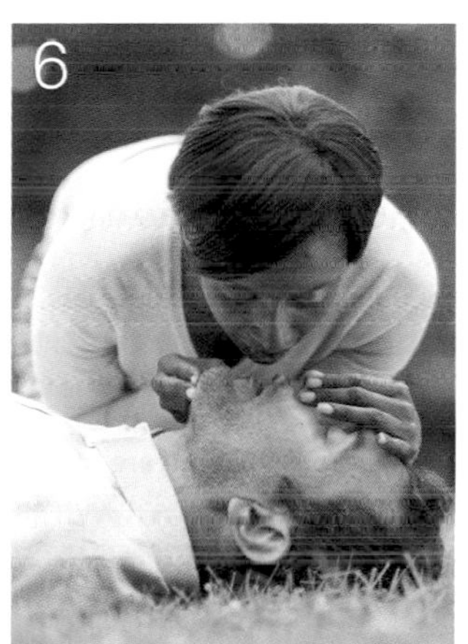

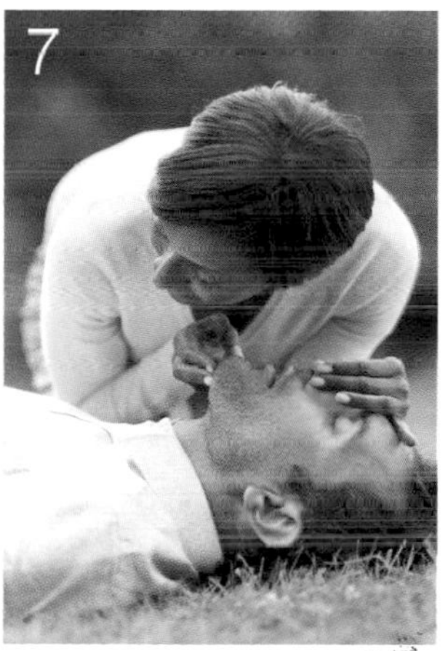

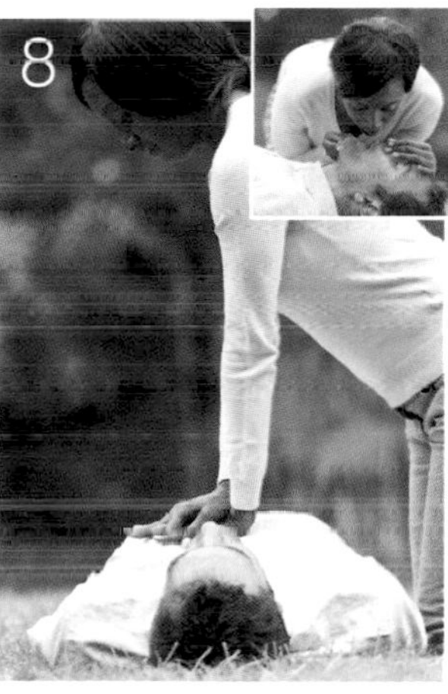

6 Take a breath and place your lips around the casualty's mouth, making sure you have a good seal. Blow into the casualty's mouth until the chest rises. A complete rescue breath should take one second. If the chest does not rise, you may need to adjust the head position (p.63).

7 Maintaining head tilt and chin lift, take your mouth off the casualty's mouth and look to see the chest fall. If the chest rises visibly as you blow and falls fully when you lift your mouth away, you have given a rescue breath – one rescue breath should take one second. Give a second rescue breath.

8 Continue the cycle of 30 chest compressions followed by TWO rescue breaths until either: emergency help arrives and takes over; the casualty shows signs of regaining consciousness, such as coughing, opening his eyes, speaking, or moving purposefully, AND starts to breathe normally; or you are too exhausted to continue.

UNCONSCIOUS CHILD (one year to puberty)

The following pages describe the techniques that may be needed for the resuscitation of an unconscious child aged between one year and puberty.

When treating a child, always approach and treat her from the same side, kneeling down next to the head or chest. You will then be in the correct position to carry out all the different stages of resuscitation: opening the airway, checking breathing and giving rescue breaths and chest compressions (together known as cardiopulmonary resuscitation, or CPR).

At each stage you will have decisions to make; for example, is the child breathing? The steps given here tell you what to do next. Your first priority is to open the child's airway, so that she can breathe, or so that you can give rescue breaths. If normal breathing resumes, place the child in the recovery position (pp.72–73).

If a child with a known heart condition collapses, call 999/112 for emergency help immediately and ask for an AED to be brought (pp.82–85). Early access to advanced care can be life-saving.

HOW TO CHECK RESPONSE

On discovering a collapsed child, you should first establish whether she is conscious or unconscious. Do this by speaking loudly and clearly to the child. Ask "What has happened?" or give a command such as, "Open your eyes". Place one hand on her shoulder, and gently tap her to see if there is a response.

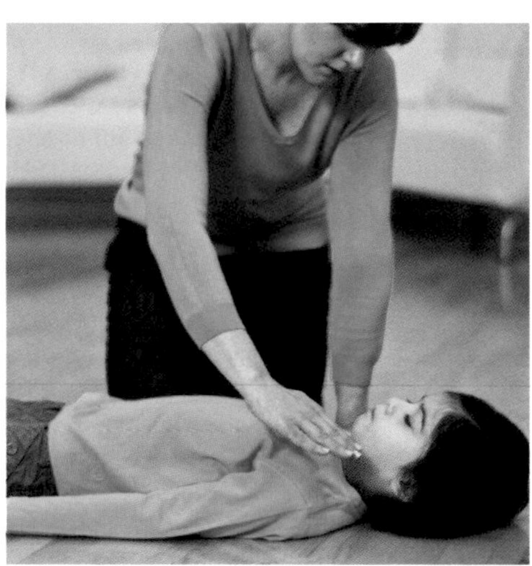

IF THERE IS A RESPONSE

1 **If there is no further danger, leave the child in the position in which she was found, check for life-threatening injuries and summon emergency help if needed.**

2 **Treat any condition found. Monitor and record vital signs – level of response, breathing and pulse (pp.52–53) – until emergency help arrives or the child recovers.**

IF THERE IS NO RESPONSE

1 **Shout for help. Leave the child in the position in which she was found, and open the airway.**

2 **If you are unable to open the airway in the position in which she was found, roll the child on to her back and open the airway. Go to *How to open the airway* (opposite).**

HOW TO OPEN THE AIRWAY

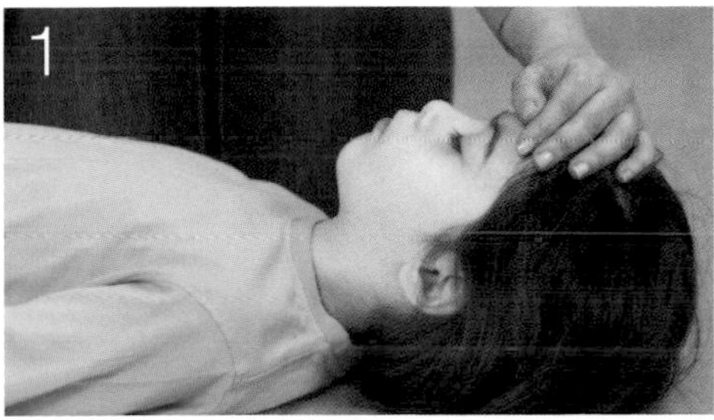

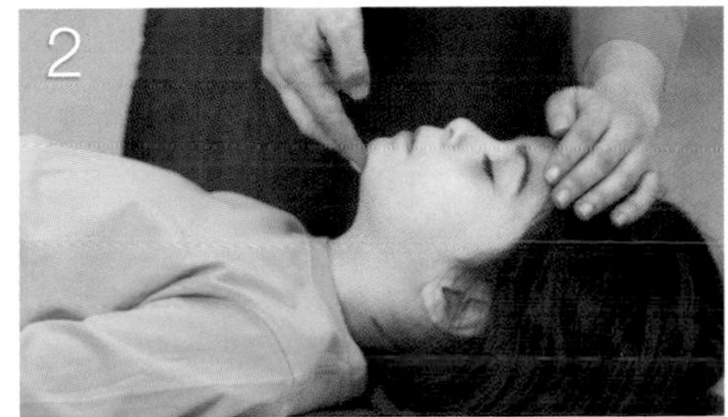

1 Place one hand on the child's forehead. Gently tilt her head back. As you do this, the mouth will fall open slightly.

2 Place the fingertips of your other hand on the point of the chin and lift. Do not push on the soft tissues under the chin since this may block the airway. Now check to see if the child is breathing. Go to *How to check breathing* (below).

HOW TO CHECK BREATHING

Keep the airway open and look, listen and feel for normal breathing – look for chest movement, listen for sounds of normal breathing and feel for breaths on your cheek. Do this for no more than ten seconds.

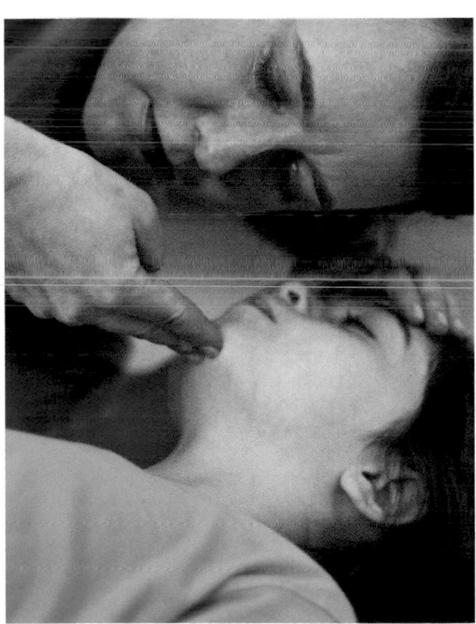

IF THE CHILD IS BREATHING

1 Check for life-threatening injuries such as severe bleeding. Treat as necessary.

2 Place the child in the recovery position and **call 999/112 for emergency help.**

3 Monitor and record vital signs – level of response, breathing and pulse (pp.52–53) – while waiting for help to arrive. Go to *How to place child in recovery position* (pp.72–73).

IF THE CHILD IS NOT BREATHING

1 Ask a helper to **call 999/112 for emergency help.** If you are on your own, perform CPR for one minute and then make the emergency call yourself.

2 Begin CPR with FIVE initial rescue breaths. Go to *How to give CPR* (pp.74–75).

UNCONSCIOUS CHILD (continued)

HOW TO PLACE CHILD IN RECOVERY POSITION

If the child is found lying on her side or front, rather than her back, not all of these steps will be necessary to place her in the recovery position. If the mechanisms of injury suggest a spinal injury, treat as on pp.171–73.

1 Kneel beside the child. Remove her spectacles and any bulky objects from her pockets, but do not search them for small items.

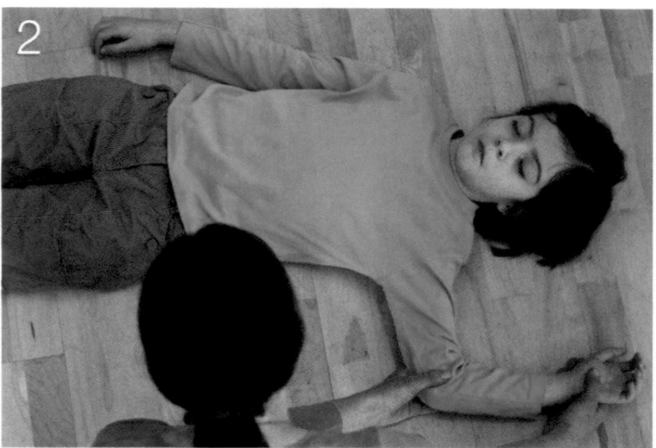

2 Make sure that both of the child's legs are straight. Place the arm nearest to you at right angles to the child's body, with the elbow bent and the palm facing upwards.

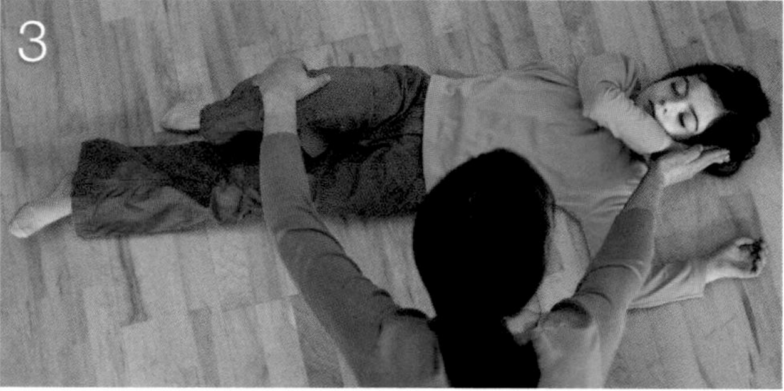

3 Bring the arm that is farthest from you across the child's chest, and hold the back of her hand against the cheek nearest to you. With your other hand, grasp the far leg just above the knee and pull it up, keeping the foot flat on the ground.

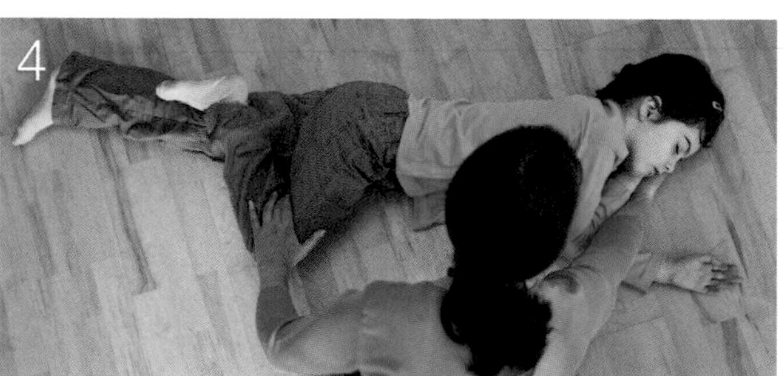

4 Keeping the child's hand pressed against her cheek, pull on the far leg and roll the child towards you and on to her side.

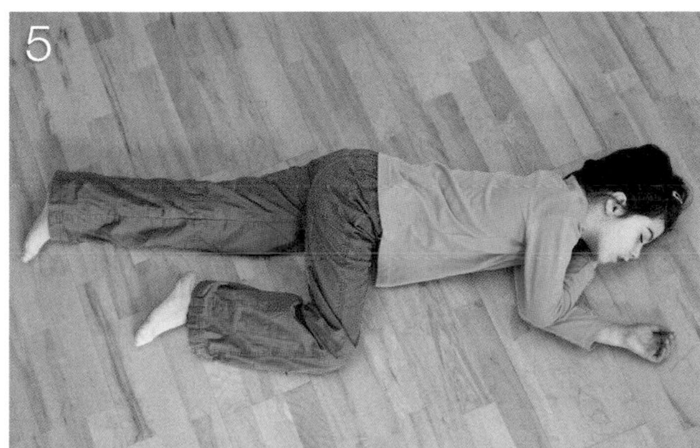
5

5 Adjust the upper leg so that both the hip and the knee are bent at right angles. Tilt the child's head back and lift the chin so that the airway remains open.

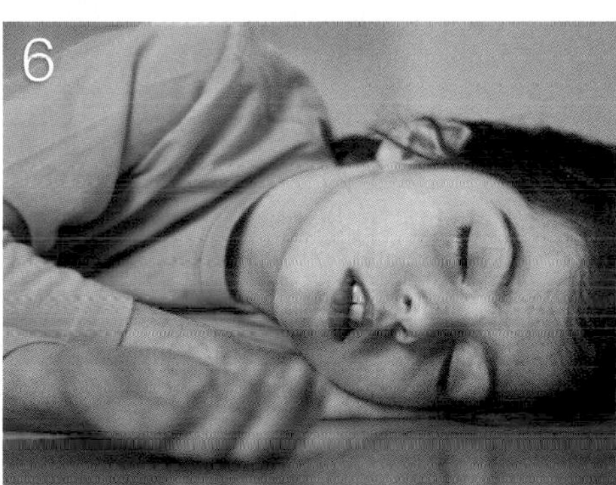
6

6 If necessary, adjust the hand under the cheek to make sure that the head remains tilted and the airway stays open. If it has not already been done, **call 999/112 for emergency help**. Monitor and record vital signs – level of response, breathing and pulse (pp.52–53) – until help arrives.

7 If the child has to be left in the recovery position for longer than 30 minutes, you should roll her on to her back, then turn her on to the opposite side – unless other injuries prevent you from doing this.

SPECIAL CASE RECOVERY POSITION FOR SUSPECTED SPINAL INJURY

If you suspect a spinal injury (p.171) and need to place the casualty in the recovery position because you can't maintain an open airway, try to keep the spine straight using the following guidelines:

- If you are alone, use the technique shown on this page.
- If there are two of you, one person should steady the head while the other turns the child.
- If there are three of you, one person should steady the head while one person turns the child. The third person should keep the child's back straight during the manoeuvre.
- If there are four or more people in total, use the log-roll technique (p.173).

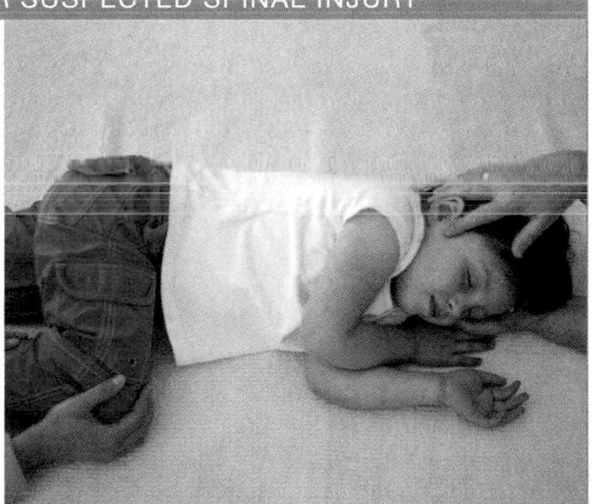

UNCONSCIOUS CHILD (continued)

HOW TO GIVE CPR

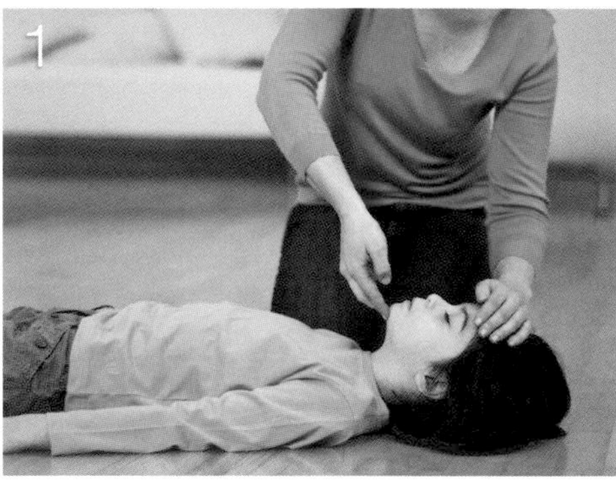

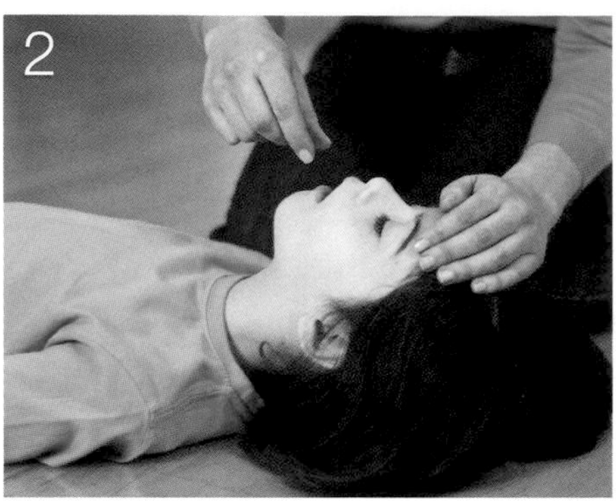

1 Ensure the airway is still open by keeping one hand on the child's forehead and two fingers of the other hand on the point of her chin.

2 Pick out any visible obstructions from the mouth. Do not sweep the mouth with your finger to look for obstructions.

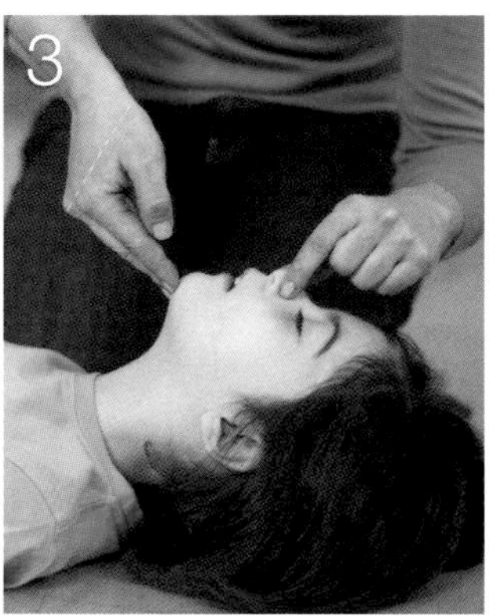

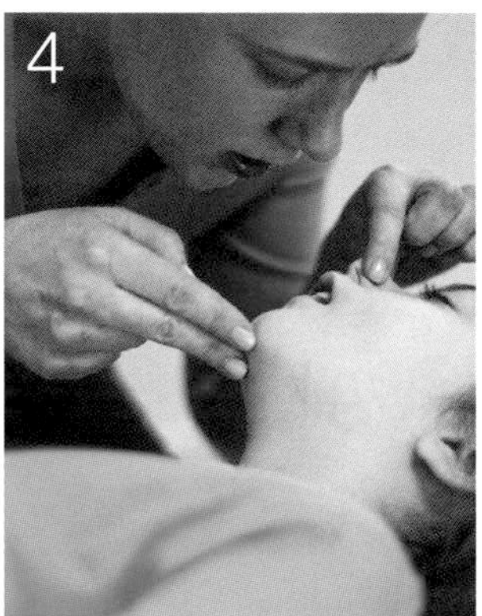

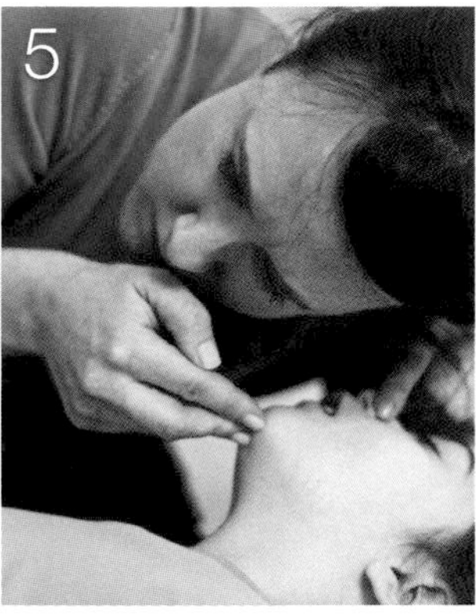

3 Pinch the soft part of the child's nose with the finger and thumb of the hand that was on the forehead. Make sure that her nostrils are closed to prevent air from escaping. Allow her mouth to fall open.

4 Take a deep breath in before placing your lips around the child's mouth, making sure that you form an airtight seal. Blow steadily into the child's mouth; the chest should rise.

5 Maintaining head tilt and chin lift, take your mouth off the child's mouth and look to see the chest fall. If the chest rises visibly as you blow and falls fully when you lift your mouth, you have given a rescue breath. Each complete rescue breath should take one second. If the chest does not rise you may need to adjust the head (p.71). Give a child FIVE initial rescue breaths.

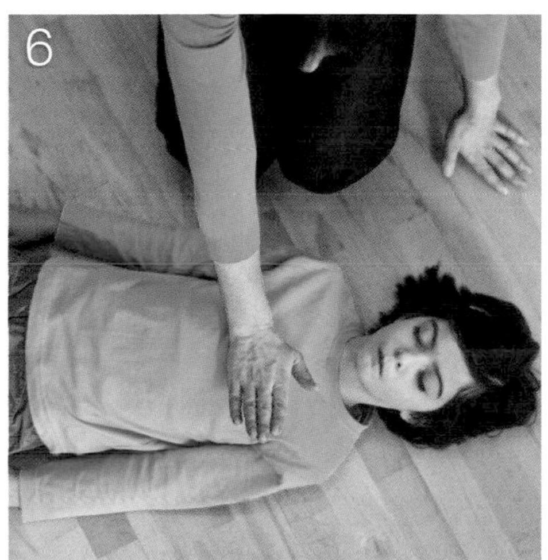

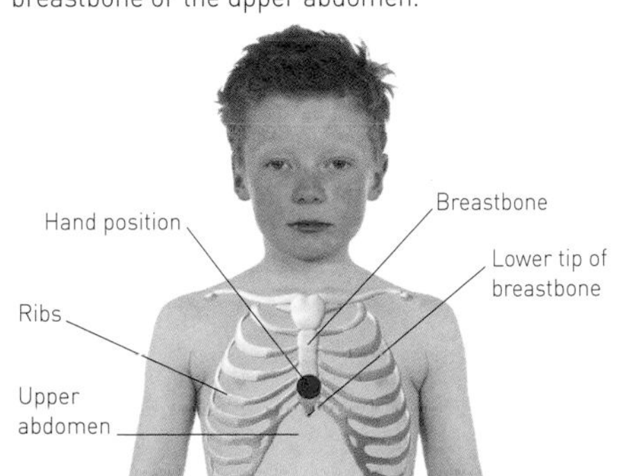

6 Kneel level with the child's chest. Place one hand on the centre of her chest. This is the point at which you will apply pressure.

CAUTION

With more than one rescuer, change every 1–2 minutes, with minimal interruption to compressions.

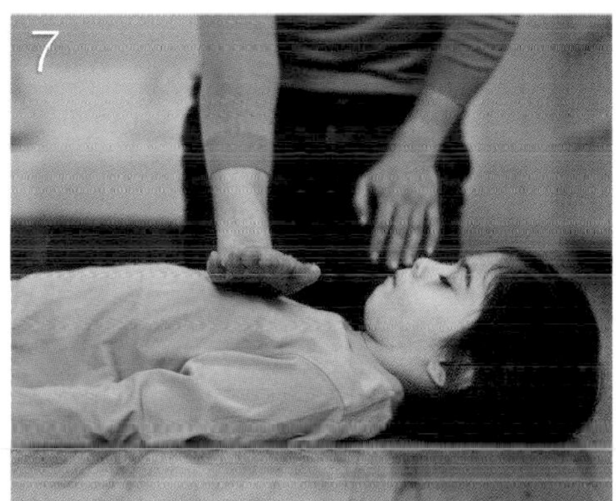

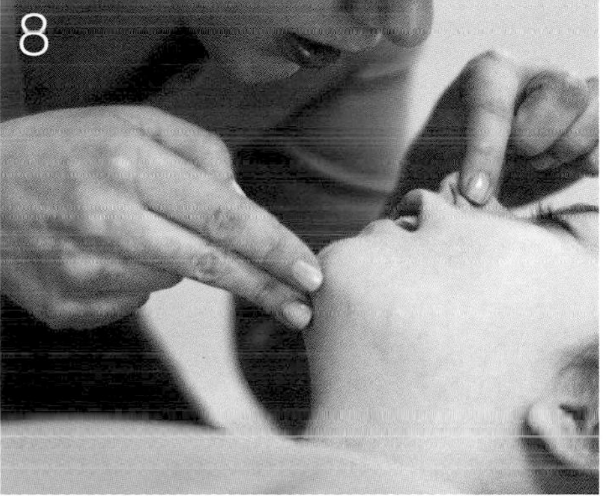

7 Lean over the child, with your arm straight, and then press down vertically on the breastbone with the heel of your hand. Depress the chest by at least one-third of its depth. Release the pressure without removing your hand from the chest. Allow the chest to come back up completely (recoil) before you give the next compression. Compress the chest 30 times, at a rate of 100–120 compressions per minute. The time taken for compression and release should be about the same.

8 Return to the child's head, open the airway and give TWO further rescue breaths.

9 If you are on your own, alternate 30 chest compressions with TWO rescue breaths for one minute, then stop to **call 999/112 for emergency help**. Continue CPR until either emergency help arrives, the child shows signs of regaining consciousness, such as coughing, opening her eyes, speaking, or moving purposefully, AND starts to breathe normally, or you become too exhausted to continue.

UNCONSCIOUS CHILD (continued)

SPECIAL CONSIDERATIONS FOR CPR

There are circumstances when it may be more difficult to deliver CPR. For example, you may not have been formally trained in CPR or you may be unwilling or unable to give rescue breaths. In this situation you can give chest compressions only. If you call an ambulance, the dispatcher will give instructions for compression-only CPR.

- **If there is more than one rescuer**, change over every 1–2 minutes, with minimal interruption to compressions.
- **If the child vomits** during CPR, roll her away from you onto her side, ensuring that her head is turned towards the floor to allow vomit to drain away. Clear the mouth, then immediately roll her onto her back again and recommence CPR.
- **If the child is large**, or the rescuer is small, give chest compressions using both hands, as for an adult casualty (pp.66–67). Place one hand on the chest, cover it with your other hand and interlock your fingers.

CHEST COMPRESSION-ONLY CPR

1 **Kneel beside the child, level with her chest. Place the heel of one hand on the centre of his chest, cover it with your other hand and interlock your fingers.**

2 **Lean over the child with your arms straight and depress the chest by at least one third of the depth, and release the pressure (but do not remove your hands).**

3 **Repeat compressions at a rate of 100–120 per minute until help arrives or the child shows signs of regaining consciousness, such as coughing, opening her eyes, speaking, or moving purposefully, AND starts to breathe normally, or you are too exhausted to continue.**

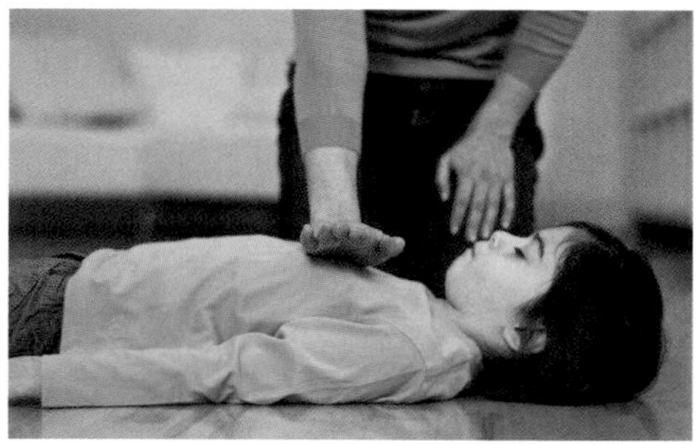

PROBLEMS WITH RESCUE BREATHING

If a child's chest does not rise when giving rescue breaths:

- **Recheck the head tilt** and chin lift;
- **Recheck the mouth.** Remove any obvious obstructions, but do not do a finger sweep of the mouth.

Make no more than two attempts to achieve rescue breaths before repeating the chest compressions.

VARIATIONS FOR RESCUE BREATHING

There are some cases where mouth-to-mouth rescue breaths are not appropriate and you will need to use a mouth-to-nose technique.

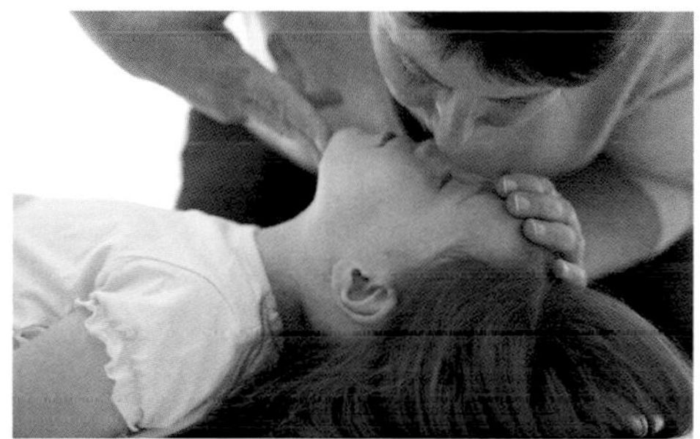

MOUTH-TO-NOSE RESCUE BREATHING
If a child has been rescued from water, or injuries to the mouth make it impossible to achieve a good seal, you can use the mouth-to-nose method for giving rescue breaths. With the child's mouth closed, form a tight seal with your lips around the nose and blow steadily into the casualty's nose. Then allow the mouth to fall open to let the air escape.

FACE SHIELDS AND POCKET MASKS

A face shield is a plastic barrier with a filter that is placed over the casualty's mouth. A pocket mask is more substantial and has a valve through which breaths are given. If you know how to use one of these aids, carry it with you and use it if you need to resuscitate a child.

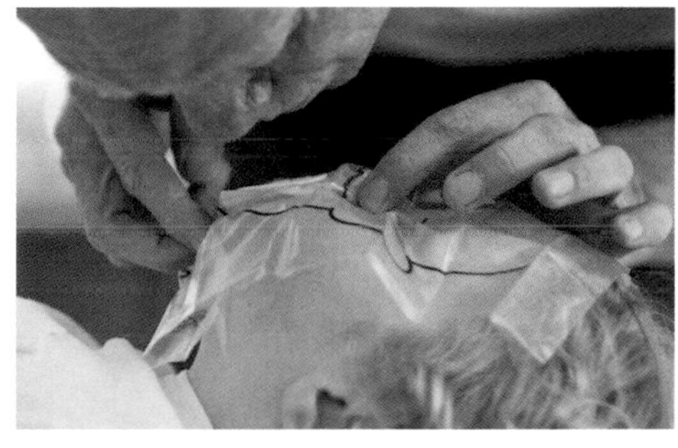

USING A FACE SHIELD
Tilt the child's head back to open the airway and lift the chin. Place the plastic shield over the child's face so that the filter is over her mouth. Pinch the nose and deliver breaths through the filter.

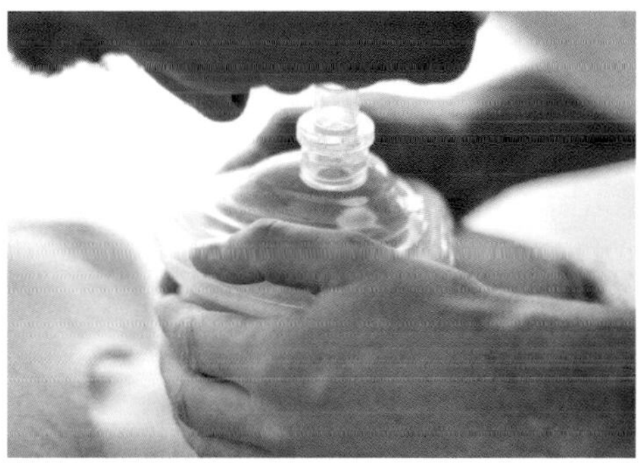

USING A POCKET MASK
Kneel behind the child's head. Open the airway and place the mask, broad end towards you, over the child's mouth and nose. Deliver breaths through the mouthpiece.

WHEN THE AMBULANCE ARRIVES

The ambulance service may initially send a sole responder in a fast response vehicle or a community first responder ahead of the ambulance. If an AED is not already attached to the casualty the ambulance personnel will do that. They will also use additional drugs and equipment to provide advanced care (p.57). If you are asked to help you should listen carefully and follow the instructions carefully (p.23). The ambulance personnel will make a decision whether to transfer the child to hospital immediately or to continue treatment at the scene. Any decision to stop resuscitation can only be made by a health care professional.

UNCONSCIOUS INFANT (under one year)

The following pages describe techniques that may be used for the resuscitation of an unconscious infant under one year. For a child over the age of one year, use the child resuscitation procedure (pp.70–77).

Always treat the infant from the side, the correct position for doing all the stages of resuscitation: opening the airway, checking breathing and giving rescue breaths and chest compressions (together known as cardiopulmonary resuscitation, or CPR). Your first priority is to ensure that the airway is open and clear. If normal breathing resumes at any stage, hold the infant in the recovery position (opposite).

Call 999/112 for emergency help if an infant with a known heart condition becomes unconscious.

HOW TO CHECK RESPONSE

Gently tap or flick the sole of the infant's foot and call his name to see if he responds. Never shake an infant.

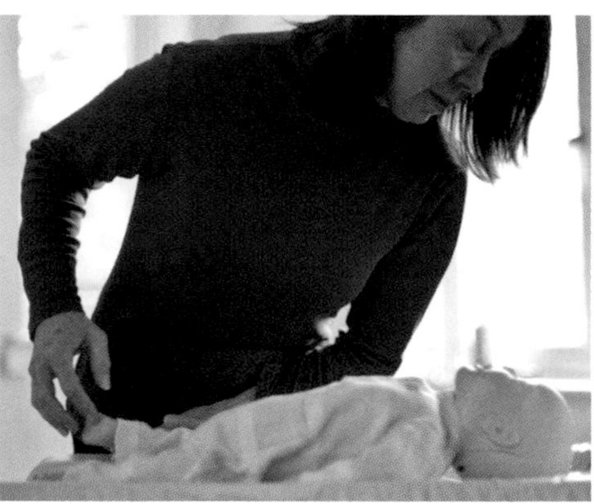

IF THERE IS A RESPONSE

Check and treat for life-threatening injuries. Take the infant with you to summon help if needed. Monitor and record vital signs – level of response, breathing and pulse (pp.52–53) – until help arrives.

IF THERE IS NO RESPONSE

Shout for help, then open the airway. Go to *How to open the airway* (below).

HOW TO OPEN THE AIRWAY

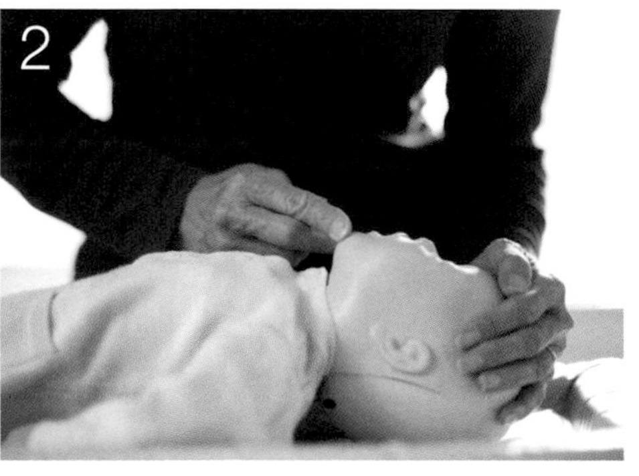

1 Place one hand on the infant's forehead and very gently tilt the head back.

2 Place one fingertip of your other hand on the point of the chin. Gently lift the point of the chin. Do not push on the soft tissues under the chin since this may block the airway.

3 Now check to see if the infant is breathing. Go to *How to check breathing* (opposite).

HOW TO CHECK BREATHING

Keep the airway open and look, listen and feel for normal breathing – look for chest movement, listen for sounds of breathing and feel for breaths on your cheek. Do this for no more than ten seconds.

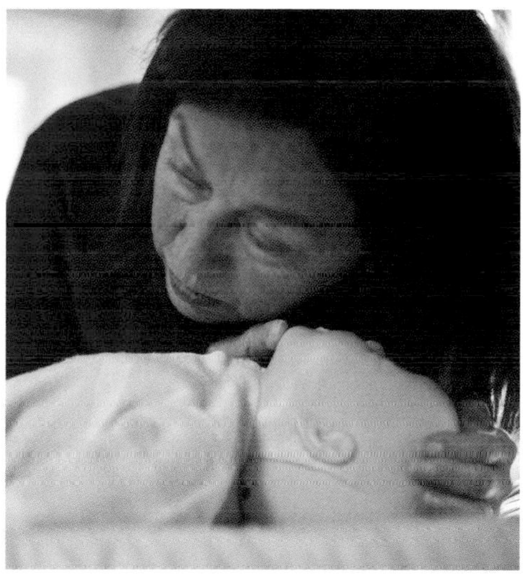

IF THE INFANT IS BREATHING

1 Check for life-threatening injuries, such as severe bleeding, and treat if necessary.

2 Hold the infant in the recovery position. Monitor and record vital signs – level of response, breathing and pulse (pp.52–53) – regularly until help arrives. Go to *How to hold in recovery position* (below).

IF THE INFANT IS NOT BREATHING

1 Ask a helper to **call 999/112 for emergency help**. If you are on your own, perform CPR for one minute before making the call yourself.

2 Begin CPR with FIVE initial rescue breaths. Go to *How to give CPR* (pp.80–81).

HOW TO HOLD IN RECOVERY POSITION

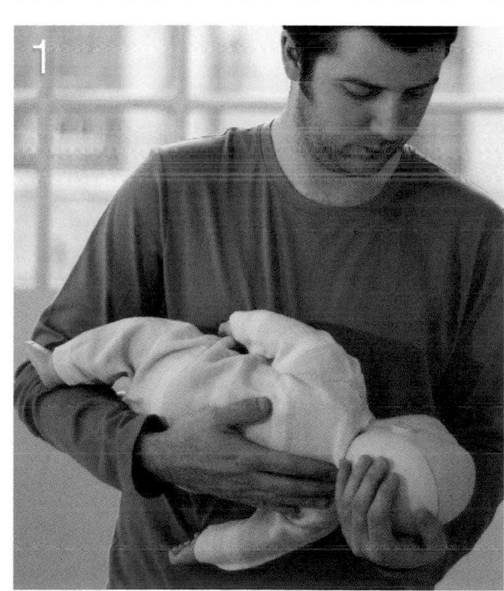

1 Cradle the infant in your arms with his head tilted downwards. This position prevents him from choking on his tongue or from inhaling vomit.

2 Monitor and record vital signs – level of response, breathing and pulse (pp.52–53) – until help arrives.

UNCONSCIOUS INFANT (continued)

HOW TO GIVE CPR

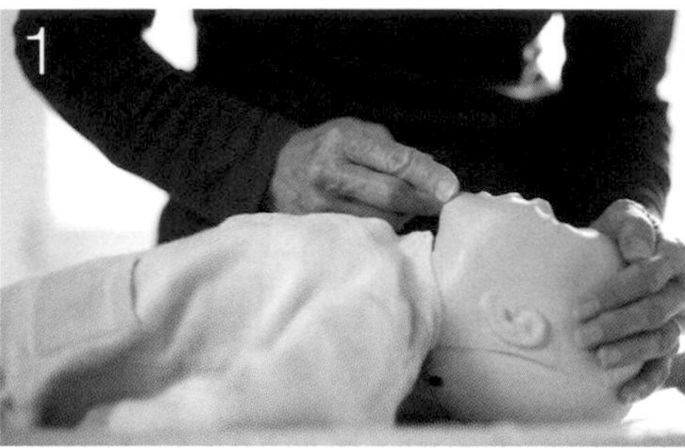

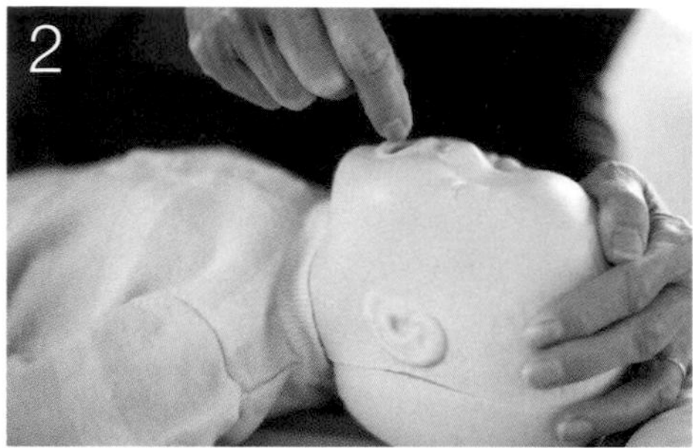

1 Place the infant on his back on a flat surface, at about waist height in front of you, or on the floor. Make sure that the airway is still open by keeping one hand on the infant's forehead and one fingertip of the other hand under the tip of his chin.

2 Pick out any visible obstructions from mouth and nose. Do not sweep the mouth with your finger looking for obstructions.

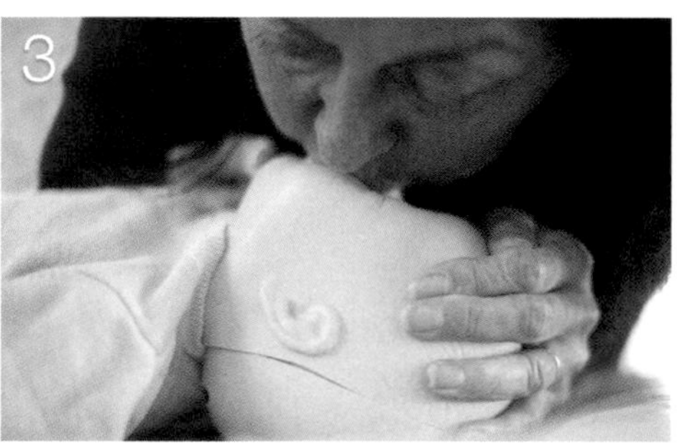

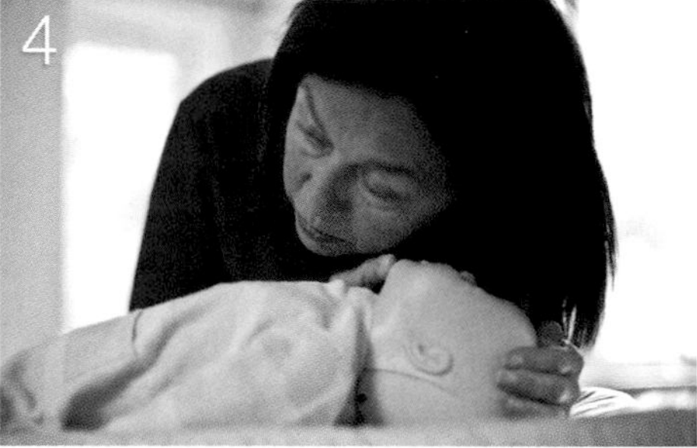

3 Take a breath. Place your lips around the infant's mouth and nose to form an airtight seal. If you cannot make a seal around the mouth and nose, close the infant's mouth and make a seal around the nose only. Take a breath and blow steadily into the infant's mouth for one second; the chest should rise.

4 Maintaining head tilt and chin lift, take your mouth off the infant's mouth and see if his chest falls. If the chest rises visibly as you blow and falls fully when you lift your mouth, you have given a breath. Each complete rescue breath should take one second. Give FIVE rescue breaths.

CAUTION

If you cannot achieve breaths:

- Recheck the head tilt and chin lift;
- Recheck the infant's mouth and nose and remove obvious obstructions. Do not do a finger sweep;
- Check that you have a firm seal around the mouth and nose;
- Make up to five attempts to achieve rescue breaths, then begin chest compressions.

If the infant vomits during CPR, roll him away from you onto his side to allow the vomit to drain. Resume CPR as soon as possible.

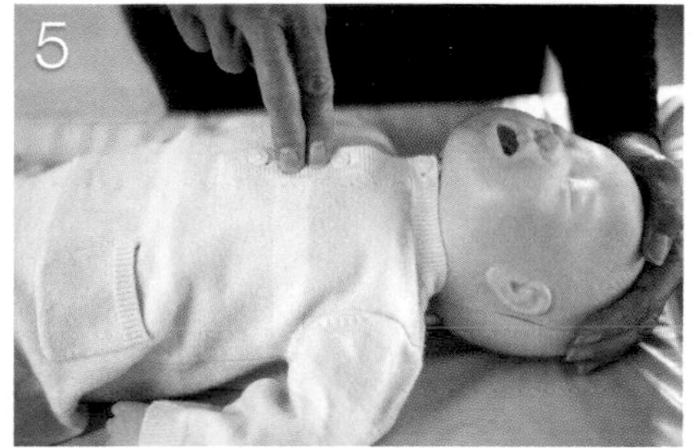

5 Place two fingertips of your lower hand on the centre of the infant's chest. Press down vertically on the infant's breastbone and depress the chest by at least one-third of its depth. Release the pressure without removing your fingers from the breastbone. Allow the chest to come back up fully (recoil) before giving the next compression. The time taken for compression and release should be about the same. Repeat to give 30 compressions at a rate of 100–120 times per minute.

6 Return to the infant's head, open the airway and give TWO further rescue breaths.

7 If you are on your own, alternate 30 chest compressions with TWO rescue breaths for one minute then stop to **call 999/112 for emergency help**. Continue CPR until either emergency help arrives and takes over, the infant shows signs of regaining consciousness, such as coughing, opening his/her eyes, speaking or moving AND starts to breathe normally or you become too exhausted to continue.

HAND POSITION

Place your fingers on the breastbone as indicated here. Make sure that you do not apply pressure over the ribs, the lower tip of the infant's breastbone or the upper abdomen.

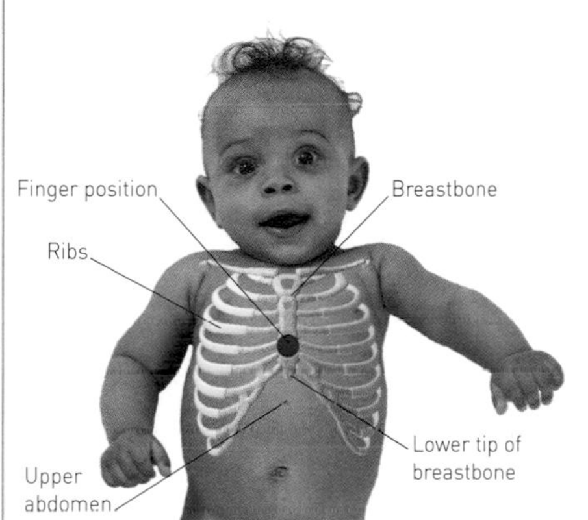

CHEST COMPRESSION-ONLY CPR

Give chest compressions only if you have not had formal training in CPR or if you are unwilling or unable to give resuc breaths. The ambulance dispatcher will give instructions for chest compression-only CPR.

HOW TO USE AN AED

CAUTION

- Make sure that no-one is touching the casualty because this will interfere with the AED readings and there is a risk of electric shock.
- Do not turn off the AED or remove the pads at any point, even if the casualty appears to have recovered.
- It does not matter if the AED pads are reversed. If you put them on the wrong way round, do not remove and replace them; it wastes time and the pads may not stick to the chest properly when they are reattached.

When the heart stops, a cardiac arrest has occurred. The most common cause is an abnormal rhythm of the heart, known as ventricular fibrillation. This abnormal rhythm can occur when the heart muscle is damaged as a result of a heart attack or when insufficient oxygen reaches the heart. A machine called an automated external defibrillator (AED) can be used to correct the heart rhythm by one or more electric "shocks". AEDs can be used safely and effectively without prior training. They are available in many public places, including shopping centres, railway stations and airports. The machine analyses the casualty's heart rhythm and shows with visual prompts – or tells you by voice prompts – what action to take at each stage. In most cases when an AED is called for, you will have already started CPR. When the AED is brought, continue with CPR while the pads are attached to the casualty.

POSITIONING THE PADS

1 Switch on the AED and take the pads out of the sealed pack. Remove or cut through clothing and wipe away sweat from the chest if necessary.

2 Remove the backing paper and attach the pads to the casualty's chest in the positions indicated. Place the first pad on the casualty's upper right side, just below his collarbone.

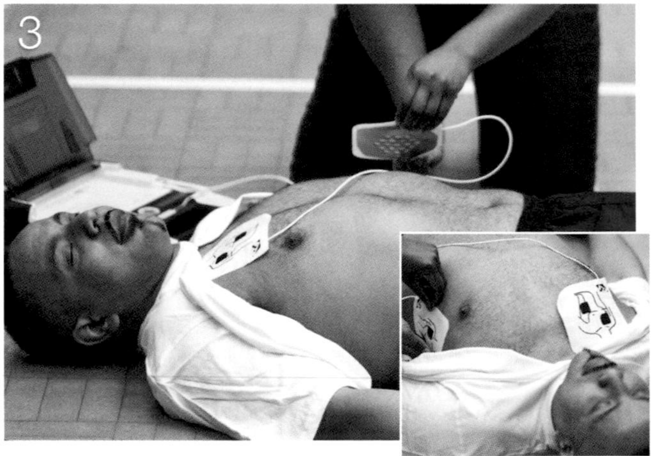

3 Place the second pad on the casualty's left side, just below his armpit (inset). Make sure the pad has its long axis along the head-to-toe axis of the casualty's body.

4 The AED will start analysing the heart rhythm. Ensure that no one is touching the casualty. Follow the voice and/or visual prompts given by the machine (opposite).

SEQUENCE OF AED INSTRUCTIONS

The AED will start to give you a series of visual and verbal prompts as soon as it is switched on. There are several different AED models available, each of which has different voice prompts. You should always follow the prompts given by the AED that you are using until advanced emergency care is available.

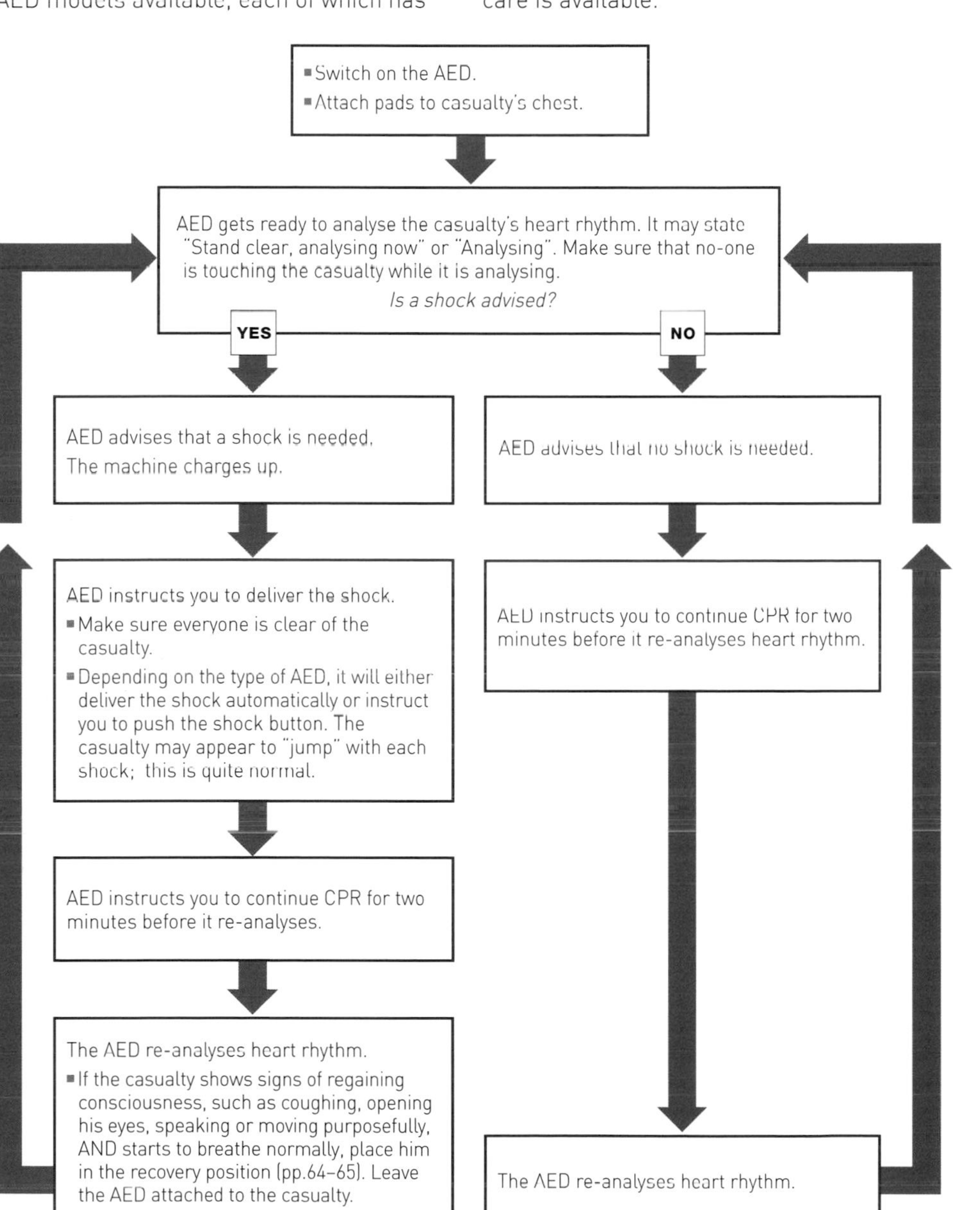

HOW TO USE AN AED (continued)

CONSIDERATIONS WHEN USING AN AED

CAUTION

Never use an AED on an infant under one year.

The use of an AED is occasionally complicated by underlying medical conditions, external factors, clothing or the cause of the cardiac arrest. Safety of all concerned should always be your first consideration.

CLOTHING AND JEWELLERY

Any clothing or jewellery that could interfere with pads should be removed or cut away. Normal amounts of chest hair are not a problem, but if it prevents good contact between the skin and the pads, it should be shaved off. Ensure any metal is removed from the area where the pads will be attached. Remove clothing containing metal, such as an underwired bra.

EXTERNAL FACTORS

Water or excessive sweat on the chest can reduce the effectiveness of the shock so the chest should be dry. If a casualty is rescued from water (p.36), dry the chest before applying the AED pads.

If the casualty is unconscious following an electric shock, start CPR immediately the contact with electricity is broken. The electric current may cause muscle paralysis, which can make rescue breaths and chest compressions more difficult to perform, however, it will not affect the use of the AED.

MEDICAL CONDITIONS

Some casualties with heart conditions have a pacemaker or an implantable cardioverter defibrillator (ICD). This should not stop you using an AED. However, if you can see or feel a device under the chest skin, do not place the pad directly over it. If a casualty has a patch such as a glyceryl trinitrate (GTN) patch on the chest, remove it before you apply the AED.

PREGNANT CASUALTIES

There are no contra-indications to using an AED during pregnancy; however, the increased breast size may present some problems. Therefore, to place the AED pads correctly, you may need to move one or both breasts. This must be carried out with respect and dignity.

POSITIONING AED PADS ON CHILDREN

Standard adult AEDs can be used on children over the age of eight years. For children between the ages of one and eight, use a paediatric AED or a standard machine and paediatric pads. If neither is available, then a standard AED and pads can be used.

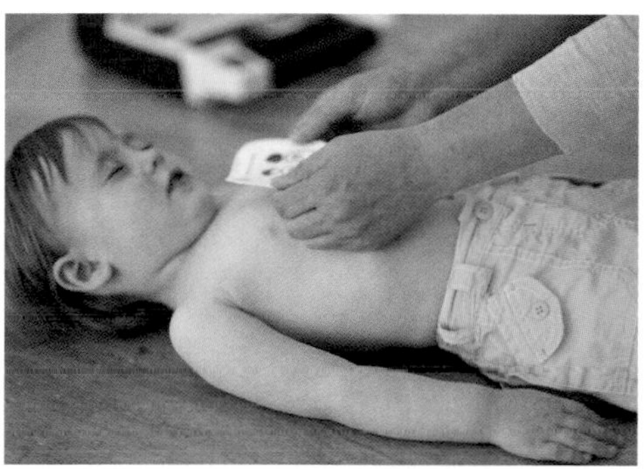

POSITIONING PAEDIATRIC AED PADS

Place one pad in the centre of the child's back. Then place the second upper pad over the centre of the child's chest. Make sure both pads are vertical. Connect the pads to the AED and proceed as described on p.83.

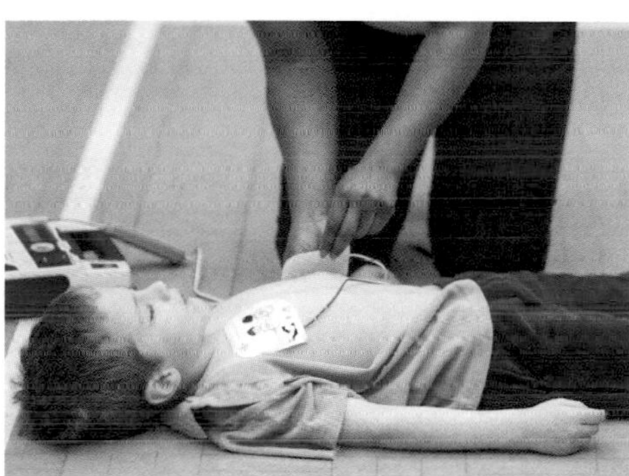

USING AED PADS ON A LARGER CHILD

Place the pads on the child's chest as for an adult – one on the child's upper right side, just below his collarbone, and the second pad on the child's left side, just below the armpit. Make sure the pad has its long axis along the head-to-toe axis of the child's body.

HANDING OVER TO THE EMERGENCY SERVICES

When the emergency services arrive continue to resuscitate the child until they take over from you. They need to know:

- **Casualty's present status;** for example, unconscious and not breathing;
- **Number of shocks** you have delivered;
- **When the casualty collapsed** and the length of time he has been unconscious;
- **Any relevant history,** if known.

If the casualty recovers at any point, leave the AED pads attached to his chest. Ensure that any used materials from the AED cabinet are disposed of as clinical waste (p.238). Inform the relevant person what has been taken out of the cabinet since it will need to be replaced.

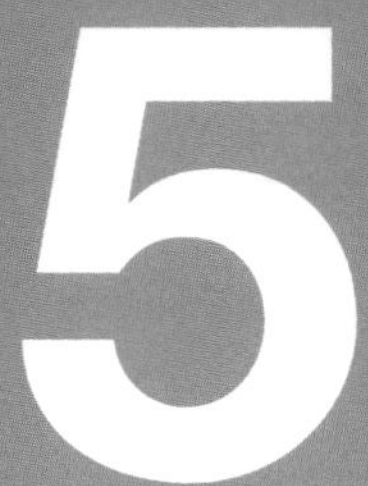

Oxygen is essential to life. Every time we breathe in, air containing oxygen enters the lungs. This oxygen is then transferred to the blood, to be transported around the body. Breathing and the exchange of oxygen and carbon dioxide (a waste product from body tissues) are described as "respiration". The structures in the body that enable us to breathe – the lungs and heart – make up the respiratory system.

Respiration can be impaired in various ways. The airways may be blocked causing choking or suffocation, the exchange of oxygen and carbon dioxide in the lungs may be affected by the inhalation of smoke or fumes, lung function may be impaired by chest injury, or the breathing mechanism may be affected by conditions such as asthma. Anxiety can also cause breathing difficulties. Problems with respiration can be life-threatening and need urgent first aid.

AIMS AND OBJECTIVES

- To assess the casualty's condition.
- To identify and remove the cause of the problem and provide fresh air.
- To comfort and reassure the casualty.
- To maintain an open airway, check breathing and be prepared to resuscitate if necessary.
- To obtain medical help if necessary. Call 999/112 for emergency help if you suspect a serious illness or injury.

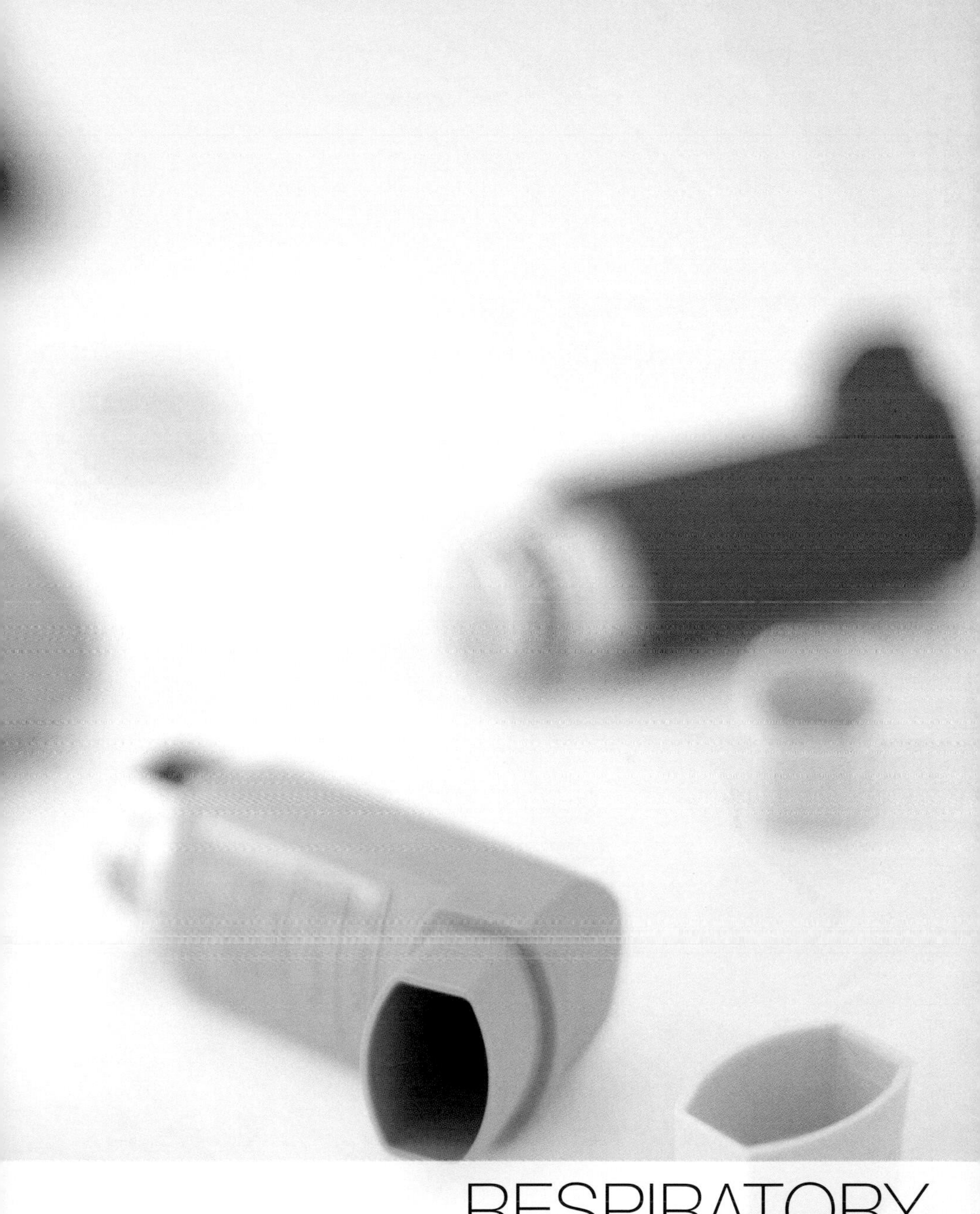

RESPIRATORY PROBLEMS

THE RESPIRATORY SYSTEM

This system comprises the mouth, nose, windpipe (trachea), lungs and pulmonary blood vessels. Respiration involves the process of breathing and the exchange of gases (oxygen and carbon dioxide) in the lungs and in cells throughout the body.

We breathe in air to take oxygen into the lungs, and we breathe out to expel the waste gas, carbon dioxide, a by-product of respiration. When we breathe, air is drawn through the nose and mouth into the airway and the lungs. In the lungs, oxygen is taken from air sacs (alveoli) into the pulmonary capillaries. At the same time, carbon dioxide is released from the capillaries into the alveoli. Carbon dioxide is then expelled as we breathe out. An average man's lungs can hold approximately 6 litres (10 pints) of air; a woman's lungs can hold about 4 litres (7 pints) of air.

Structure of the respiratory system
The lungs form the central part of the respiratory system. Together with the circulatory system, they perform the vital function of gas exchange in order to distribute oxygen around the body and remove carbon dioxide.

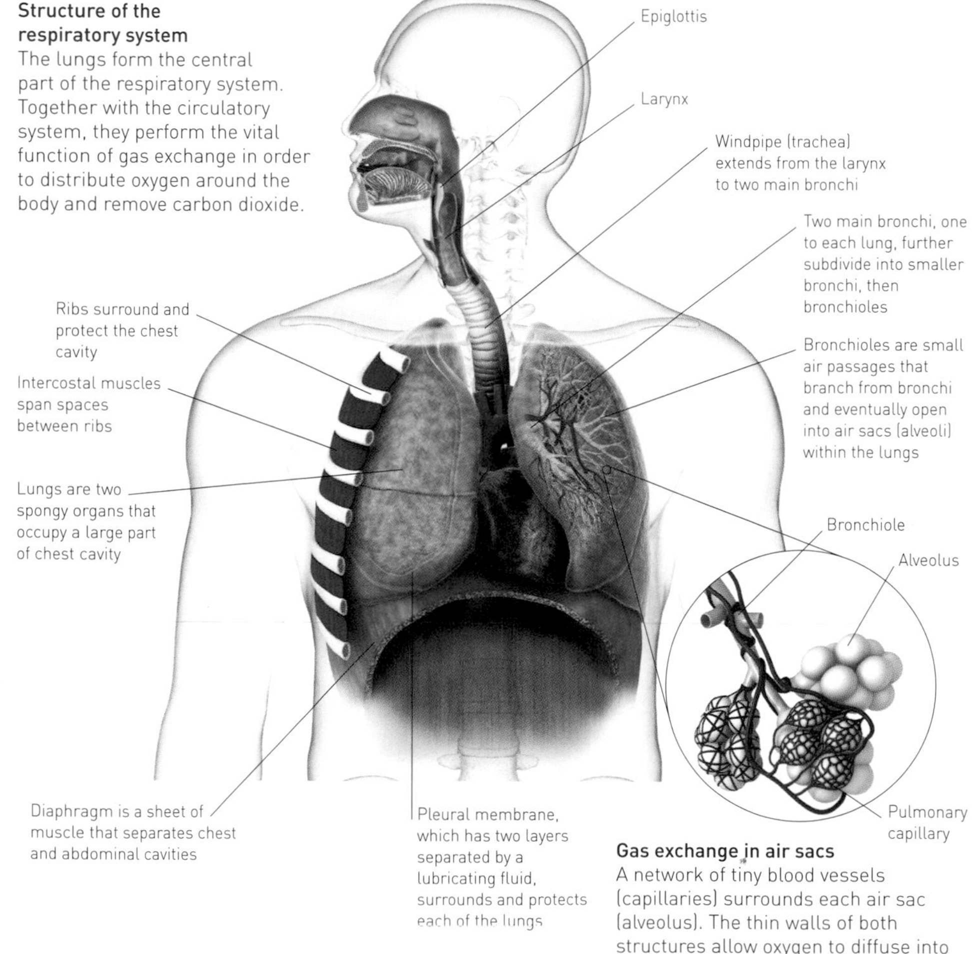

Gas exchange in air sacs
A network of tiny blood vessels (capillaries) surrounds each air sac (alveolus). The thin walls of both structures allow oxygen to diffuse into the blood and carbon dioxide to leave it.

HOW BREATHING WORKS

The breathing process consists of the actions of breathing in (inspiration) and breathing out (expiration), followed by a pause. Pressure differences between the lungs and the air outside the body determine whether air is drawn in or expelled. When the air pressure in the lungs is lower than outside, air is drawn in; when pressure is higher, air is expelled. The pressure within the lungs is altered by the movements of the two main sets of muscles involved in breathing: the intercostal muscles and the diaphragm.

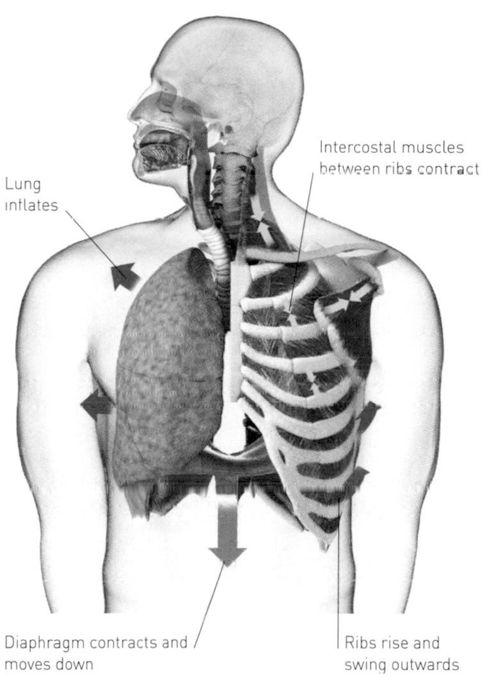

Breathing in
The intercostal muscles (the muscles between the ribs) and the diaphragm contract, causing the ribs to move up and out, the chest cavity to expand, and the lungs to expand to fill the space. As a result, the pressure inside the lungs is reduced, and air is drawn into the lungs.

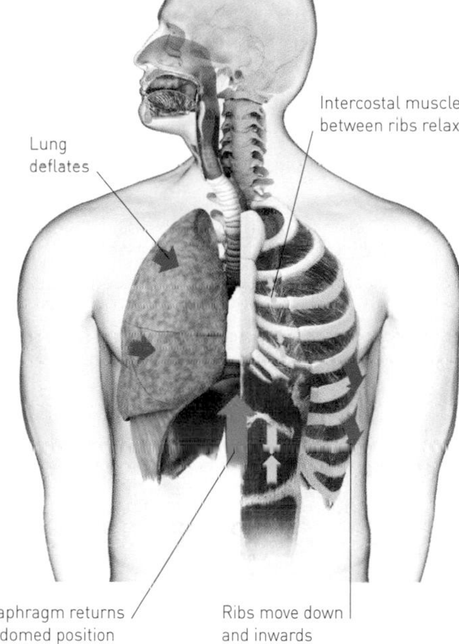

Breathing out
The intercostal muscles relax, and the ribcage returns to its resting position, while the diaphragm relaxes and resumes its domed shape. As a result, the chest cavity becomes smaller, and pressure inside the lungs increases. Air flows out of the lungs to be exhaled.

HOW BREATHING IS CONTROLLED

Breathing is regulated by a group of nerve cells in the brain called the respiratory centre. This centre responds to changes in the level of carbon dioxide in the blood. When the level rises, the respiratory centre responds by stimulating the intercostal muscles and the diaphragm to contract, and a breath occurs. Our breathing rate can be altered consciously under normal conditions or in response to abnormal levels of carbon dioxide, low levels of oxygen, or with stress, exercise, injury or illness.

HYPOXIA

RECOGNITION

In moderate and severe hypoxia, there will be:

- Rapid breathing;
- Breathing that is distressed or gasping;
- Difficulty speaking;
- Grey-blue skin (cyanosis). At first, this is more obvious in the extremities, such as lips, nailbeds and earlobes, but as the hypoxia worsens cyanosis affects the rest of the body;
- Anxiety;
- Restlessness;
- Headache;
- Nausea and possibly vomiting;
- Cessation of breathing if the hypoxia is not quickly reversed.

This condition arises when there is insufficient oxygen in the body tissues. There are a number of causes of hypoxia, ranging from suffocation, choking or poisoning to impaired lung or brain function. The condition is accompanied by a variety of symptoms, depending on the degree of hypoxia. If not treated quickly, hypoxia is potentially fatal because a sufficient level of oxygen is vital for the normal function of all the body organs and tissues, but especially the brain.

In a healthy person, the amount of oxygen in the air is more than adequate for the body tissues to function normally. However, in an injured or ill person, a reduction in oxygen reaching the tissues results in deterioration of body function.

Mild hypoxia reduces a casualty's ability to think clearly, but the body responds to this by increasing the rate and depth of breathing (p.89). However, if the oxygen supply to the brain cells is cut off for as little as three minutes, the brain cells will begin to die. All the conditions covered in this chapter can result in hypoxia.

See also
Anaphylactic shock **p.221**
Asthma **p.100**
Burns to the airway **p.185**
Croup **p.101**
Drowning **p.98**
Hanging and strangulation **p.95**
Inhalation of fumes **pp.96–97**
Penetrating chest wound **p.102**
Stroke **pp.174–75**

INJURIES OR CONDITIONS CAUSING LOW BLOOD OXYGEN (HYPOXIA)

INJURY OR CONDITION	CAUSES
Insufficient oxygen in inspired air	▪ Suffocation by smoke or gas ▪ Changes in atmospheric pressure, for example, at high altitude or in a depressurised aircraft
Airway obstruction	▪ Blocking or swelling of the airway ▪ Hanging or strangulation ▪ Something covering the mouth and nose ▪ Asthma ▪ Choking ▪ Anaphylaxis
Conditions affecting the chest wall	▪ Crushing, for example, by a fall of earth or sand or pressure from a crowd ▪ Chest wall injury with multiple rib fractures or constricting burns
Impaired lung function	▪ Lung injury ▪ Collapsed lung ▪ Lung infections, such as pneumonia
Damage to the brain or nerves that control respiration	▪ A head injury or stroke that damages the breathing centre in the brain ▪ Some forms of poisoning ▪ Paralysis of nerves controlling the muscles of breathing, as in spinal cord injury
Impaired oxygen uptake by the tissues	▪ Carbon monoxide or cyanide poisoning ▪ Shock

CHOKING ADULT

RECOGNITION

Ask the casualty:
"Are you choking?"

Mild obstruction:

- Casualty able to speak, cough and breathe.

Severe obstruction:

- Casualty unable to speak, cough or breathe, with eventual loss of consciousness.

YOUR AIMS

- To remove the obstruction.
- To arrange urgent removal to hospital if necessary.

CAUTION

- If at any stage the casualty loses consciousness, open the airway and check breathing (p.63). If she is not breathing, begin CPR (pp.66–67) to try to relieve the obstruction.

See also
Unconscious adult **pp.62–69**

A foreign object that is stuck in the throat may block it and cause muscular spasm. If blockage of the airway is mild, the casualty should be able to clear it; if it is severe, she will be unable to speak, cough or breathe, and will eventually lose consciousness. If she loses consciousness, the throat muscles may relax and the airway may open enough to do rescue breathing. Be prepared to begin rescue breaths and chest compressions.

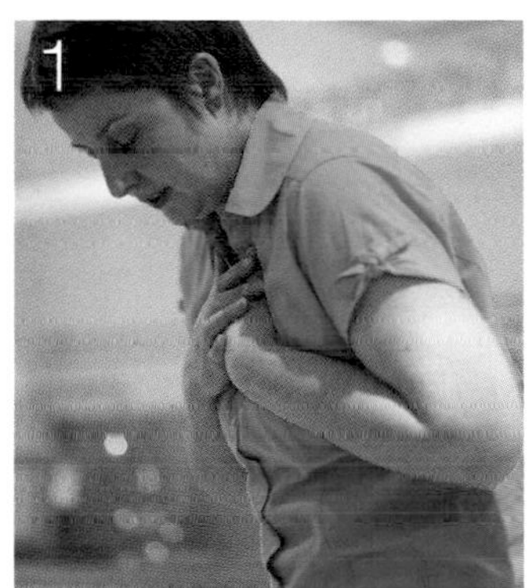

1 If the casualty is breathing, encourage her to continue coughing. Remove any obvious obstruction from the mouth.

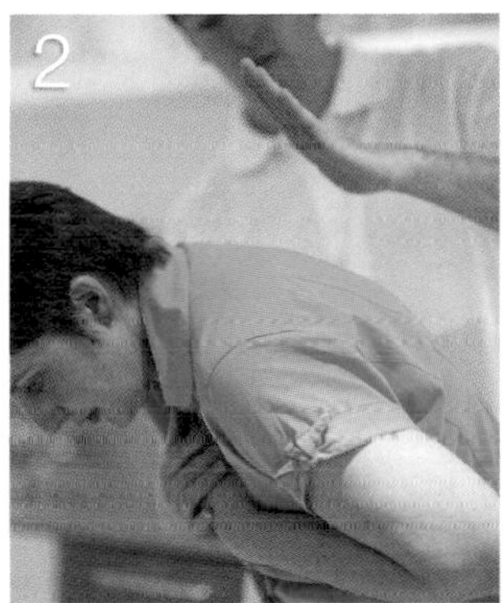

2 If the casualty cannot speak or stops coughing or breathing, carry out back blows. Support her upper body with one hand, and help her to lean well forward. Give up to five sharp blows between her shoulder blades with the heel of your hand. Stop if the obstruction clears. Check her mouth.

3 If back blows fail to clear the obstruction, try abdominal thrusts. Stand behind the casualty and put both arms around the upper part of her abdomen. Make sure that she is still bending well forwards. Clench your fist and place it between the navel and the bottom of her breastbone. Grasp your fist firmly with your other hand. Pull sharply inwards and upwards up to five times.

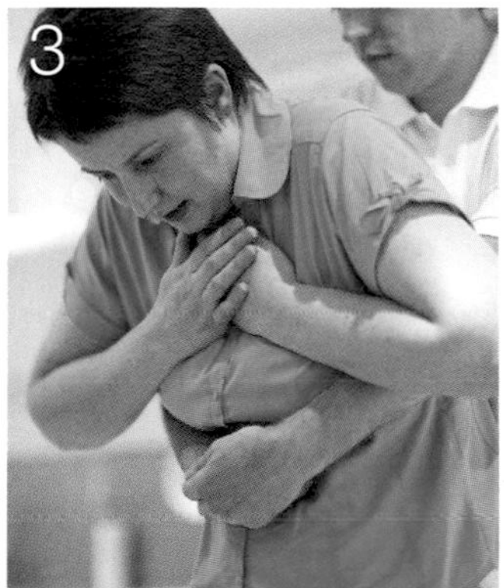

4 Check her mouth. If the obstruction has not cleared, repeat steps 2 and 3 up to three times, checking the mouth after each step.

5 If the obstruction still has not cleared, **call 999/112 for emergency help.** Continue until help arrives or the casualty loses consciousness.

CHOKING CHILD (one year to puberty)

RECOGNITION

Ask the child:
"Are you choking?"

Mild obstruction:

- Child able to speak, cough and breathe.

Severe obstruction:

- Child unable to speak, cough or breathe, with eventual loss of consciousness.

YOUR AIMS

- To remove the obstruction.
- To arrange urgent removal to hospital if necessary.

CAUTION

- If the child loses consciousness at any stage, open the airway and check breathing (p.71). If the child is not breathing, begin CPR to try to relieve the obstruction (pp.74–75).

See also
Unconscious child **pp.70–77**

Young children especially are prone to choking. A child may choke on food, or may put small objects into her mouth and cause a blockage of the airway.

If a child is choking, you need to act quickly. If she loses consciousness, the throat muscles may relax and the airway may open enough to do rescue breathing. Be prepared to begin rescue breaths and chest compressions.

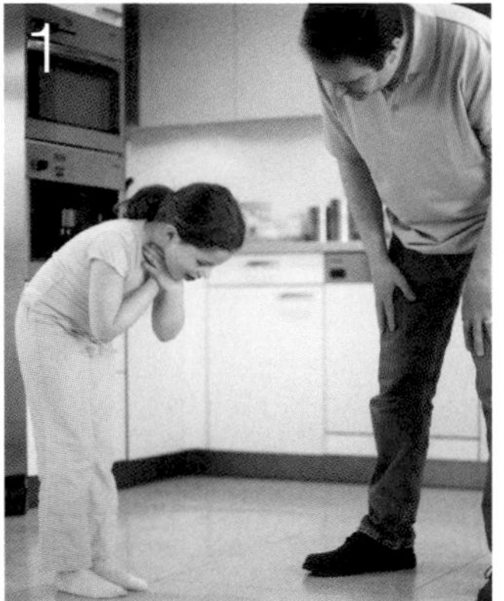

1 If the child is breathing, encourage her to cough; this may clear the obstruction. Remove any obvious obstruction from her mouth.

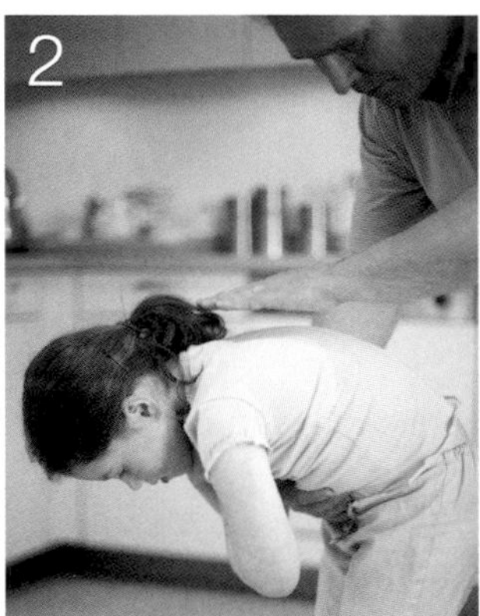

2 If the child cannot speak, or stops coughing or breathing, carry out back blows. Bend her well forward and give up to five blows between her shoulder blades using the heel of your hand. Check her mouth but do not sweep the mouth with your finger.

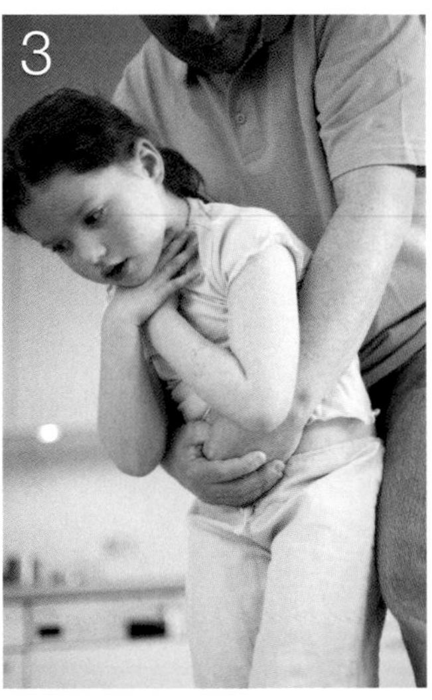

3 If the back blows fail, try abdominal thrusts. Put your arms around the child's upper abdomen. Make sure that she is bending well forwards. Place your fist between the navel and the bottom of her breastbone, and grasp it with your other hand. Pull sharply inwards and upwards up to five times. Stop if the obstruction clears. Check her mouth again.

4 If the obstruction has not cleared, repeat steps 2 and 3 up to three times. Keep checking the mouth.

5 If the obstruction still has not cleared, **call 999/112 for emergency help**. Continue until help arrives or the child loses consciousness.

CHOKING INFANT (under one year)

RECOGNITION

Mild obstruction:

- Infant able to cough, but has difficulty crying or making any other noise.

Severe obstruction:

- Unable to make any noise or breathe, with eventual loss of consciousness.

YOUR AIMS

- To remove the obstruction.
- To arrange urgent removal to hospital if necessary.

CAUTION

- If the infant loses consciousness at any stage, open the airway and check breathing (pp.78–79). If the infant is not breathing, begin CPR (pp.80–81) to try to relieve the obstruction.

See also
Unconscious infant **pp.78–81**

An infant is more likely to choke on food or small objects than an adult. The infant will rapidly become distressed, and you need to act quickly to clear any obstruction. If the infant loses consciousness, the throat muscles may relax and the airway may open enough to do rescue breathing. Be prepared to begin rescue breaths and chest compressions.

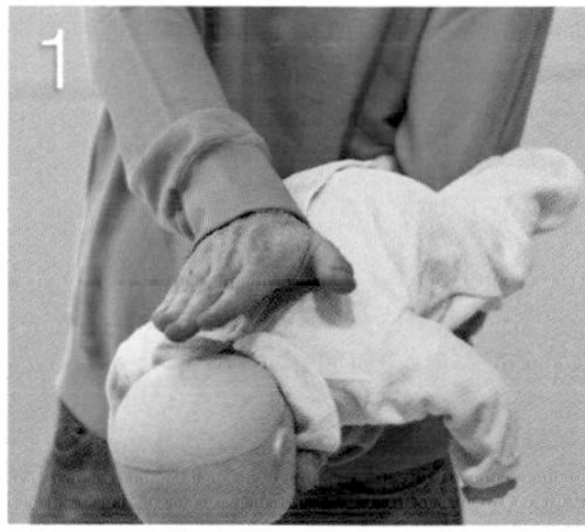

1 If the infant is distressed, is unable to cry, cough or breathe, lay him face down along your forearm, with his head low, and support his back and head. Give up to five back blows, with the heel of your hand.

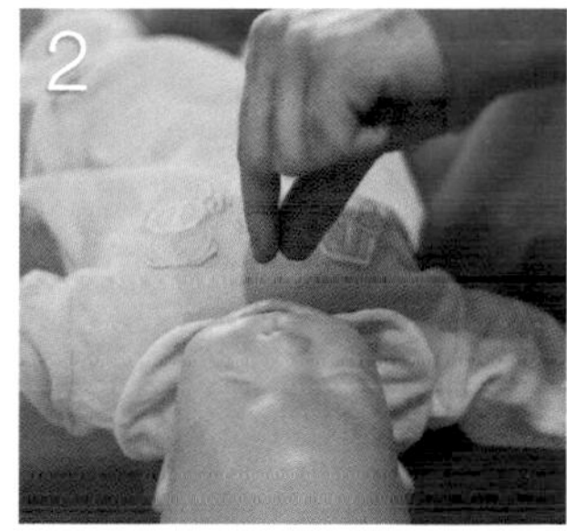

2 Check the infant's mouth; remove any obvious obstructions with your fingertips. Do not sweep the mouth with your finger as this may push the object further down the throat.

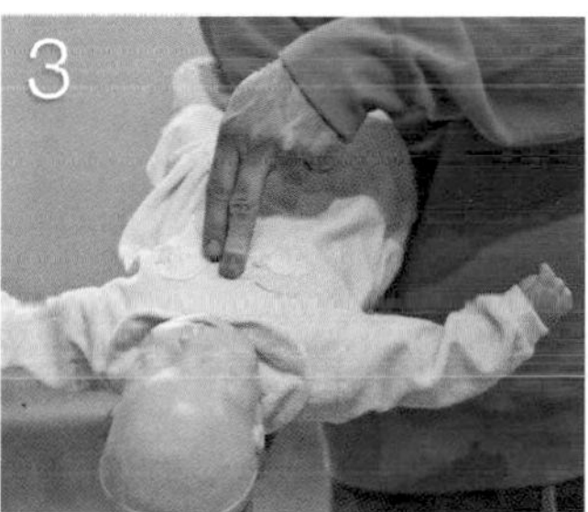

3 If back blows fail to clear the obstruction, turn the infant on to his back and give chest thrusts. Using two fingers, push inwards and upwards (towards the head) against the infant's breastbone, one finger's breadth below the nipple line.

4 Perform up to five chest thrusts. The aim is to relieve the obstruction with each chest thrust rather than necessarily doing all five. Check the mouth. If the obstruction still has not cleared, repeat steps 1–4 three times.

5 If the obstruction still has not cleared, take the infant with you to **call 999/112 for emergency help.** Continue until help arrives or the infant loses consciousness.

AIRWAY OBSTRUCTION

RECOGNITION

- Features of hypoxia (p.90), such as grey-blue tinge to the lips, earlobes and nailbeds (cyanosis).
- Difficulty speaking and breathing.
- Noisy breathing.
- Red, puffy face.
- Signs of distress from the casualty, who may point to the throat or grasp the neck.
- Flaring of the nostrils.
- A persistent cough.

YOUR AIMS

- To remove the obstruction.
- To restore normal breathing.
- To arrange removal to hospital.

CAUTION

If the casualty is unconscious, open the airway and check breathing (The unconscious casualty pp.54–85).

The airway may be obstructed externally or internally, for example, by an object that is stuck at the back of the throat (pp.91–93). The main causes of obstruction are:

- **Inhalation** of an object, such as food;
- **Blockage** by the tongue, blood or vomit while a casualty is unconscious (p.58);
- **Internal swelling** of the throat occurring with burns, scalds, stings or anaphylaxis;
- **Injuries** to the face or jaw;
- **An asthma attack** in which the small airways in the lungs constrict (p.100);
- **External pressure** on the neck, as in hanging or strangulation;
- **Peanuts,** which can swell up when in contact with body fluids. These pose a particular danger in young children because they can completely block the airway.

Airway obstruction requires prompt action; be prepared to give chest compressions and rescue breaths if the casualty stops breathing (The unconscious casualty pp.54–85).

The information on this page is appropriate for all causes of airway obstruction, but if you need detailed instructions for specific situations, refer to the relevant pages given below.

See also
Asthma **p.100**
Burns to the airway **p.185**
Choking adult **p.91**
Choking child **p.92**
Choking infant **p.93**
Drowning **p.98**
Hanging and strangulation **opposite**
Inhalation of fumes **p.96–97**

1 Remove the obstruction if it is external or visible in the mouth.

2 If the casualty is conscious and breathing normally, reassure him, but keep him under observation.

3 Even if the casualty appears to have made a complete recovery, **call 999/112 for emergency help.** Monitor and record his vital signs – level of response, breathing and pulse (pp.52–53) – until help arrives.

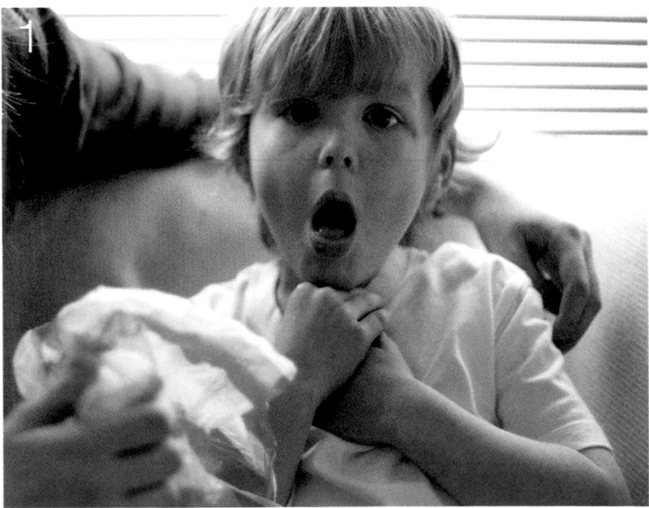

HANGING AND STRANGULATION

RECOGNITION

- A constricting article around the neck.
- Marks around the casualty's neck.
- Rapid, difficult breathing; impaired consciousness; grey–blue skin (cyanosis).
- Congestion of the face, with prominent veins and, possibly, tiny red spots on the face or on the whites of the eyes.

YOUR AIMS

- To restore adequate breathing.
- To arrange urgent removal to hospital.

CAUTION

- Do not move the casualty unnecessarily, in case of spinal injury.
- Do not destroy or interfere with any material that has been constricting the neck, such as knotted rope; police may need it as evidence.
- If the casualty is unconscious, open the airway and check breathing (The unconscious casualty pp.54–85).

See also
Spinal injury **pp.171–73**

If pressure is exerted on the outside of the neck, the airway is squeezed and the flow of air to the lungs is cut off. The main causes of such pressure are:

- **Hanging** – suspension of the body by a noose around the neck;
- **Strangulation** – constriction or squeezing around the neck or throat.

Sometimes, hanging or strangulation may occur accidentally – for example, by ties or clothing becoming caught in machinery. Hanging may cause a broken neck; for this reason, a casualty in this situation must be handled extremely carefully.

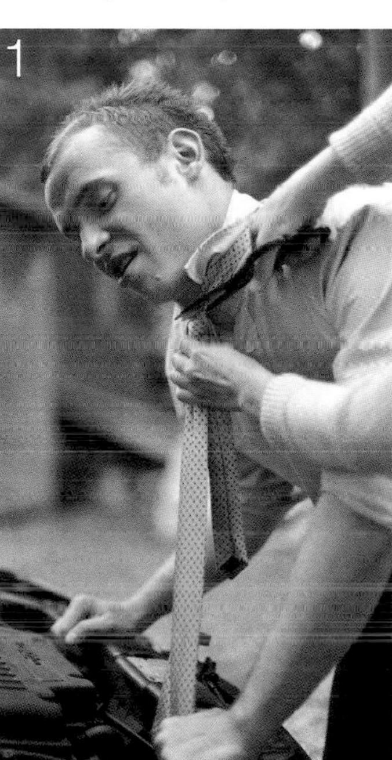

1 Quickly remove any constriction from around the casualty's neck.

2 If the casualty is hanging, support the body while you relieve the constriction. Be aware that the body will be very heavy if he is unconscious.

3 If conscious, help the casualty to lie down while supporting his head and neck.

4 **Call 999/112 for emergency help**, even if he appears to recover fully. Monitor and record his vital signs – level of response, breathing and pulse (pp.52–53) – until help arrives.

INHALATION OF FUMES

The inhalation of smoke, gases (such as carbon monoxide) or toxic vapours can be lethal. A casualty who has inhaled fumes is likely to have low levels of oxygen in his body tissues (Hypoxia p.90) and therefore needs urgent medical attention. Do not attempt to carry out a rescue if it is likely to put your own life at risk; fumes that have built up in a confined space will quickly overcome anyone who is not wearing protective equipment.

SMOKE INHALATION

Any person who has been enclosed in a confined space during a fire should be assumed to have inhaled smoke. Smoke from burning plastics, foam padding and synthetic wall coverings is likely to contain poisonous fumes. Casualties who have suffered from fume inhalation should also be examined for other injuries due to the fire, such as external burns.

INHALATION OF CARBON MONOXIDE

Carbon monoxide is a poisonous gas that is produced by burning, but it has no taste or smell. The gas acts directly on red blood cells, preventing them from carrying oxygen to the body tissues. If inhaled in large quantities – for example, from smoke or vehicle exhaust fumes in a confined space – it can very quickly prove fatal. Lengthy exposure to even a small amount of carbon monoxide – for example, due to a leakage of fumes from a defective heater or flue – may also result in severe, or possibly fatal, poisoning.

EFFECTS OF FUME INHALATION

FUMES	SOURCE	EFFECTS
Carbon monoxide	▪ Exhaust fumes of motor vehicles ▪ Smoke from most fires ▪ Back-draughts from blocked chimney flues ▪ Emissions from defective gas or paraffin heaters and poorly maintained boilers	Prolonged exposure to low levels: ▪ Headache ▪ Confusion ▪ Aggression ▪ Nausea and vomiting ▪ Incontinence Brief exposure to high levels: ▪ Grey-blue skin coloration ▪ Rapid, difficult breathing ▪ Impaired consciousness, leading to unconsciousness
Smoke	▪ Fires: smoke is a bigger killer than fire itself. Smoke is low in oxygen (which is used up by the burning of the fire) and may contain toxic fumes from burning materials	▪ Rapid, noisy and difficult breathing ▪ Coughing and wheezing ▪ Burning in the nose or mouth ▪ Soot around the mouth and nose ▪ Unconsciousness
Carbon dioxide	▪ Tends to accumulate and become dangerously concentrated in deep enclosed spaces, such as coal pits, wells and underground tanks	▪ Breathlessness ▪ Headache ▪ Confusion ▪ Unconsciousness
Solvents and fuels	▪ Glues ▪ Cleaning fluids ▪ Lighter fuels ▪ Camping gas and propane-fuelled stoves (Solvent abusers may use a plastic bag to concentrate the vapour, especially with glues)	▪ Headache and vomiting ▪ Impaired consciousness ▪ Airway obstruction from using a plastic bag or from choking on vomit may result in death ▪ Solvent abuse is a potential cause of cardiac arrest

YOUR AIMS

- To restore adequate breathing.
- To **call 999/112 for emergency help** and obtain urgent medical attention.

CAUTION

- If the casualty is in a garage filled with vehicle exhaust fumes, open the doors wide and let the gas escape before you enter.
- If the casualty is found unconscious, open the airway and check breathing (The unconscious casualty pp.54–85).

See also
Burns to the airway **p.185**
Fires **pp.32–33**
Hypoxia **p.90**
The unconscious casualty **pp.54–85**

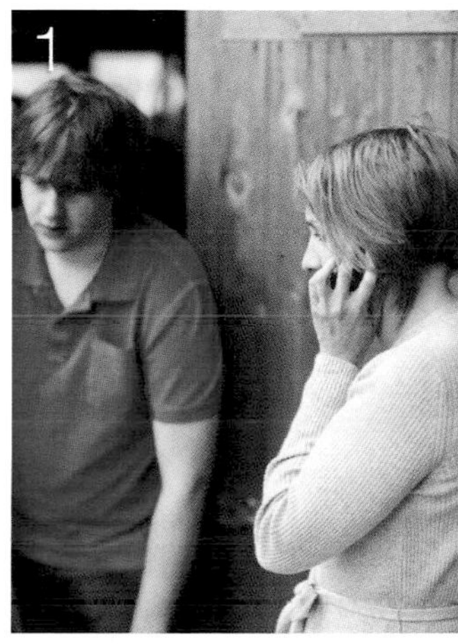

1 **Call 999/112 for emergency help**. Tell ambulance control that you suspect fume inhalation.

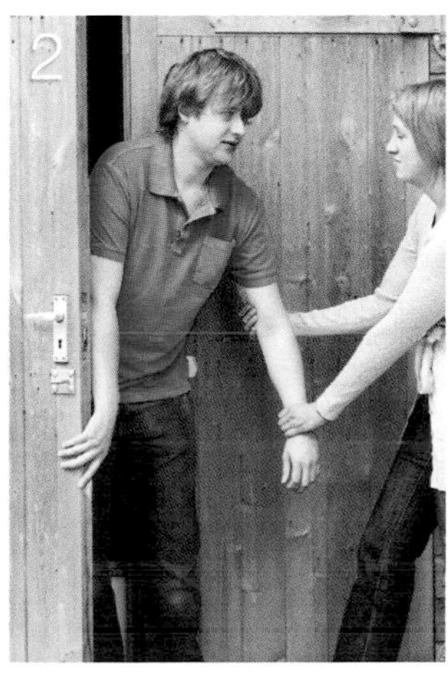

2 If it is necessary to escape from the source of the fumes, help the casualty away from the fumes into fresh air. Do not enter the fume-filled area yourself.

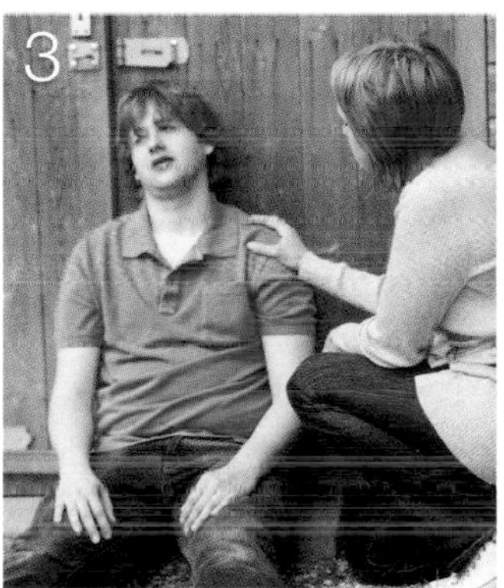

3 Support the casualty and encourage him to breathe normally. If the casualty's clothing is still burning, try to extinguish the flames (p.33). Treat any obvious burns (pp.182–88) or other injuries.

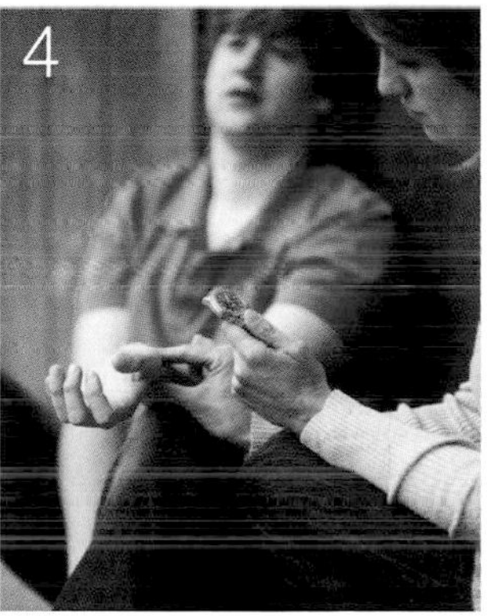

4 Stay with the casualty until help arrives. Monitor and record the casualty's vital signs – level of response, breathing and pulse (pp.52–53) – while waiting for help.

DROWNING

YOUR AIMS

- To restore adequate breathing.
- To keep the casualty warm.
- To arrange urgent removal to hospital.

CAUTION

- If the casualty is unconscious, open the airway and check breathing (The unconscious casualty pp.54–85).
- If the casualty is not breathing give FIVE initial rescue breaths before you start chest compressions. If you are alone, give CPR for one minute before you call for emergency help.
- Give chest compressions only if you have not had formal training in CPR or you are unwilling or unable to give rescue breaths. The ambulance dispatcher will give instructions for chest compression-only CPR.

See also
Hypothermia **pp.194–96**
The unconscious casualty **pp.54–85**
Water incidents **p.36**

Drowning can result in death from hypothermia due to immersion in cold water, sudden cardiac arrest due to cold water, spasm of the throat blocking the airway and/or inhalation of water and consequent airway obstruction.

A casualty rescued from a drowning incident should always receive medical attention even if he seems to have recovered at the time. Any water entering the lungs causes them to become irritated, and the air passages may begin to swell several hours later – a condition known as secondary drowning. The casualty may also need to be treated for hypothermia (pp.194–96).

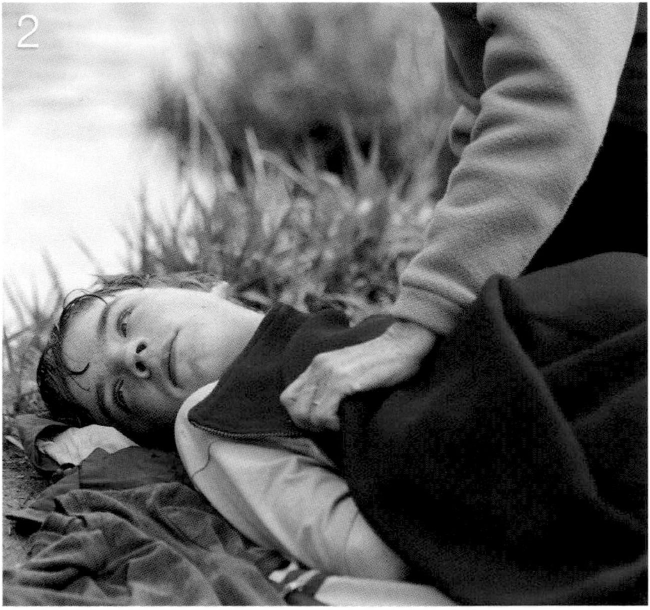

1 If you have rescued the casualty from the water, help him to lie down on a rug or coat with his head lower than the rest of the body so that water can drain from his mouth. This reduces the risk of inhaling water (p.36).

2 Treat the casualty for hypothermia; replace wet clothing with dry clothes if possible and cover him with dry blankets or coats. If the casualty is fully conscious, give him chocolate and/or a warm drink.

3 **Call 999/112 for emergency help** even if he appears to recover fully because of the risk of secondary drowning. Monitor and record his vital signs – level of response, breathing and pulse (pp.52–53) – until help arrives.

HYPERVENTILATION

RECOGNITION

- Unnaturally fast breathing.
- Fast pulse rate.
- Apprehension.

There may also be:

- Attention-seeking behaviour;
- Dizziness or faintness;
- Trembling, sweating and dry mouth, or marked tingling in the hands;
- Tingling and cramps in the hands and feet and around the mouth.

YOUR AIMS

- To remove the casualty from the cause of distress.
- To reassure the casualty and calm her down.

CAUTION

- Do not advise the casualty to rebreathe her own air from a paper bag since this may cause a more serious illness.
- Hyperventilation due to acute anxiety is rare in children. Look for other causes.

This is commonly a manifestation of acute anxiety and may accompany a panic attack. It may occur in susceptible individuals who have recently experienced an emotional upset or those with a history of panic attacks.

Hyperventilation causes an increased loss of carbon dioxide from the blood, leading to chemical changes within the blood. These changes lead to symptoms such as unnaturally fast breathing, dizziness and trembling, as well as tingling in the hands. As breathing returns to normal, these symptoms will gradually subside.

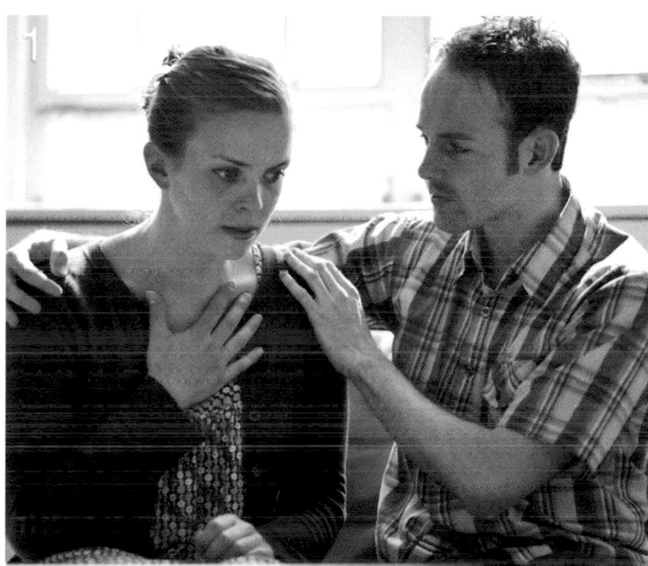

1 When speaking to the casualty, be firm, but kind and reassuring. If possible, lead the casualty away to a quiet place where she may be able to regain control of her breathing more easily and quickly. If this is not possible, ask any bystanders to leave.

2 Encourage the casualty to seek medical advice on preventing and controlling panic attacks in the future.

ASTHMA

RECOGNITION

- Difficulty breathing.
- Wheezing.
- Difficulty speaking, leading to short sentences and whispering.
- Coughing.
- Distress and anxiety.
- Features of hypoxia (p.90), such as a grey-blue tinge to the lips, earlobes and nailbeds (cyanosis).
- Exhaustion in a severe attack. If the attack worsens the casualty may stop breathing and lose consciousness.

YOUR AIMS

- To ease breathing.
- To obtain medical help if necessary.

CAUTION

- If this is a first attack and the casualty has no medication **call 999/112 for emergency help** immediately.
- If the casualty is unconscious, open the airway and check breathing (The unconscious casualty pp.54–85).

In an asthma attack, the muscles of the air passages in the lungs go into spasm. As a result, the airways become narrowed, which makes breathing difficult.

Sometimes, there is a recognised trigger for an attack, such as an allergy, a cold, a particular drug or cigarette smoke. At other times, there is no obvious trigger. Many sufferers have sudden attacks.

People with asthma usually deal with their own attacks by using a "reliever" inhaler at the first sign of an attack. Most reliever inhalers have blue caps. Preventer inhalers have brown or white caps and are used to help prevent attacks. They should not be used during an asthma attack.

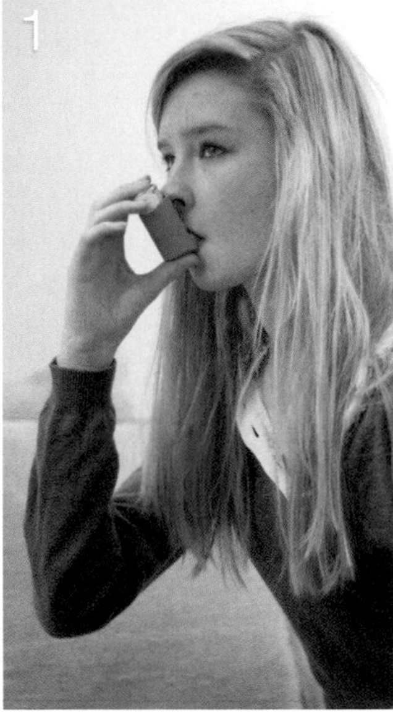

1 **Keep calm and reassure the casualty. Get her to take a puff of her reliever inhaler; use a spacer if she has one. Ask her to breathe slowly and deeply.**

2 **Sit her down in the position she finds most comfortable; do not let her lie down.**

3 **A mild attack should ease within a few minutes. If it does not, ask the casualty to take another dose from her inhaler.**

4 **Call 999/112 for emergency help** if the attack is severe and one of the following occurs: the inhaler has no effect; the casualty is getting worse; breathlessness makes talking difficult; she is becoming exhausted.

5 **Help the casualty to use her inhaler as required. Monitor her vital signs – level of response, breathing and pulse (pp.52–53) – until help arrives.**

SPECIAL CASE USING A SPACER

A plastic diffuser, known as a spacer, can be fitted to an asthma inhaler to help a casualty breathe in the medication more effectively. They are especially useful when giving medication to young children.

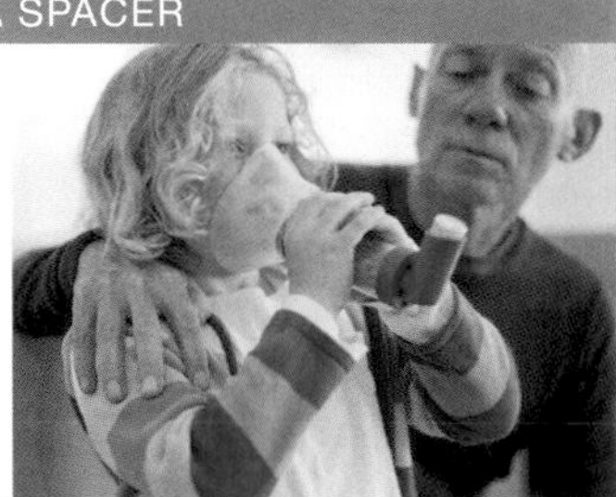

CROUP

RECOGNITION

- Distressed breathing in a young child.

There may also be:

- A short, barking cough;
- A rasping noise, especially on breathing in (stridor);
- Croaky voice;
- Blue-grey skin (cyanosis);
- In severe cases, the child using muscles around the nose, neck and upper arms in trying to breathe.

Suspect epiglottitis if:

- A child is in respiratory distress and not improving;
- The child has a high temperature.

YOUR AIMS

- To comfort and support the child.
- To obtain medical help if necessary.

CAUTION

Do not put your fingers down the child's throat. This can cause the throat muscles to go into spasm and block the airway.

An attack of breathing difficulty in young children is known as croup. It is caused by inflammation in the windpipe and larynx. Croup can be alarming but usually passes without lasting harm. Attacks of croup usually occur at night and and are made worse by the child crying and parental anxiety.

If an attack of croup persists, or is severe, and accompanied by fever, call for emergency help. There is a small risk that the child is suffering from a rare, croup-like condition called epiglottitis, in which the epiglottis (p.88), a small, flap-like structure in the throat, becomes infected and swollen and may block the airway completely. The child then needs urgent medical attention.

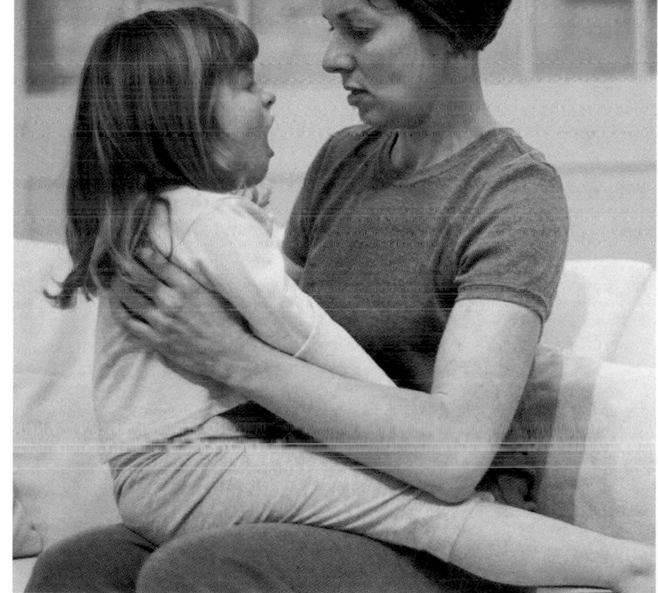

1 Sit your child on your knee, supporting her back. Calmly reassure the child. Try not to panic since this will only alarm her and is likely to make the attack worse.

2 If it is safe to do so, creating a steamy atmosphere may help. This can be done by taking the child into the bathroom and running a hot tap or shower, or going into the kitchen and boiling some water. Keep the child clear of hot running water or steam.

3 Call medical help or, if the croup is severe, **call 999 /112 for emergency help**. Keep monitoring her vital signs – level of response, breathing and pulse (pp.52–53) – while waiting for help.

PENETRATING CHEST WOUND

RECOGNITION

- Difficult and painful breathing, possibly rapid, shallow and uneven.
- Casualty feels an acute sense of alarm.
- Features of hypoxia (p.90), including grey-blue skin coloration (cyanosis).

There may also be:

- Coughed-up frothy, red blood;
- A crackling feeling of the skin around the site of the wound, caused by air collecting in the tissues;
- Blood bubbling out of the wound;
- Sound of air being sucked into the chest as the casualty breathes in;
- Veins in the neck becoming prominent.

See also
Hypoxia **p.90**
The unconscious casualty **pp.54–85**
Shock **pp.116–17**

The heart and lungs, and the major blood vessels around them, lie in the chest, protected by the breastbone and the 12 pairs of ribs that make up the ribcage. The ribcage extends far enough downwards to protect organs such as the liver and spleen in the upper part of the abdomen.

If a sharp object penetrates the chest wall, there may be severe damage to the organs in the chest and the upper abdomen and this will lead to shock. The lungs are particularly susceptible to injury, either by being damaged themselves or from wounds that perforate the two-layered membrane (pleura) that surrounds and protects each lung. Air can then enter between the membranes and exert pressure on the lung, and the lung may collapse – a condition called pneumothorax.

Pressure around the affected lung may build up to such an extent that it affects the uninjured lung. As a result, the casualty becomes increasingly breathless. This build-up of pressure may prevent the heart from refilling with blood properly, impairing the circulation and causing shock – a condition known as a tension pneumothorax. Sometimes, blood collects in the pleural cavity and puts pressure on the lungs.

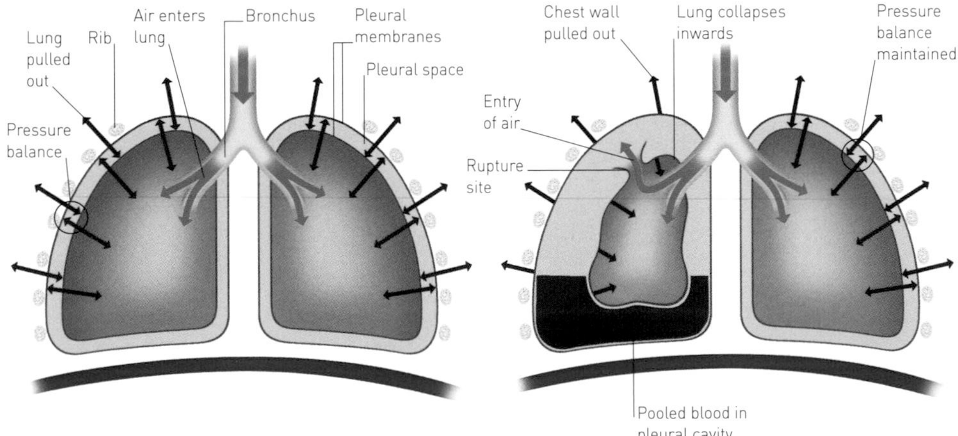

Normal breathing
The lungs inflate by being pulled out as they "suck" onto the chest wall. Pressure is maintained within the fluid-filled pleural space.

Collapsed (right) lung
Air from the right lung enters the surrounding pleural space and changes the pressure balance. The lung shrinks away from the chest wall.

YOUR AIMS

- To seal the wound and maintain breathing.
- To minimise shock.
- To arrange urgent removal to hospital.

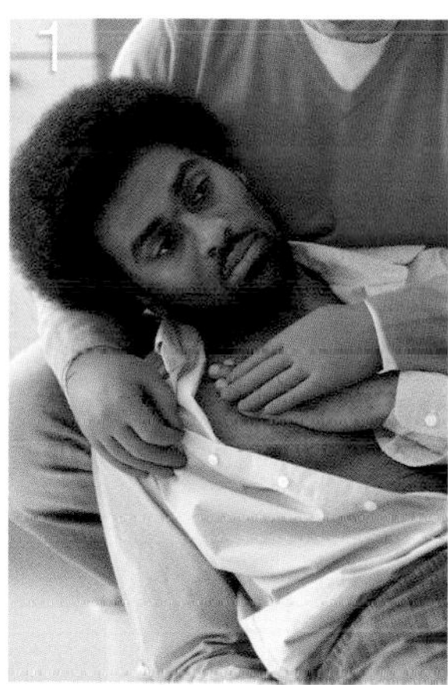

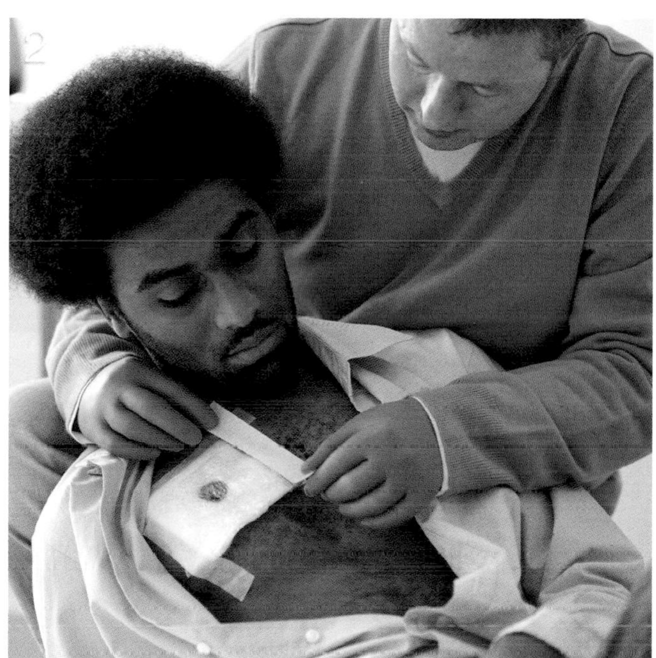

1 Help the casualty to sit down. Encourage him to lean towards the injured side and cover the wound with the palm of his hand.

2 Place a sterile dressing or clean non-fluffy pad over the wound and surrounding area. Cover with a plastic bag, foil or kitchen film. Secure firmly with adhesive tape on three edges only so that the dressing is taut.

3 **Call 999/112 for emergency help.** While waiting for help, continue to support the casualty in the same position as long as he remains conscious.

4 Monitor and record the casualty's vital signs – level of response, breathing and pulse (pp.52–53) – until emergency help arrives.

SPECIAL CASE IF THE CASUALTY IS UNCONSCIOUS

If the casualty is unconscious, open the airway and check breathing (The unconscious casualty pp.54–85). If you need to place a breathing casualty in the recovery position, roll him on to his injured side to help the healthy lung to work effectively (pp.54–85).

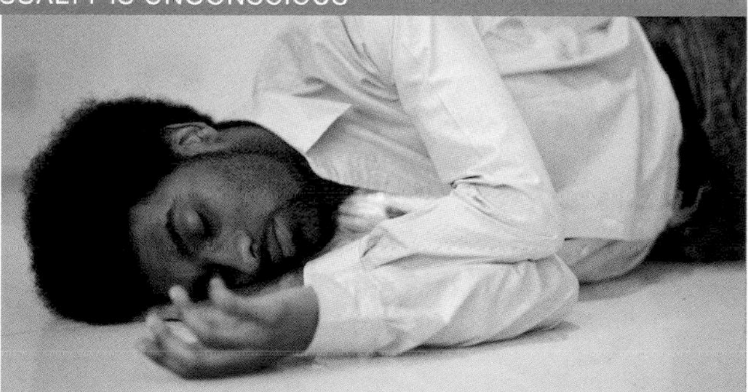

6

The heart and blood vessels are collectively known as the circulatory (cardiovascular) system. This system keeps the body supplied with blood, which carries oxygen and nutrients to all body tissues. The circulatory system may be disrupted by severe internal or external bleeding or fluid loss, for example from burns (pp.182–87). The techniques described in this section show how you can help to maintain an adequate blood supply to the heart and brain following injury or illness affecting the circulatory system.

A break in the skin or the internal body surfaces is known as a wound. Wounds can be daunting, particularly if there is a lot of bleeding, but prompt action reduces the amount of blood loss and minimises shock. Treatments for all circulatory conditions and types of wound are covered in this chapter.

AIMS AND OBJECTIVES

- To assess the casualty's condition quickly and calmly.
- To control blood loss by applying pressure and elevating the injured part.
- To minimise the risk of shock.
- To comfort and reassure the casualty.
- To call 999/112 for emergency help if you suspect a serious injury or illness.
- To be aware of your own needs, including the need to protect yourself against blood-borne infections.

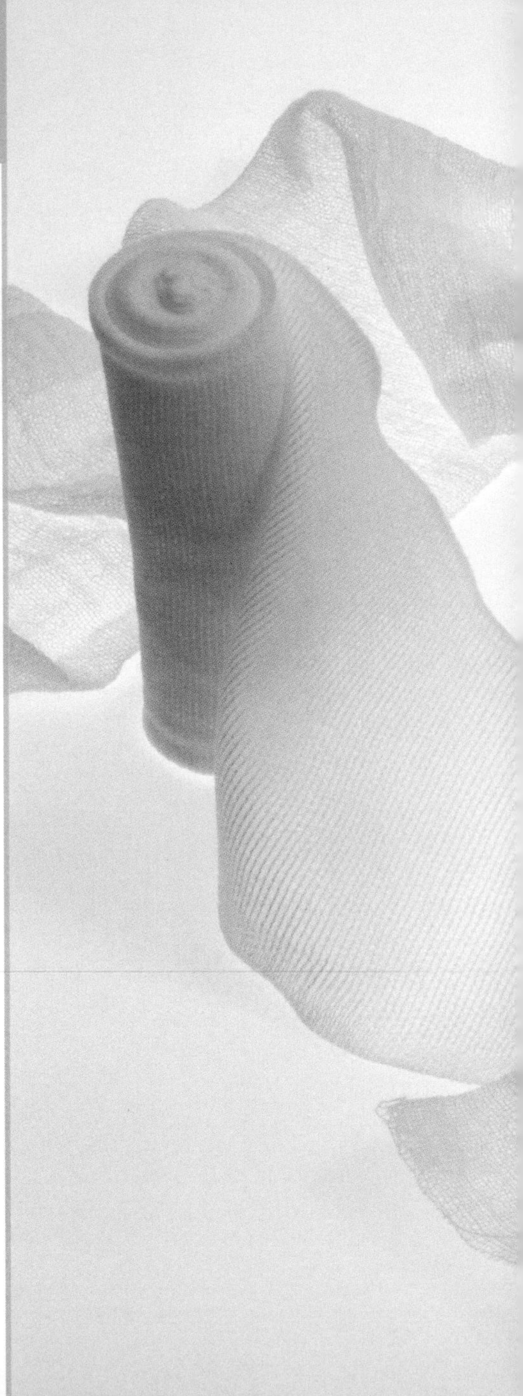

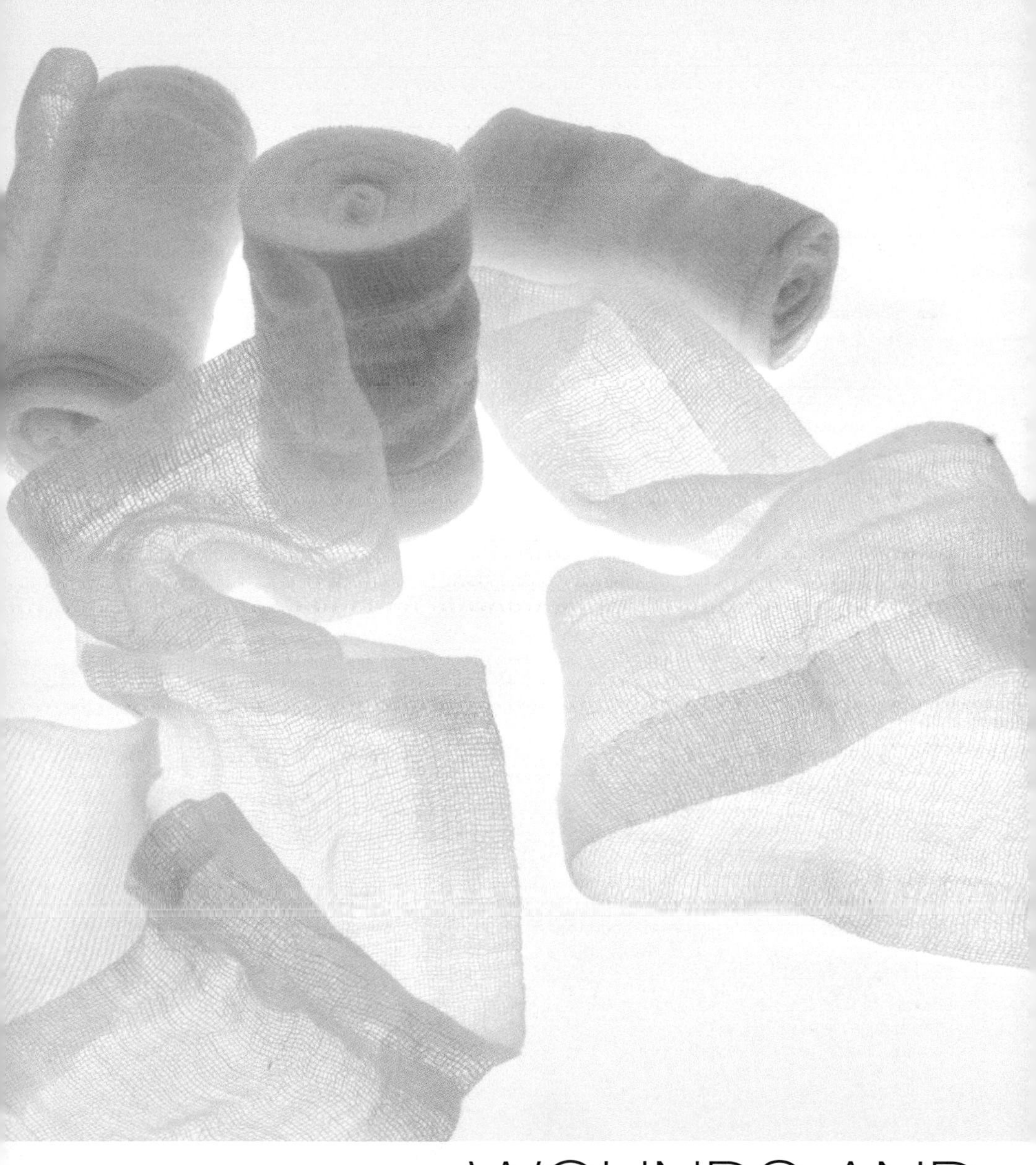

WOUNDS AND CIRCULATION

THE HEART AND BLOOD VESSELS

The heart and the blood vessels make up the circulatory system. These structures supply the body with a constant flow of blood, which brings oxygen and nutrients to the tissues and carries waste products away.

Blood is pumped around the body by rhythmic contractions (beats) of the heart muscle. The blood runs through a network of vessels, divided into three types: arteries, veins and capillaries. The force that is exerted by the blood flow through the main arteries is called blood pressure. It varies with the strength and phase of the heartbeat, the elasticity of the arterial walls and the volume and thickness of the blood.

How blood circulates
Oxygenated blood passes from the lungs to the heart, then travels to body tissues via the arteries. Blood that has given up its oxygen (deoxygenated blood) returns to the heart through the veins.

Brachial artery

Aorta carries oxygenated blood to body tissues

Vena cava carries deoxygenated blood from body tissues to heart

Radial artery

Femoral artery

Carotid artery

Jugular vein

Brachial vein

Pulmonary arteries carry deoxygenated blood to lungs

Pulmonary veins carry oxygenated blood from lungs to heart

Heart pumps blood around body

Radial vein

Femoral vein

Capillary

Small vein (venule)

Small artery (arteriole)

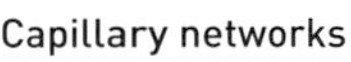

Capillary networks
A network of fine blood vessels (capillaries) links arteries and veins within body tissues. Oxygen and nutrients pass from the blood into the tissues; waste products pass from the tissues into the blood, through capillaries.

KEY
- Vessels carrying oxygenated blood
- Vessels carrying deoxygenated blood

Aorta

Pulmonary artery

Superior vena cava

Coronary artery

Heart muscle

Inferior vena cava

The heart
This muscular organ pumps blood around the body and then to the lungs to pick up oxygen. Coronary blood vessels supply the heart muscle with oxygen and nutrients.

HOW THE HEART FUNCTIONS

The heart pumps blood by muscular contractions called heartbeats, which are controlled by electrical impulses generated in the heart. Each beat has three phases: diastole, when the blood enters the heart; atrial systole, when it is squeezed out of the atria (collecting chambers); and ventricular systole, when blood leaves the heart.

In diastole, the heart relaxes. Oxygenated blood from the lungs flows via the pulmonary veins into the left atrium. Blood that has given up its oxygen to body tissues (deoxygenated blood) flows from the venae cavae (large veins that enter the heart) into the right atrium.

In atrial systole, the two atria contract and the valves between the atria and the ventricles (pumping chambers) open so that blood flows into the ventricles.

During ventricular systole, the ventricles contract. The thick-walled left ventricle forces blood into the aorta (main artery), which carries it to the rest of the body. The right ventricle pumps blood into the pulmonary arteries, which carry it to the lungs to collect more oxygen.

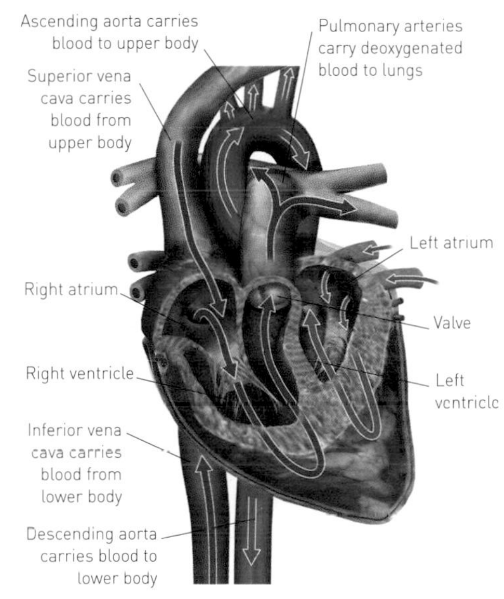

Blood flow through the heart
The heart's right side pumps deoxygenated blood from the body to the lungs. The left side pumps oxygenated blood to the body via the aorta.

KEY
- Vessels carrying oxygenated blood
- Vessels carrying deoxygenated blood

COMPOSITION OF BLOOD

There are about 6 litres (10 pints), or 1 litre per 13kg of body weight (1 pint per stone), of blood in the average adult body. Roughly 55 per cent of the blood is clear yellow fluid (plasma). In this fluid are suspended the red and white blood cells and the platelets, all of which make up the remaining 45 per cent.

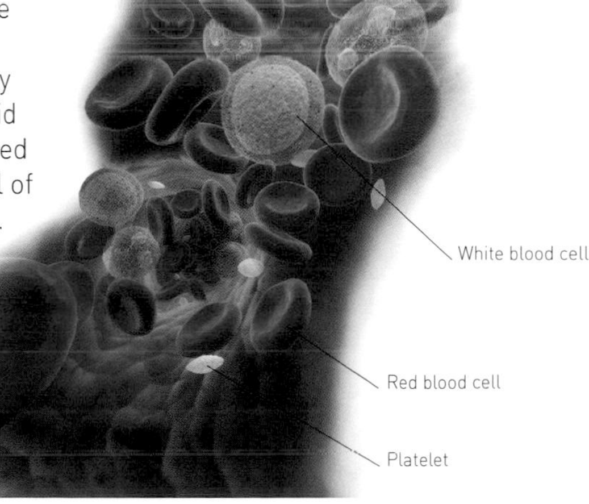

The blood cells
Red blood cells contain haemoglobin, a red pigment that enables the cells to carry oxygen. White blood cells play a role in defending the body against infection. Platelets help blood to clot.

BLEEDING AND TYPES OF WOUND

When a blood vessel is damaged, the vessel constricts, and a series of chemical reactions occur to form a blood clot – a "plug" over the damaged area (below). If large blood vessels are torn or severed, uncontrolled blood loss may occur before clotting can take place, and shock (pp.116–17) may develop.

TYPES OF BLEEDING

Bleeding (haemorrhage) is classified by the type of blood vessel that is damaged. Arteries carry oxygenated blood under pressure from the heart. If an artery is damaged, bleeding will be profuse. Blood will spurt out in time with the heartbeat. If a main artery is severed, the volume of circulating blood will fall rapidly.

Blood from veins, having given up its oxygen into the tissues, is darker red. It is under less pressure than arterial blood, but vein walls can widen greatly and the blood can "pool" inside them (varicose vein). If a large or varicose vein is damaged, blood will gush from it profusely.

Bleeding from capillaries occurs with any wound. At first, bleeding may be brisk, but blood loss is usually slight. A blow may rupture capillaries under the skin, causing bleeding into the tissues (bruising).

HOW WOUNDS HEAL

When a blood vessel is severed or damaged, it constricts (narrows) in order to prevent excessive amounts of blood from escaping. Injured tissue cells at the site of the wound, together with specialised blood cells called platelets, then trigger a series of chemical reactions that result in the formation of a substance that forms a mesh. This mesh traps blood cells to make a blood clot. The clot releases a fluid known as serum, which contains antibodies and specialised cells; this serum begins the process of repairing the damaged area.

At first, the blood clot is a jelly-like mass. Fibroblast cells form a plug within the clot. Later, this dries into a crust (scab) that seals and protects the site of the wound until the healing process is complete.

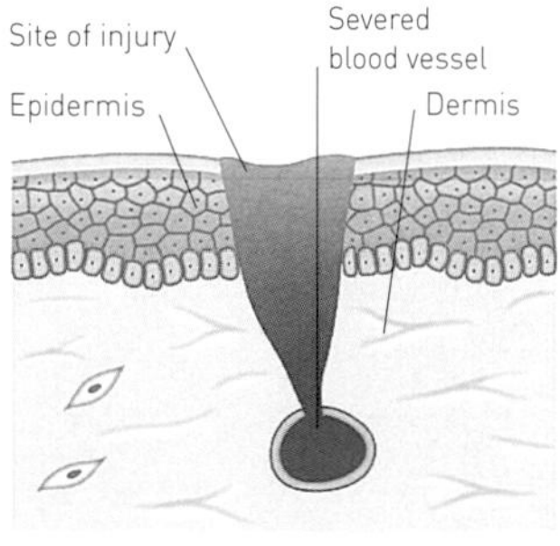

Injury
At the site of injury, platelets in the blood arrive to begin formation of a clot. Other cells are attracted to the site to help with repair.

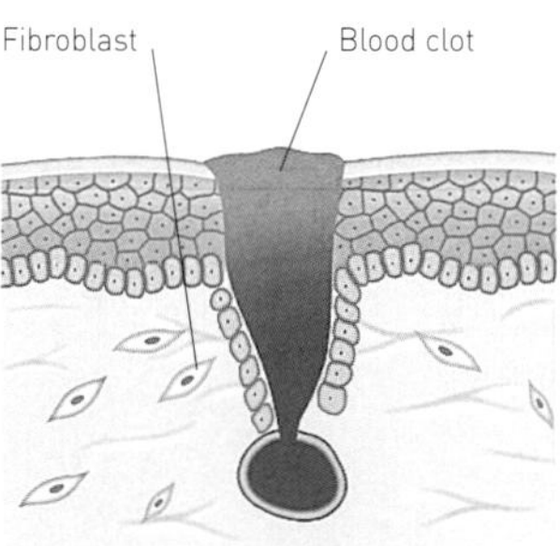

Clotting
A clot is formed by platelets in the blood and blood-clotting protein. Tissue-forming cells migrate to the damaged area to start repair.

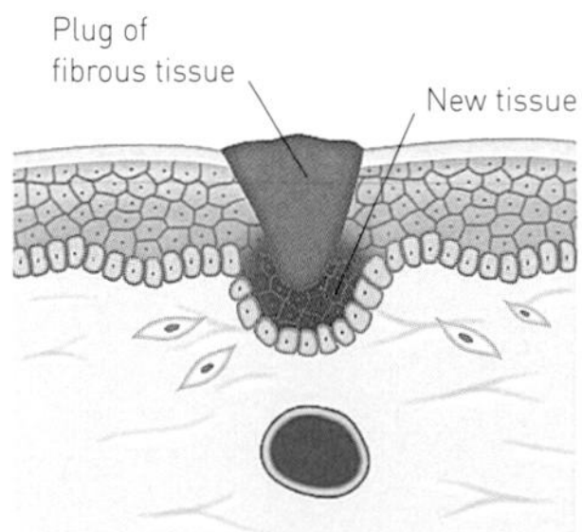

Plugging and scabbing
A plug of fibrous tissue is formed within the clot. The plug hardens and forms a scab that eventually drops off when skin beneath it is healed.

TYPES OF WOUND

Wounds can be classified into a number of different types, depending on the object that produces the wound – such as a knife or a bullet – and the manner in which the wound has been inflicted.

Each of these types of wound carries specific risks associated with surrounding tissue damage and infection.

INCISED WOUND

This is caused by a clean surface cut from a sharp-edged object such as a razor. Blood vessels are cut straight across, so bleeding may be profuse. Structures such as tendons or nerves may be damaged.

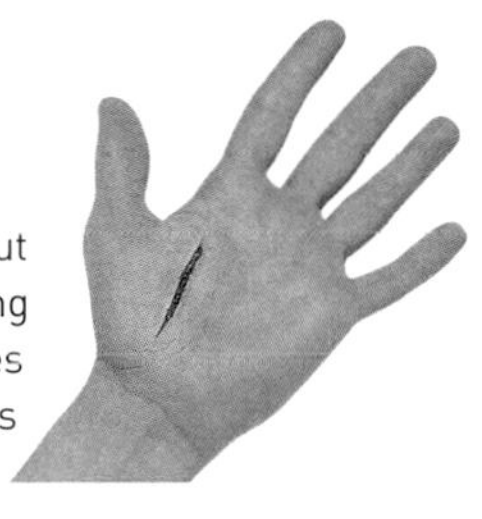

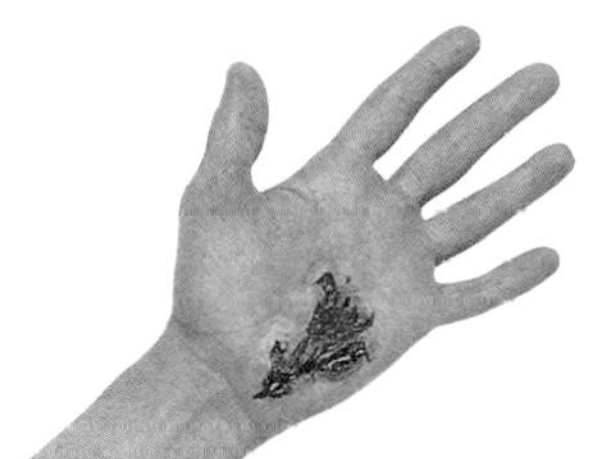

LACERATION

Crushing or ripping forces result in tears or lacerations. These wounds may bleed less profusely than incised wounds, but there is likely to be more tissue damage. Lacerations are often contaminated with germs, so the risk of infection is high.

ABRASION (GRAZE)

This is a superficial wound in which the topmost layers of skin are scraped off, leaving a raw, tender area. Abrasions are often caused by a sliding fall or a friction burn. They can contain embedded foreign particles that may cause infection.

CONTUSION (BRUISE)

A blunt blow can rupture capillaries beneath the skin, causing blood to leak into the tissues. This process results in bruising. The skin may also split. Extensive contusion may indicate deeper damage, such as a fracture or an internal injury.

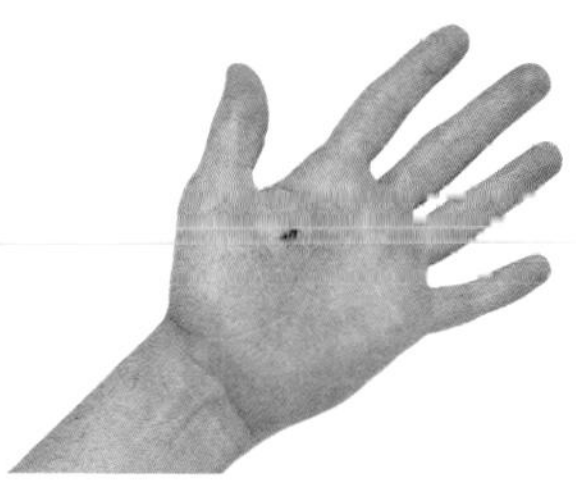

PUNCTURE WOUND

An injury such as standing on a nail or being pricked by a needle will result in a puncture wound. It has a small entry site but a deep track of internal damage. Since germs and dirt can be carried far into the body, the infection risk with this kind of wound is high.

STAB WOUND

This type of wound can be caused by a long or bladed instrument, usually a knife, penetrating the body. Stab wounds to the trunk must always be treated seriously because of the danger of injury to vital organs and life-threatening internal bleeding.

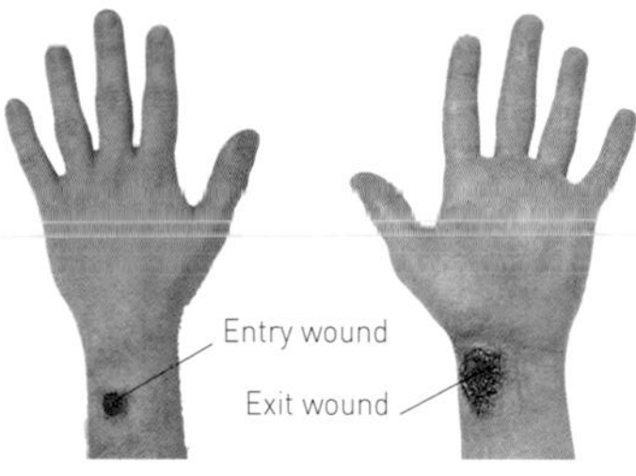

GUNSHOT WOUND

This type of wound is caused by a bullet or missile being driven into or through the body, causing serious internal injury and sucking in clothing and contaminants from the air. The entry wound may be small and neat; any exit wound may be large and ragged.

HEART ATTACK

RECOGNITION

- Persistent, vice-like central chest pain, which may spread to the jaw and down one or both arms. Unlike angina (opposite), the pain does not ease when the casualty rests.
- Breathlessness.
- Discomfort occurring high in the abdomen, which may feel similar to severe indigestion.
- Collapse, often without any warning.
- Sudden faintness or dizziness.
- Casualty feels a sense of impending doom.
- "Ashen" skin and blueness at the lips.
- A rapid, weak or irregular pulse.
- Profuse sweating.
- Extreme gasping for air ("air hunger").

YOUR AIMS

- To ease the strain on the heart by ensuring that the casualty rests.
- To call for urgent medical help without delay.

CAUTION

- If the casualty loses consciousness, open the airway and check breathing (The unconscious casualty pp.54–85).
- Do not give the casualty aspirin if you know that he is allergic to it.

A heart attack is most commonly caused by a sudden obstruction of the blood supply to part of the heart muscle – for example, because of a clot in a coronary artery (coronary thrombosis). It can also be called a myocardial infarction. The main risk is that the heart will stop beating.

The effects of a heart attack depend largely on how much of the heart muscle is affected; many casualties recover completely. Aspirin can be used to try to limit the extent of damage to the heart muscle.

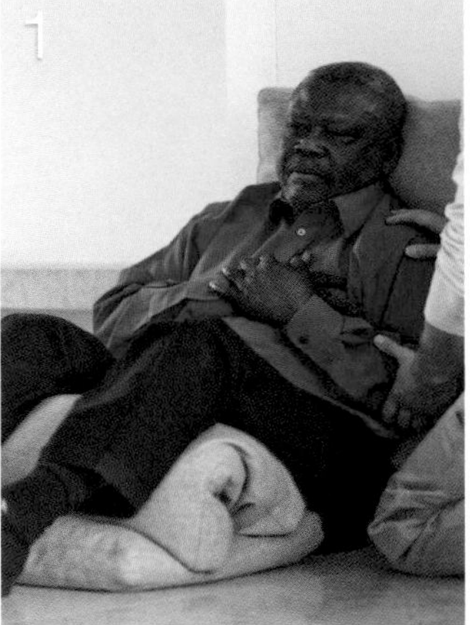

1 **Make the casualty as comfortable as possible to ease the strain on his heart. A half-sitting position, with his head and shoulders supported and his knees bent, is often best. Place cushions behind him and under his knees.**

2 **Call 999/112 for emergency help.** Tell ambulance control that you suspect a heart attack. If the casualty asks you to do so, call his own doctor too.

3 Assist the casualty to take one full dose aspirin tablet (300mg in total). Advise him to chew it slowly.

4 If the casualty has angina medication, such as tablets or a pump-action or aerosol spray, let him administer it; help him if necessary. Encourage him to rest.

5 Monitor and record vital signs – level of response, breathing and pulse (pp.52–53) – while waiting for help to arrive.

6 Avoid undue stress by staying calm.

ANGINA

RECOGNITION

- Vice-like central chest pain, which may spread to the jaw and down one or both arms.
- Pain easing with rest.
- Shortness of breath.
- Tiredness, which is often sudden and extreme.
- Feeling of anxiety.

YOUR AIMS

- To ease strain on the heart by ensuring that the casualty rests.
- To help the casualty with any medication.
- To obtain medical help if necessary.

CAUTION

- If the casualty loses consciousness, open the airway and check breathing, (The unconscious casualty pp.54 85).

The term angina means literally a constriction of the chest. Angina occurs when coronary arteries that supply the heart muscle with blood become narrowed and cannot carry sufficient blood to meet increased demands during exertion or excitement. An attack forces the casualty to rest; the pain should ease soon afterwards.

2

1 **Help the casualty to stop what he is doing and sit down. Make sure that he is comfortable and reassure him; this should help the pain to ease.**

2 **If the casualty has angina medication, such as tablets or a pump-action or aerosol spray, let him administer it himself. If necessary, help him to take it.**

3 **Encourage the casualty to rest, and keep any bystanders away. The pain should ease within a few minutes.**

4 **If the pain subsides after rest and/or medication, the casualty will usually be able to resume what he was doing. If he is concerned tell him to seek medical advice.**

5 If the pain persists, or returns, suspect a heart attack (opposite). **Call 999/112 for emergency help.**

FAINTING

RECOGNITION

- Brief loss of consciousness that causes the casualty to fall to the ground.
- A slow pulse.
- Pale, cold skin and sweating.

YOUR AIMS

- To improve blood flow to the brain.
- To reassure the casualty and make her comfortable.

CAUTION

- If the casualty does not regain consciousness quickly open the airway and check breathing (The unconscious casualty pp.54–85).

A faint is a brief loss of consciousness caused by a temporary reduction of the blood flow to the brain. It may be a reaction to pain, exhaustion, lack of food or emotional stress. Fainting is also common after long periods of physical inactivity, such as standing or sitting still, especially in a warm atmosphere. This inactivity causes blood to pool in the legs, reducing the amount of blood reaching the brain.

When a person faints, the pulse rate becomes very slow. However, the rate soon picks up and returns to normal. A casualty who has fainted usually makes a rapid and complete recovery. Do not advise a person who feels faint to sit on a chair with her head between her knees because if she faints she may fall.

See also
The unconscious casualty pp.54–85

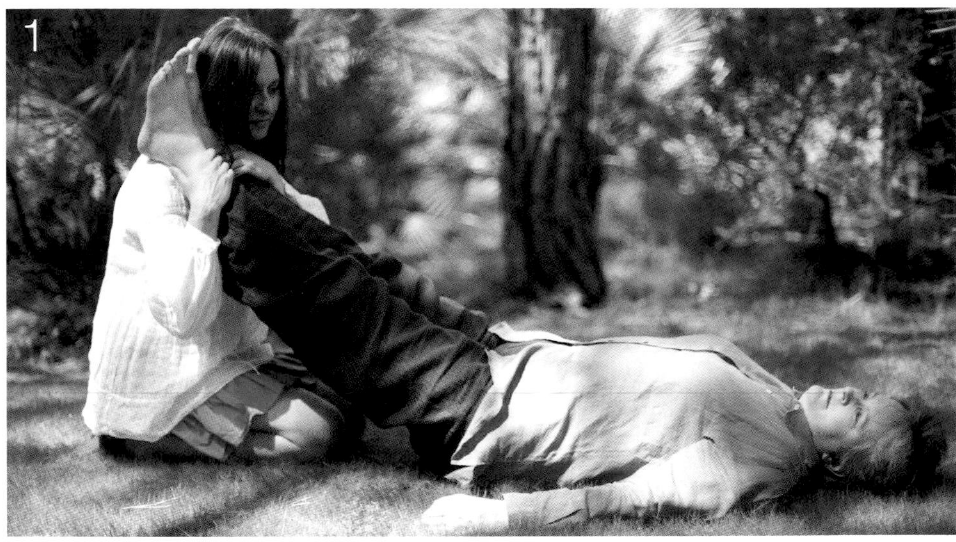

1 When a casualty feels faint, advise her to lie down. Kneel down, raise her legs, supporting her ankles on your shoulders to improve blood flow to the brain. Watch her face for signs of recovery.

2 Make sure that the casualty has plenty of fresh air; ask someone to open a window if you are indoors. In addition, ask any bystanders to stand clear.

3 As the casualty recovers, reassure her and help her to sit up gradually. If she starts to feel faint again, advise her to lie down once again, and raise and support her legs until she recovers fully.

INTERNAL BLEEDING

RECOGNITION

- Initially, pale, cold, clammy skin. If bleeding continues, the skin may turn blue-grey (cyanosis).
- Rapid, weak pulse.
- Thirst.
- Rapid, shallow breathing.
- Confusion, restlessness and irritability.
- Possible collapse and unconsciousness.
- Bleeding from body openings (orifices).
- In cases of violent injury, "pattern bruising" – an area of discoloured skin with a shape that matches the pattern of clothes or crushing or restraining objects.
- Pain.
- Information from casualty that indicates recent injury, illness, or operation.

Bleeding inside body cavities may follow an injury, such as a fracture or a blow from a blunt object, but it can also occur spontaneously – for example, bleeding from a stomach ulcer. The main risk from internal bleeding is shock (pp.116–17). In addition, blood can build up around organs such as the lungs or brain and exert damaging pressure on them.

Suspect internal bleeding if a casualty develops signs of shock without obvious blood loss. Check for any bleeding from body openings (orifices) such as the ear, mouth and nose. There may also be bleeding from the urethra or anus (below).

The signs of bleeding vary depending on the site of the blood loss (below), but the most obvious is a discharge of blood from a body opening. Blood loss from any orifice is significant and can lead to shock. In addition, bleeding from some orifices can indicate a serious underlying injury or illness. Follow treatment for shock (pp.116–17).

See also
Cerebral compression p.167
Crush injury p.119
Head injury p.165
Shock pp.116–17

POSSIBLE SIGNS OF INTERNAL BLEEDING

SITE	APPEARANCE OF BLOOD	CAUSE OF BLOOD LOSS
Mouth	▪ Bright red, frothy, coughed-up blood	▪ Bleeding in the lungs
	▪ Vomited blood, red or dark reddish-brown, resembling coffee grounds	▪ Bleeding within the digestive system
Ear	▪ Fresh, bright red blood	▪ Injury to the inner or outer ear or perforated eardrum
	▪ Thin, watery blood	▪ Leakage of fluid from around the brain due to head injury
Nose	▪ Fresh, bright red blood	▪ Ruptured blood vessel in the nostril
	▪ Thin, watery blood	▪ Leakage of fluid from around the brain due to head injury
Anus	▪ Fresh, bright red blood	▪ Piles or injury to the anus or lower intestine
	▪ Black, tarry, offensive-smelling stool (melaena)	▪ Disease or injury to the intestine
Urethra	▪ Red or smoky appearance to urine, occasionally containing clots	▪ Bleeding from the bladder, kidneys or urethra
Vagina	▪ Either fresh or dark blood	▪ Menstruation ▪ Miscarriage ▪ Pregnancy ▪ Recent childbirth ▪ Assault

SEVERE EXTERNAL BLEEDING

YOUR AIMS

- To control bleeding.
- To prevent and minimise the effects of shock.
- To minimise infection.
- To arrange urgent removal to hospital.

CAUTION

- Do not allow the casualty to eat or drink because an anaesthetic may be needed.
- If the casualty loses consciousness, open the airway and check breathing (The unconscious casualty pp.54–85).

See also
Foreign object in a wound **p.122**
Shock **pp.116–17**

When bleeding is severe, it can be dramatic and distressing. If bleeding is not controlled shock will develop and the casualty may lose consciousness.

Bleeding from the mouth or nose may affect breathing. When treating severe bleeding, check first whether there is an object embedded in the wound; take care not to press directly on the object. Do not let the casualty have anything to eat or drink as he may need an anaesthetic later.

1 Remove or cut clothing as necessary to expose the wound (p.232).

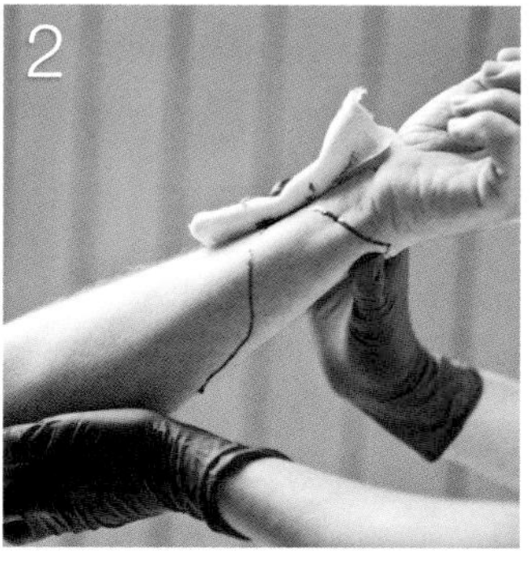

2 Apply direct pressure over the wound with your fingers using a sterile dressing or clean, non-fluffy pad. If you do not have a dressing, ask the casualty to apply direct pressure himself. If there is an object in the wound, apply pressure on either side of the object (opposite).

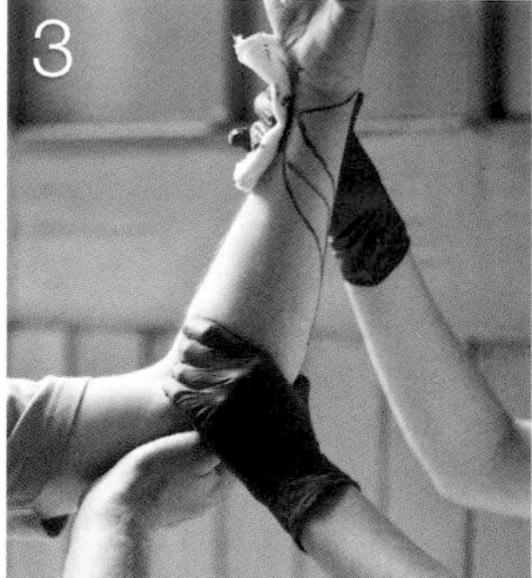

3 Maintain direct pressure on the wound to control bleeding. Raise and support the injured limb above the level of the casualty's heart to reduce blood loss.

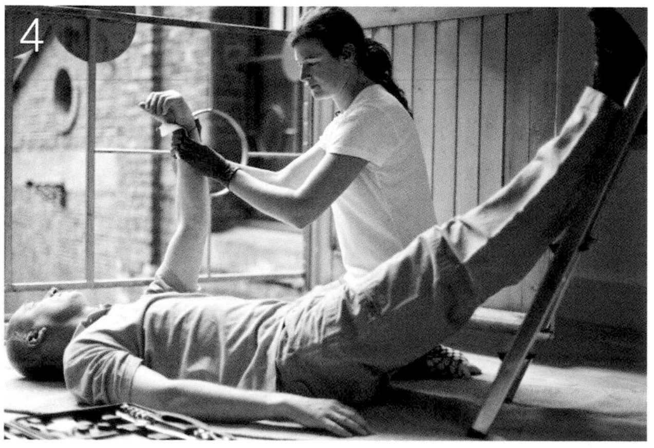

4 Help the casualty to lie down – on a rug or blanket if there is one, as this will protect him from the cold. As shock is likely to develop (pp.116–17), raise and support his legs so that they are above the level of his heart.

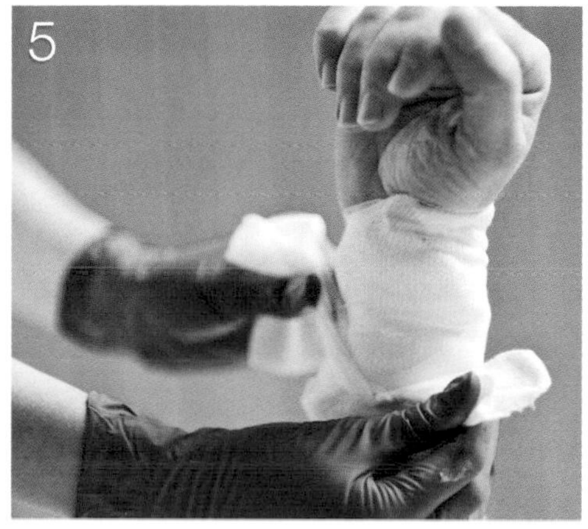

5 Secure the dressing with a bandage that is firm enough to maintain pressure, but not so tight that it impairs circulation (p.243).

6 If bleeding shows through the dressing, apply a second one on top of the first. If blood seeps through this, remove both dressings and apply a fresh one, ensuring that pressure is applied accurately at the point of bleeding.

7 Support the injured part in a raised position with a sling and/or bandage. Check the circulation beyond the bandage every ten minutes (p.243). If the circulation is impaired, loosen the bandage and reapply.

8 **Call 999/112 for emergency help.** Monitor and record vital signs – level of response, breathing and pulse (pp.52–53) – while waiting for help to arrive.

SPECIAL CASE IF THERE IS AN OBJECT IN THE WOUND

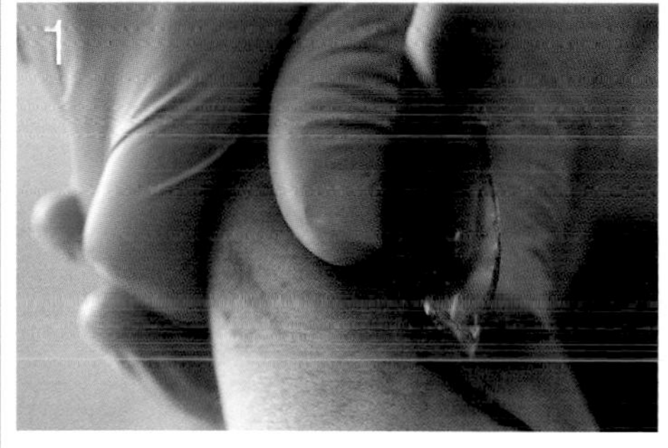

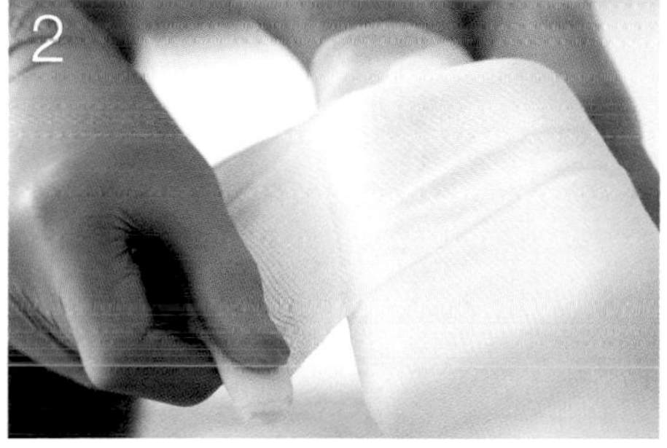

1 Control bleeding by pressing firmly on either side of the embedded object to push the edges of the wound together. Do not press directly on the object, or try to remove it. Raise the injury above the level of the heart.

2 To protect the wound, drape a piece of gauze over the object. Build up padding on either side, then carefully bandage over the object and pads without pressing on the object (p.122). Check the circulation beyond the bandage every ten minutes (p.243). If the circulation is impaired, loosen the bandage and reapply.

3 Treat for shock (pp.116–17). **Call 999/112 for emergency help.** Monitor and record vital signs – level of response, breathing and pulse (pp.52–53) – while waiting for help to arrive.

SHOCK

RECOGNITION

Initially:

- A rapid pulse;
- Pale, cold, clammy skin;
- Sweating.

As shock develops:

- Rapid, shallow breathing;
- A weak, "thready" pulse. When the pulse at the wrist disappears, about half of the blood volume will have been lost;
- Grey-blue skin (cyanosis), especially inside the lips. A fingernail or earlobe, if pressed, will not regain its colour immediately;
- Weakness and dizziness;
- Nausea, and possibly vomiting;
- Thirst.

As the brain's oxygen supply weakens:

- Restlessness and aggressiveness;
- Yawning and gasping for air;
- Unconsciousness;
- Finally, the heart will stop.

This life-threatening condition occurs when the circulatory system (which distributes oxygen to the body tissues and removes waste products) fails and, as a result, vital organs such as the heart and brain are deprived of oxygen. It requires immediate emergency treatment. Shock can be made worse by fear and pain. Minimise the risk of shock developing by reassuring the casualty and making him comfortable.

The most common cause of shock is severe blood loss. If this exceeds 1.2 litres (2 pints), which is about one-fifth of the normal blood volume, shock will develop. This degree of blood loss may result from external bleeding. It may also be caused by: hidden bleeding from internal organs (p.113), blood escaping into a body cavity (p.113) or bleeding from damaged blood vessels due to a closed fracture (p.137). Loss of other body fluids can also result in shock. Conditions that can cause severe fluid loss include diarrhoea, vomiting, bowel obstruction and serious burns.

In addition, shock may occur when there is sufficient blood volume but the heart is unable to pump the blood around the body. This problem can be due to severe heart disease, heart attack or acute heart failure. Other causes of shock include overwhelming infection, low blood sugar (hypoglycaemia), hypothermia, severe allergic reaction (anaphylactic shock), drug overdose and spinal cord injury.

See also
Anaphylactic shock p.221
Internal bleeding p.113
Severe burns and scalds pp.182–83
Severe external bleeding pp.114–15
The unconscious casualty pp.54–85

EFFECTS OF BLOOD OR FLUID LOSS

APPROXIMATE VOLUME LOST	EFFECTS ON THE BODY
0.5 litre (about 1 pint)	■ Little or no effect; this is the quantity of blood normally taken in a blood-donor session
Up to 2 litres (3½ pints)	■ Hormones such as adrenaline are released, quickening the pulse and inducing sweating ■ Small blood vessels in non-vital areas, such as the skin, shut down to divert blood and oxygen to the vital organs ■ Shock becomes evident
2 litres (3½ pints) or more (over a third of the normal volume in the average adult)	■ As blood or fluid loss approaches this level, the pulse at the wrist may become undetectable ■ Casualty will usually lose consciousness ■ Breathing may cease and the heart may stop

YOUR AIMS

- To recognise shock.
- To treat any obvious cause of shock.
- To improve the blood supply to the brain, heart and lungs.
- To arrange urgent removal to hospital.

CAUTION

- Do not allow the casualty to eat or drink because an anaesthetic may be needed. If he complains of thirst, moisten his lips with a little water.
- Do not leave the casualty unattended, unless you have to call emergency help.
- Do not warm the casualty with a hot-water bottle or any other direct source of heat.
- If the casualty is in the later stages of pregnancy, help her to lie down leaning towards her left side to prevent the baby restricting blood flow back to the heart.
- If the casualty loses consciousness, open the airway and check breathing (The unconscious casualty pp.54–85).

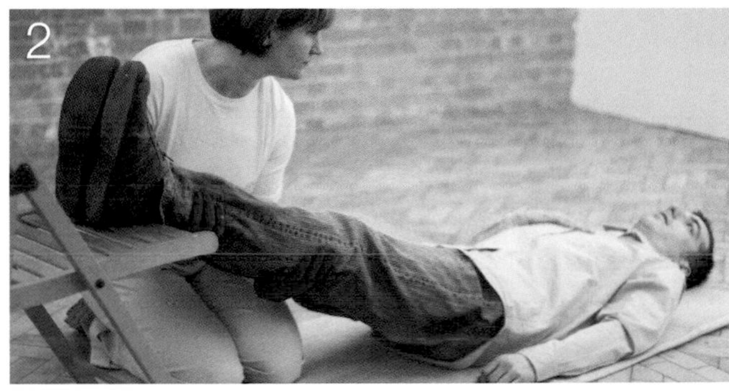

1 Treat any possible cause of shock that you can detect, such as severe bleeding (pp.114–15) or serious burns (pp.182–83). Reassure the casualty.

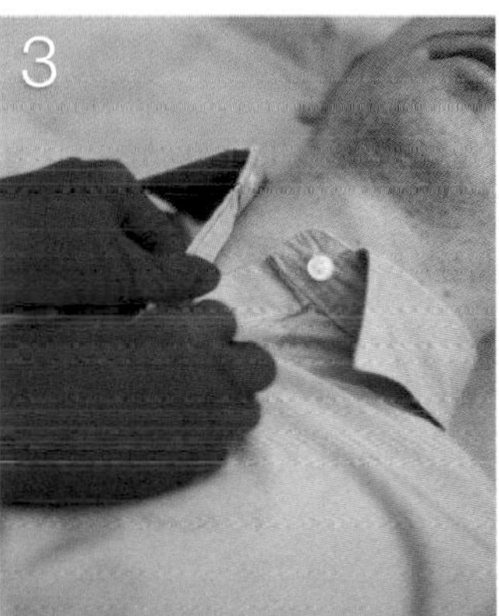

2 Help the casualty to lie down – on a rug or blanket if there is one, as this will protect him from the cold. Raise and support his legs above the level of his heart to improve blood supply to the vital organs. Keeping his head low may also prevent him from losing consciousness. Stop him from making any unnecessary movements.

3 Loosen tight clothing at the neck, chest and waist to reduce constriction.

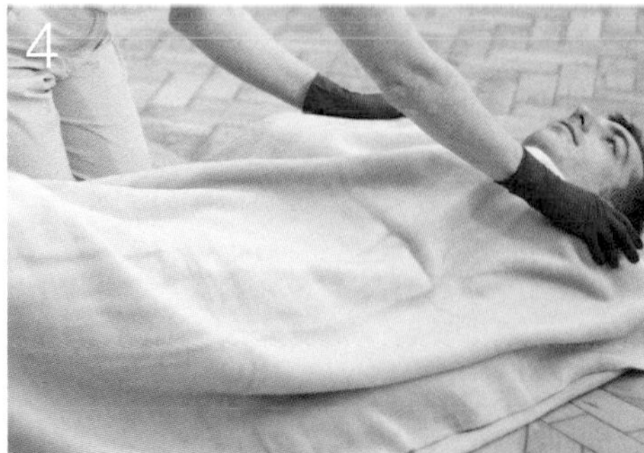

4 Keep the casualty warm by covering his body and legs with coats or blankets. **Call 999/112 for emergency help.**

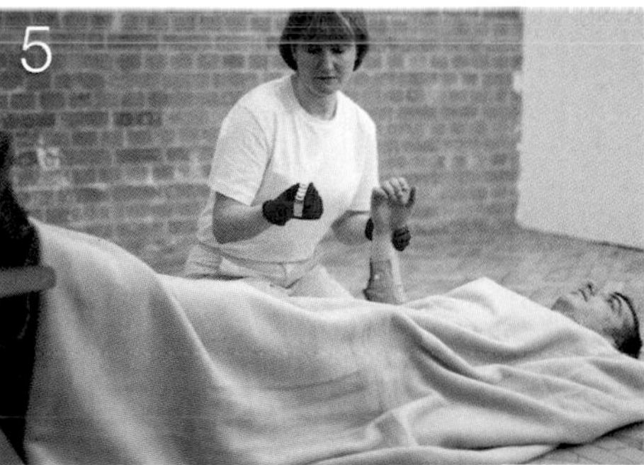

5 Monitor and record vital signs – level of response, breathing and pulse (pp.52–53) – while waiting for help to arrive.

IMPALEMENT

YOUR AIMS

- To prevent further injury.

CAUTION

- Do not allow the casualty to eat or drink because an anaesthetic may be needed.

If someone has been impaled, for example by falling onto railings, never attempt to lift the casualty off the object involved since this may worsen internal injuries. Call the emergency services immediately, giving clear details about the incident. They will bring special cutting equipment with them to free the casualty.

1 **Call 999/112 for emergency help.** Send a helper to make the call, if possible. Explain the situation clearly to ambulance control, so that the right equipment can be brought.

2 Support the casualty's body weight until the emergency services arrive and take over. Reassure the casualty while you wait for emergency help.

AMPUTATION

YOUR AIMS

- To control bleeding.
- To minimise the effects of shock.
- To arrange urgent removal to hospital.
- To prevent deterioration of the injured part.

CAUTION

- Do not wash the severed part.
- Do not let the severed part touch the crushed ice when packing it.
- Do not allow the casualty to eat or drink because an anaesthetic may be needed.

See also
Severe external bleeding **pp.114–15**
Shock **pp.116–17**

A limb that has been partially or completely severed can, in many cases, be reattached by microsurgery. The operation will require a general anaesthetic, so do not allow the casualty to eat or drink. It is vital to get the casualty and the amputated part to hospital as soon as possible. Shock is likely, and needs to be treated.

1 Control blood loss by applying direct pressure and raising the injured part above the casualty's heart.

2 Place a sterile dressing or a non-fluffy, clean pad on the wound, and secure it with a bandage. Treat the casualty for shock (pp.116–17).

3 **Call 999/112 for emergency help.** Tell ambulance control that amputation is involved. Monitor and record vital signs – level of response, breathing and pulse (pp.52–53) – while waiting for help to arrive.

4 Wrap the severed part in kitchen film or a plastic bag. Wrap the package in gauze or soft fabric and place it in a container full of crushed ice. Mark the container with the time of injury and the casualty's name. Give it to the emergency service personnel yourself.

CRUSH INJURY

YOUR AIMS

- To obtain specialist medical aid urgently, taking any steps possible to treat the casualty.

CAUTION

- Do not release a casualty who has been crushed for more than 15 minutes.
- Do not lift heavy objects.
- Do not allow the casualty to eat or drink because an anaesthetic may be needed.

See also
Fractures **pp.136–38**
Shock **pp.116–17**

Traffic and building site incidents are the most common causes of crush injuries. Other possible causes include explosions, earthquakes and train crashes.

A crush injury may include a fracture, swelling and internal bleeding. The crushing force may also cause impaired circulation, which results in numbness at or below the site of injury. You may not be able to detect a pulse in a crushed limb.

DANGERS OF PROLONGED CRUSHING

If the casualty is trapped for any length of time, two serious complications may result. First, prolonged crushing may cause extensive damage to body tissues, especially to muscles. Once the pressure is removed, shock may develop rapidly as tissue fluid leaks into the injured area.

Secondly, and more dangerously, toxic substances will build up in damaged muscle tissue around a crush injury. If released suddenly into the circulation, these toxins may cause kidney failure. This process, called "crush syndrome", is extremely serious and can be fatal.

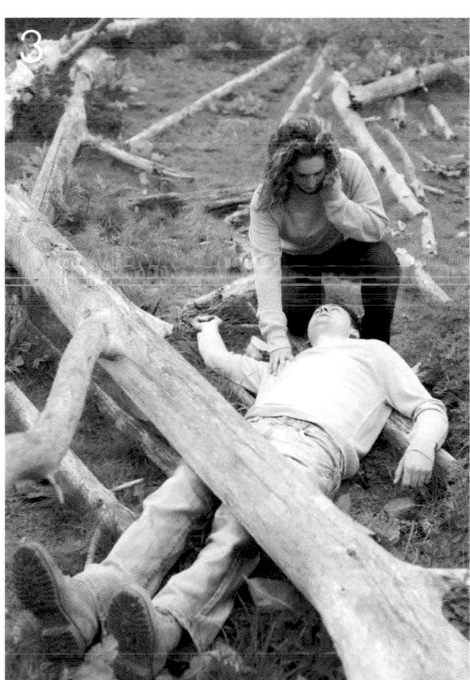

1 **If you know the casualty has been crushed for less than 15 minutes and you can release him, do this as quickly as possible. Control external bleeding and steady and support any suspected fracture (pp.136–38). Treat the casualty for shock (pp.116–17).**

2 **If the casualty has been crushed for more than 15 minutes, or you cannot move the cause of injury, leave him in the position found and comfort and reassure him.**

3 **Call 999/112 for emergency help,** giving clear details of the incident to ambulance control.

4 Monitor and record vital signs – level of response, breathing and pulse (pp.52–53) – while waiting for help to arrive.

FOREIGN OBJECT IN A WOUND

YOUR AIMS

- To control bleeding without pressing the object further into the wound.
- To minimise the risk of infection.
- To arrange transport to hospital if necessary.

CAUTION

- Ask the casualty about tetanus immunisation. Seek medical advice if: he has a dirty wound; he has never been immunised; he is uncertain about the number or timings of injections; he has not had at least five injections previously.

See also
Cuts and grazes **p.120**
Embedded fish hook **p.203**
Severe external bleeding **pp.114–15**
Splinter **p.202**

It is important to remove foreign objects, such as small pieces of glass or grit, from a wound before beginning treatment. If left in a wound, they may cause infection or delay healing. The best way to remove superficial pieces of glass or grit from the skin is to pick them out with tweezers. Alternatively, rinse loose pieces off with cold water. Do not try to remove pieces that are firmly embedded in the wound because you may damage the surrounding tissue and aggravate bleeding. Instead, cover the object with a dressing and bandage around it.

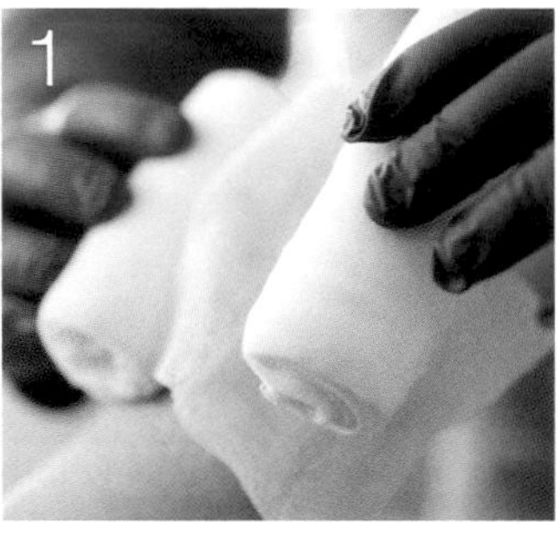

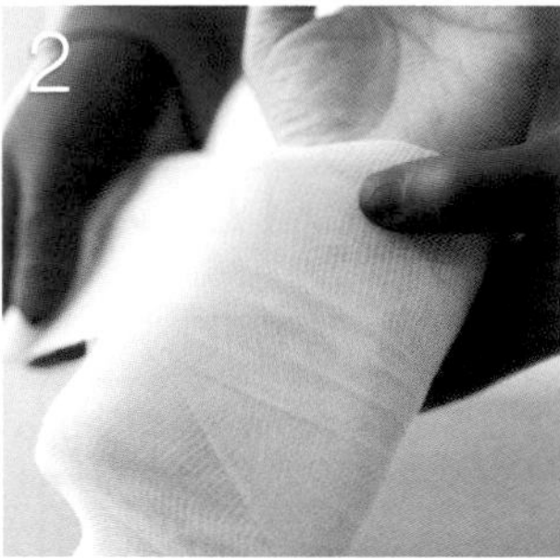

1 Control bleeding by applying pressure on either side of the object (see p.115) and raising the area above the casualty's heart level. Drape a piece of gauze over the wound and object.

2 Build up padding on either side of the object (rolled bandages make good padding) until it is high enough for you to be able to bandage over the object without pressing it further into the wound. Hold the padding in place until the bandaging is complete.

3 Arrange to take or send the casualty to hospital.

SPECIAL CASE BANDAGING AROUND A LARGER OBJECT

If you cannot build padding high enough to bandage over the top of an object, drape a clean piece of gauze over it. Place padding on either side of the object, then secure it in place by bandaging above and below the object.

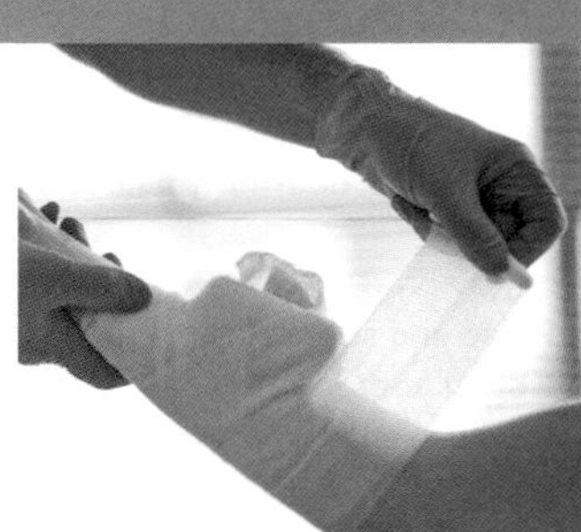

SCALP AND HEAD WOUNDS

YOUR AIMS

- To control bleeding.
- To arrange transport to hospital.

CAUTION

- If at any stage the person loses consciousness, open the airway and check breathing (The unconscious casualty pp.54–85).

The scalp has many small blood vessels running close to the skin surface, so any cut can result in profuse bleeding, which often makes a scalp wound appear worse than it is.

In some cases, however, a scalp wound may form part of a more serious underlying head injury, such as a skull fracture, or may be associated with a head or neck injury. For these reasons, you should examine a casualty with a scalp wound very carefully, particularly if it is possible that signs of a serious head injury are being masked by alcohol or drug intoxication. If you are in any doubt, follow the treatment for head injury (p.165). In addition, bear in mind the possibility of a neck (spinal) injury.

See also
Head injury **p.165**
Shock **pp.116–17**
Spinal injury **pp.171–73**

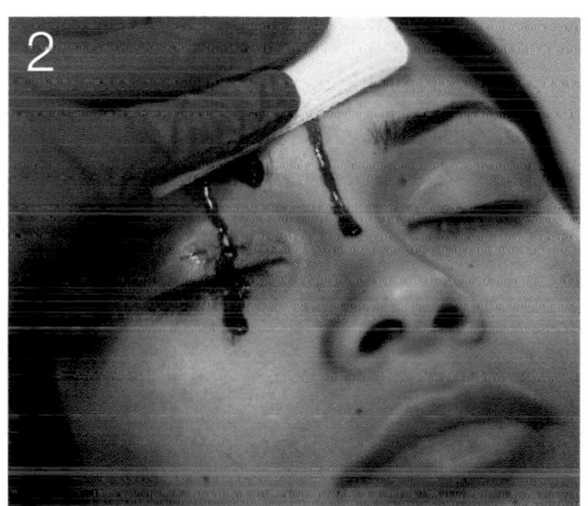

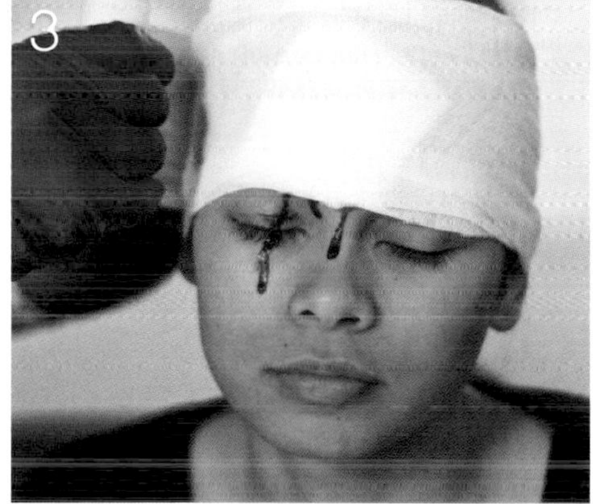

1 If there are any displaced flaps of skin at the injury site, carefully replace them over the wound. Reassure the casualty.

2 Cover the wound with a sterile dressing or a large clean, non-fluffy pad. Apply firm, direct pressure on the pad to help control bleeding to reduce blood loss, and minimise the risk of shock.

3 Keep the pad in place with a roller bandage to secure the pad and maintain pressure.

4 Help the casualty to lie down with her head and shoulders slightly raised. If she feels faint or dizzy or shows any signs of shock, **call 999/112 for emergency help**. Monitor and record vital signs – level of response, breathing and pulse (pp.52–53) – while waiting for help.

KNOCKED-OUT ADULT TOOTH

CAUTION

- Do not clean a knocked-out tooth since you may damage the tissues, reducing the chance of re-implantation.

If a secondary (adult) tooth is knocked out, it should be replanted in its socket as soon as possible. If this is not possible, ask the casualty to keep the tooth inside his cheek if he feels able to do this. Alternatively, place it in a small container of milk to prevent it from drying out.

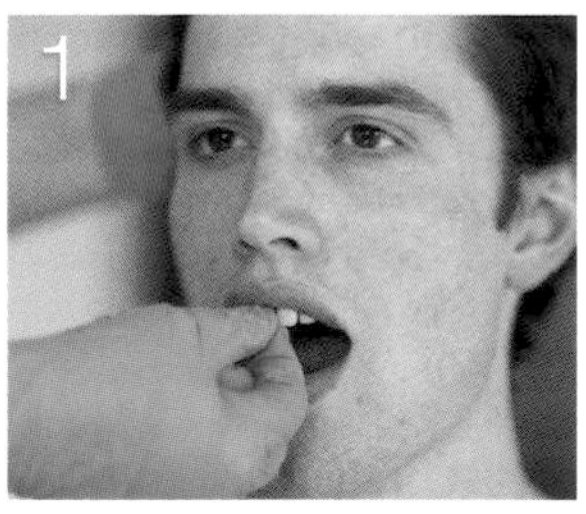

1 **Gently push the tooth into the socket. Then press a gauze pad between the bottom and top teeth to help keep the tooth in place.**

2 **Ask the casualty to hold the tooth firmly in place. Send him to a dentist or hospital.**

BLEEDING FROM THE MOUTH

YOUR AIMS

- To control bleeding.
- To safeguard the airway by preventing any inhalation of blood.

CAUTION

- If the wound is large, or bleeding lasts longer than 30 minutes or restarts, seek medical or dental advice.

Cuts to the tongue, lips or lining of the mouth range from trivial injuries to more serious wounds. The cause is usually the casualty's own teeth or dental extraction. Bleeding from the mouth may be profuse and can be alarming. In addition, there is a danger that blood may be inhaled into the lungs, causing problems with breathing.

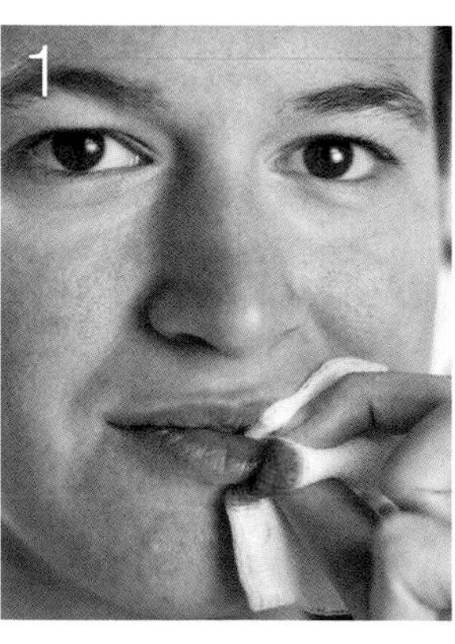

1 **Ask the casualty to sit down, with her head forwards and tilted slightly to the injured side, to allow blood to drain from her mouth. Place a sterile gauze pad over the wound. Ask the casualty to squeeze the pad between finger and thumb and press on the wound for ten minutes.**

2 **If bleeding persists, replace the pad. Tell the casualty to let the blood dribble out; if she swallows it, it may induce vomiting. Do not wash the mouth out because this may disturb a clot. Advise her to avoid drinking anything hot for 12 hours.**

SPECIAL CASE
BLEEDING SOCKET

To control bleeding from a tooth socket, roll a gauze pad thick enough to stop the casualty's teeth meeting, place it across the empty socket, and tell him to bite down on it.

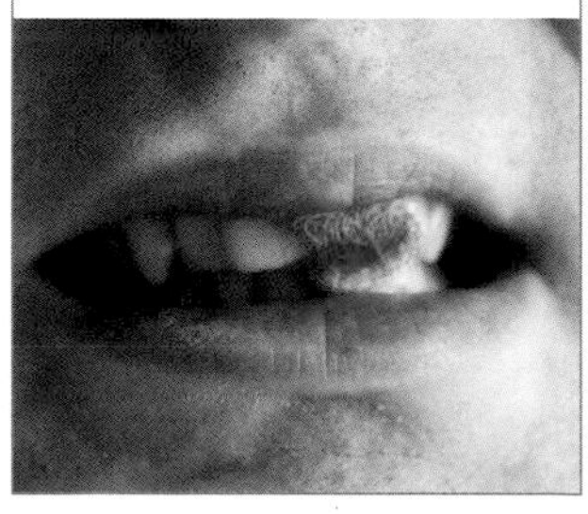

WOUND TO THE PALM

YOUR AIMS

- To control bleeding and the effects of shock.
- To minimise the risk of infection.
- To arrange transport to hospital.

See also
Foreign object in a wound **p.122**
Shock **pp.116–17**

The palm of the hand has a good blood supply, which is why a wound there may cause profuse bleeding. A deep wound to the palm may sever tendons and nerves in the hand and result in loss of feeling or movement in the fingers.

Bandaging the fist can be an effective way to control bleeding. If, however, a casualty has a foreign object embedded in a palm wound, it will be impossible to clench the fist. In such cases, treat the injury using the method described on p.122.

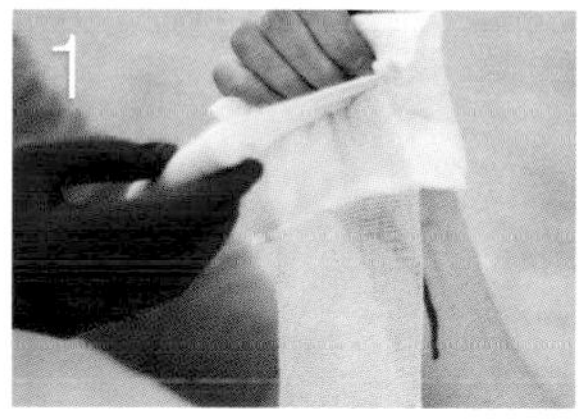

1 Press a sterile dressing or clean pad firmly into the palm, and ask the casualty to clench his fist over it or to grasp his fist with his other hand.

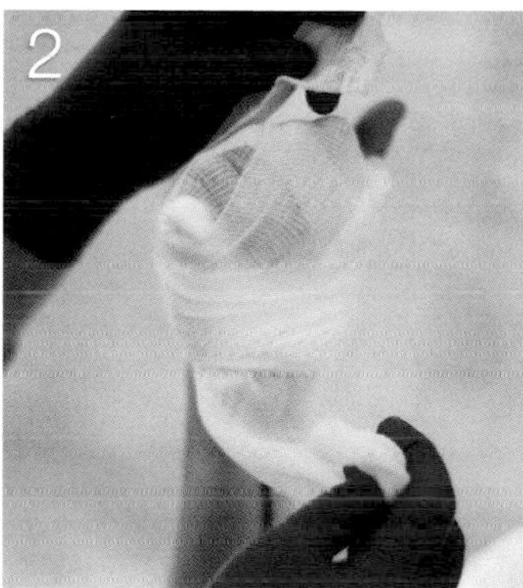

2 Raise and support the hand. Bandage the casualty's fingers so that they are clenched over the pad; leave the thumb free so that you can check circulation. Tie the ends of the bandage over the top of the fingers to help maintain pressure.

3 Support the arm in an elevation sling (p.252). Arrange to take or send him to hospital.

WOUND AT A JOINT CREASE

YOUR AIMS

- To control bleeding.
- To prevent and minimise the effects of shock.
- To arrange transport to hospital.

Large blood vessels pass across the inside of the elbow and back of the knee. If severed, these vessels will bleed profusely. The steps given below help to control bleeding and shock. However, this action also impedes the flow of blood to the lower part of the limb, so you must ensure adequate circulation to this area.

1 Press a sterile dressing or clean, non-fluffy pad on the injury. Bend the joint firmly to hold the pad in place and keep pressure on the wound.

2 Raise and support the limb. If possible, help the casualty to lie down with his legs raised and supported. Take or send the casualty to hospital.

3 Every ten minutes, check the circulation (p.243) in the lower part of the limb. If necessary, release the pressure on the wound briefly to restore normal blood flow, then reapply pressure.

ABDOMINAL WOUND

YOUR AIMS

- To minimise shock.
- To arrange urgent removal to hospital.

CAUTION

- Do not touch any protruding intestine. Cover the area with a clean plastic bag or kitchen film to prevent the intestine surface from drying out.
- If the casualty loses consciousness, open the airway and check breathing (The unconscious casualty pp.54–85). If he is breathing, support the abdomen as you put him in the recovery position. Do not allow the casualty to eat or drink because an anaesthetic may be needed.

See also
Shock **pp.116–17**

A stab wound, gunshot or crush injury to the abdomen may cause a serious wound. Organs and large blood vessels can be punctured, lacerated or ruptured. There may be external bleeding, protruding abdominal contents and internal injury and bleeding, so this is an emergency.

1 **Help the casualty to lie down on a firm surface, on a blanket if available. Loosen any tight clothing, such as a belt or a shirt.**

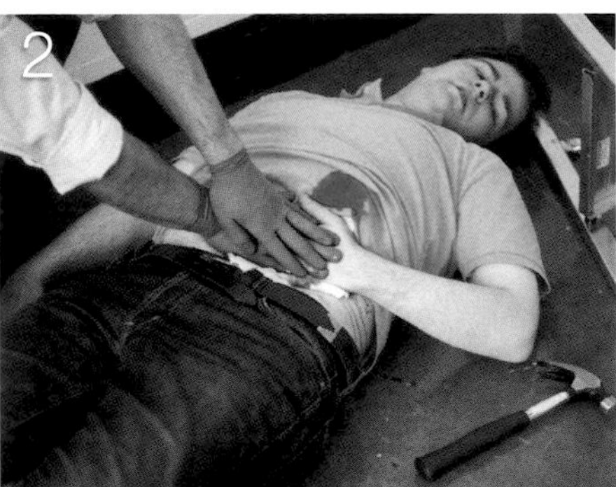

2 **Cover wound with a sterile dressing and hold it firmly; the casualty may be able to help. Raise and support the casualty's knees to ease strain on injury.**

3 **Call 999/112 for emergency help.** Treat the casualty for shock (pp.116–17). Monitor and record vital signs (pp.52–53) while waiting for help to arrive.

VAGINAL BLEEDING

YOUR AIMS

- To make the woman comfortable and reassure her.
- To arrange removal to hospital if necessary.

CAUTION

- If bleeding is severe, **call 999/112 for emergency help**.
- Treat for shock (pp.116–17). Monitor and record vital signs (pp.52–53) while waiting for help.

See also
Shock **pp.116–17**

Be sensitive to the woman's feelings. The bleeding is most likely to be menstrual bleeding, but it can also indicate a more serious condition such as miscarriage, pregnancy, recent termination of pregnancy, childbirth or injury as a result of sexual assault. If the bleeding is severe, shock may develop.

If a woman has been sexually assaulted, it is vital to preserve the evidence if possible. Gently advise her to refrain from washing or using the toilet until a forensic examination has been performed. If she wishes to remove clothing, keep it intact in a clean plastic bag if possible. Be aware that she may feel vulnerable and will prefer to be treated by a woman.

1 **Allow the woman privacy and give her a sanitary towel. Make her as comfortable as possible in whichever position she prefers.**

2 **If she has period pains, she may take the recommended dose of paracetamol or her own painkillers.**

BLEEDING VARICOSE VEIN

YOUR AIMS

- To control bleeding.
- To minimise shock.
- To arrange urgent removal to hospital.

See also
Shock **pp.116–17**

Veins contain one-way valves that keep the blood flowing towards the heart. If these valves fail, blood collects (pools) behind them and makes the veins swell. This problem, called varicose veins, usually develops in the legs.

A varicose vein has taut, thin walls and is often raised, typically producing knobbly skin over the affected area. The vein can be burst by a gentle knock, and this may result in profuse bleeding. Shock will quickly develop if bleeding is not controlled.

1 Help the casualty to lie down on his back. Raise and support the injured leg as high as possible to immediately reduce the amount of bleeding.

2 Rest the injured leg on your shoulder or on a chair. Apply firm, direct pressure on the injury, using a sterile dressing, or a clean, non-fluffy pad, until the blood loss is under control. If necessary, carefully cut away clothing to expose the site of the bleeding.

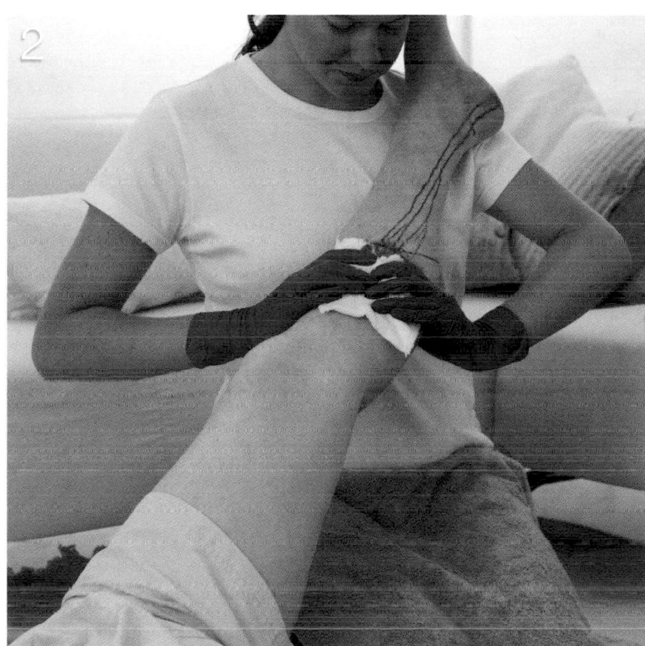

3 Remove garments such as garters or elastic-topped stockings because these may cause the bleeding to continue.

4 Keeping the leg raised, put another large, soft pad over the dressing. Bandage it firmly enough to exert even pressure, but not so tightly that the circulation in the limb is impaired.

5 **Call 999/112 for emergency help.** Keep the injured leg raised and supported until the ambulance arrives. Monitor and record vital signs – level of response, breathing and pulse (pp.52–53) – regularly until help arrives. In addition, check the circulation in the limb beyond the bandage (p.243) every ten minutes.

7

The skeleton is the supporting framework around which the body is constructed. It is jointed in many places, and muscles attached to the bones enable us to move. Most of our movements are controlled at will and coordinated by impulses that travel from the brain via the nerves to every muscle and joint in the body.

It is difficult for a first aider to distinguish between different bone, joint and muscle injuries, so this chapter begins with an overview of how bones, muscles and joints function and how damage occurs. First aid treatments for most injuries, from serious fractures to sprains, strains and dislocations, are included here in this section. First aid for head and spinal injuries is covered in the chapter that deals with the nervous system (pp.160–75) because of the potential damage these injuries can have on the brain and spinal cord.

AIMS AND OBJECTIVES

- To assess the casualty's condition quickly and calmly.
- To steady and support the injured part of the body.
- To minimise shock.
- To call 999/112 for emergency help if you suspect a serious injury.
- To comfort and reassure the casualty.
- To be aware of your own needs.

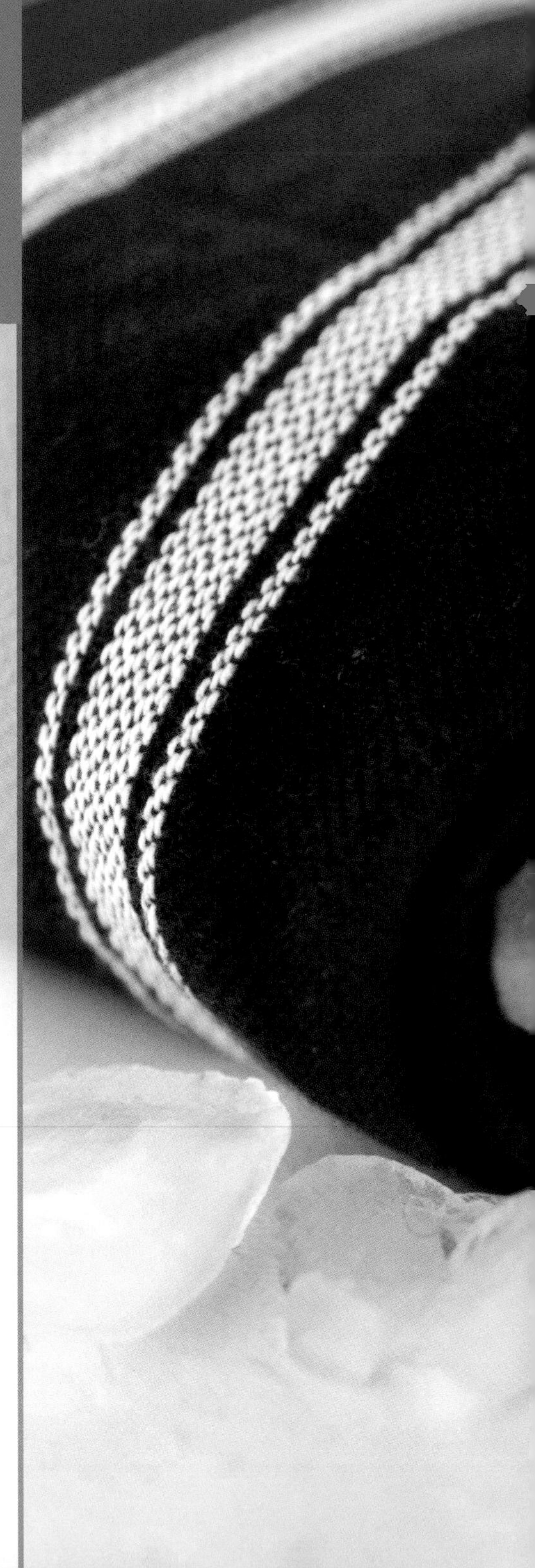

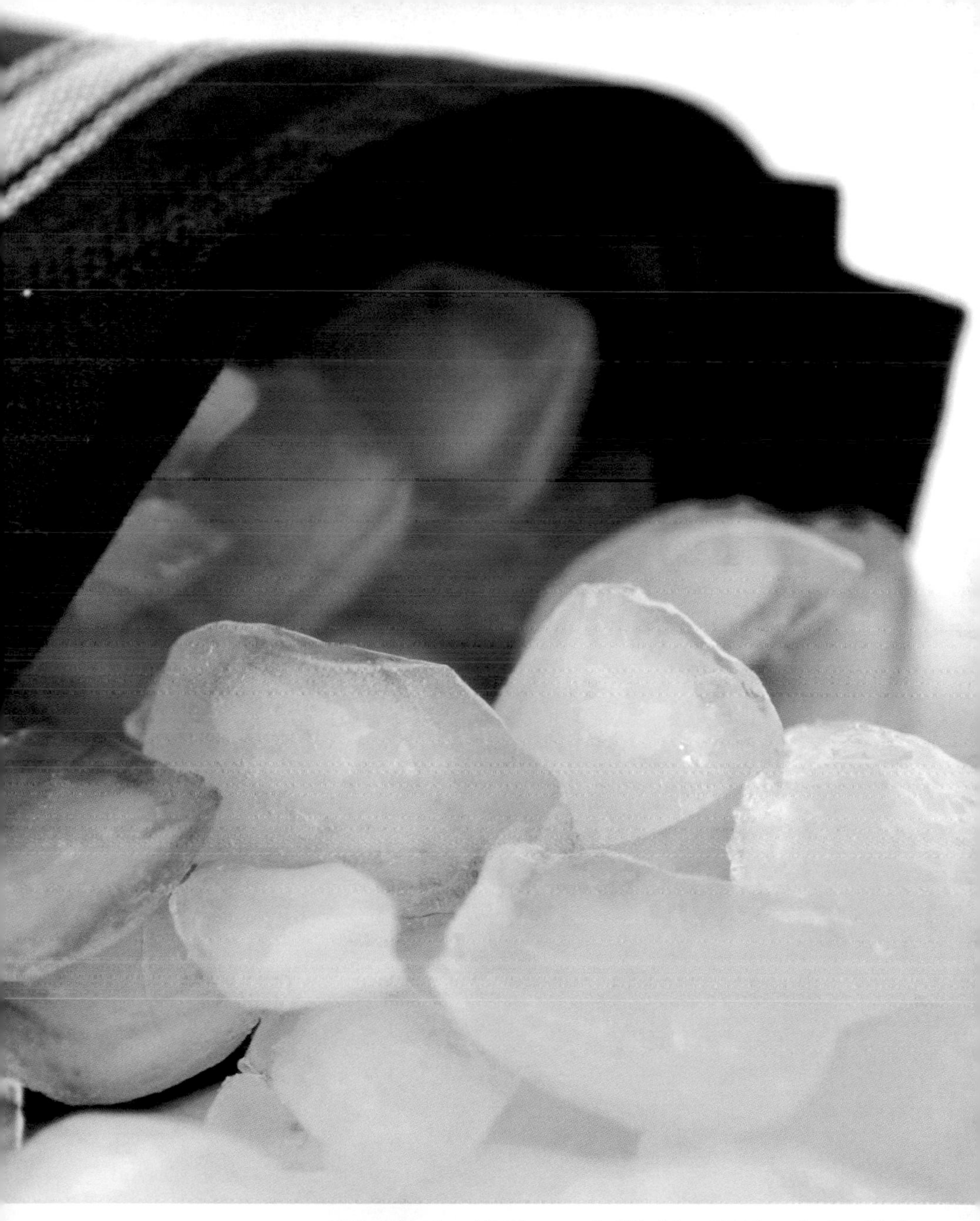

BONE, JOINT AND MUSCLE INJURIES

THE SKELETON

The body is built on a framework of bones called the skeleton. This structure supports the muscles, blood vessels and nerves of the body. Many bones of the skeleton also protect important organs such as the brain and heart. At many points on the skeleton, bones articulate with each other by means of joints. These are supported by ligaments and moved by muscles that are attached to the bones by tendons.

The skeleton
There are 206 bones in the skeleton, providing a protective framework for the body. The skull, spine and ribcage protect vital body structures; the pelvis supports the abdominal organs; and the bones and joints of the arms and legs enable the body to move.

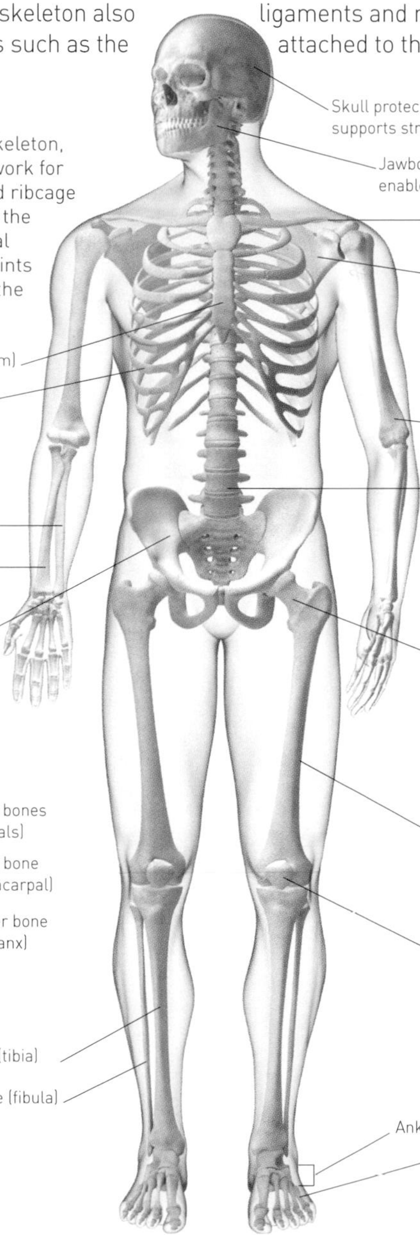

Skull protects brain and supports structures of face
Jawbone (mandible) is hinged and enables mouth to open and close
Collar bone (clavicle)
Shoulder blade (scapula)
Collar bones and shoulder blades form shoulder girdle, to which arms are attached
Breastbone (sternum)
Twelve pairs of ribs form ribcage, which protects vital organs in chest and moves with lungs during breathing
Upper arm bone (humerus)
Forearm bones
Ulna
Radius
Spine, which is formed from 33 bones (vertebrae), protects spinal cord and enables back to move
Pelvis is attached to lower part of spine and protects lower abdominal organs
Hip joint is point at which leg bones are connected to pelvis
Scaphoid
Wrist bones (carpals)
Hand bone (metacarpal)
Finger bone (phalanx)
BONES OF THE HAND
Thigh bone (femur)
Kneecap (patella)
Lower leg bones
Shin bone (tibia)
Splint bone (fibula)
Ankle bones (tarsals)
Foot bones (metatarsals)

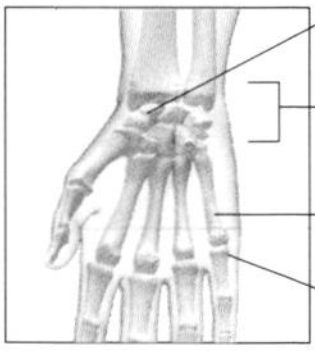

THE SPINE

Also known as the backbone, the spine has a number of functions. It supports the head, makes the upper body flexible, helps to support the body's weight and protects the spinal cord (p.171). The spine is a column made up of 33 bones called vertebrae, which are connected by joints.

Between individual vertebrae are discs of fibrous tissue, called intervertebral discs, which help to make the spine flexible and cushion it from jolts. Muscles and ligaments attached to the vertebrae help to stabilise the spine and control the movements of the back.

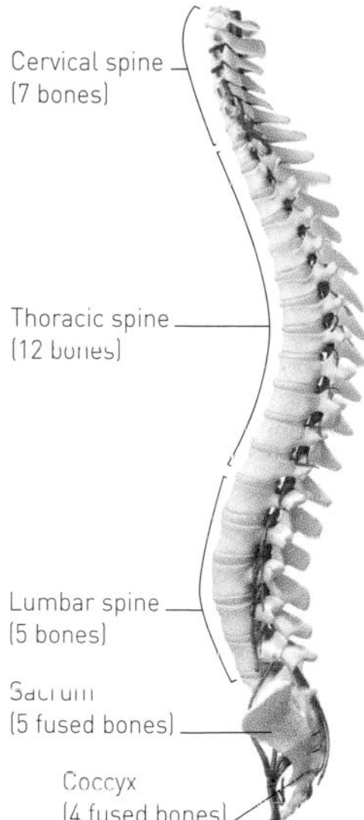

Spinal column
The vertebrae form five groups: the cervical vertebrae support the head and neck; the thoracic vertebrae form an anchor for the ribs; the lumbar vertebrae help to support the body's weight and give stability; the sacrum supports the pelvis; and the coccyx forms the end of the spine.

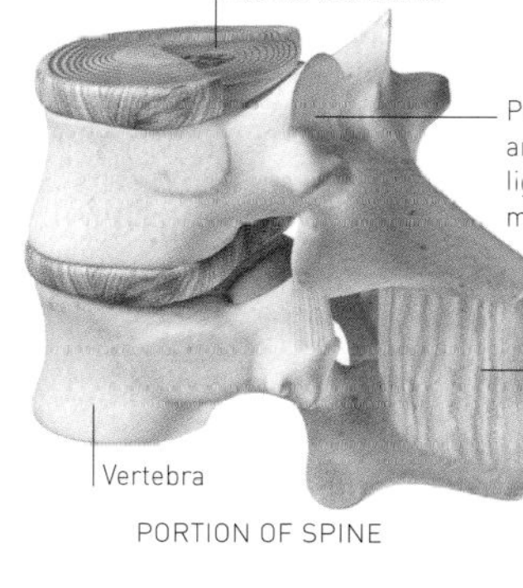

PORTION OF SPINE

Structures that make the spine flexible
The joints connecting the vertebrae, and the discs between the vertebrae, allow the spine to move. There is only limited movement between adjacent vertebrae, but together the vertebrae, discs and ligaments allow a range of movements in the spine as a whole.

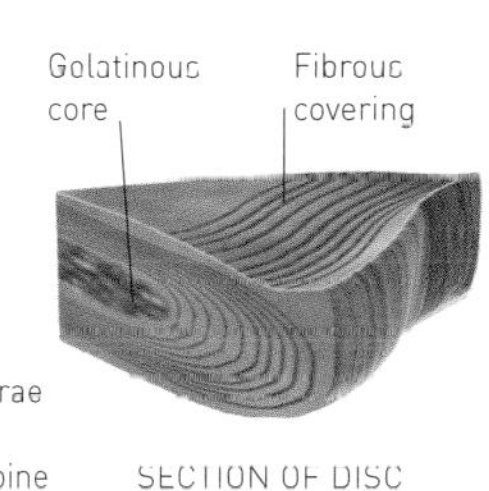

SECTION OF DISC

THE SKULL

This bony structure protects the brain and the top of the spinal cord. It also supports the eyes and other facial structures. The skull is made up of several bones, most of which are fused at joints called sutures. Within the bone are air spaces (sinuses), which lighten the skull. The bones covering the brain form a dome called the cranium. Several other bones form the eye sockets, nose, cheeks and jaw.

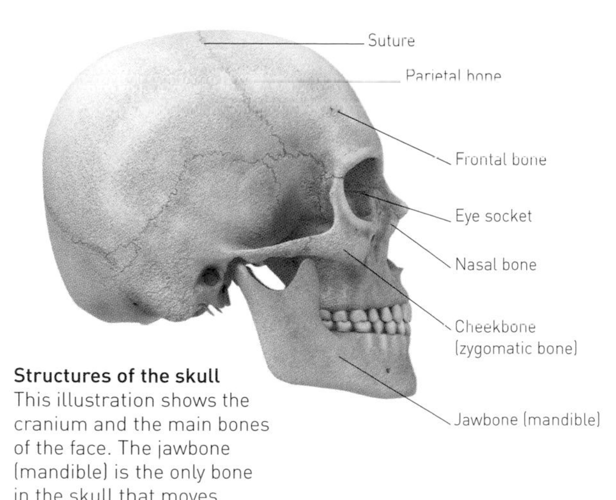

Structures of the skull
This illustration shows the cranium and the main bones of the face. The jawbone (mandible) is the only bone in the skull that moves.

BONES, MUSCLES AND JOINTS

THE BONES

Bone is a living tissue containing calcium and phosphorus; minerals that make it hard, rigid and strong. From birth to early adulthood, bones grow by laying down calcium on the outside. They are also able to generate new tissue after injury. Age and certain diseases can weaken bones, making them brittle and susceptible to breaking or crumbling, either under stress or spontaneously. Inherited problems, or bone disorders such as rickets, cancer and infections, can cause bones to become distorted and weakened. Damage to the bones during adolescence can shorten a bone or impair movement. In older people, a disorder called osteoporosis can cause the bones to lose density, making them brittle and prone to breaking.

Parts of a bone
Each bone is covered by a membrane (periosteum), which contains nerves and blood vessels. Under this membrane is a layer of compact, dense bone; at the core is spongy bone. In some bones, there is a cavity at the centre containing soft tissue called bone marrow.

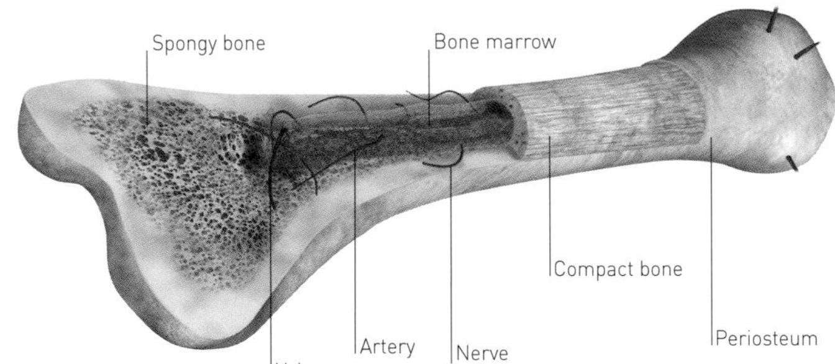

THE MUSCLES

Muscles cause various parts of the body to move. Skeletal (voluntary) muscles control movement and posture. They are attached to bones by bands of strong, fibrous tissue (tendons), and many operate in groups. As one group of muscles contracts, its paired group relaxes.

Involuntary muscles operate the internal organs, such as the heart, and work constantly, even while we are asleep. They are controlled by the autonomic nervous system (p.163).

Straightening the arm
The triceps muscle, at the back of the upper arm, shortens (contracts) to pull down the bones of the forearm. The biceps muscle, at the front of the arm, relaxes.

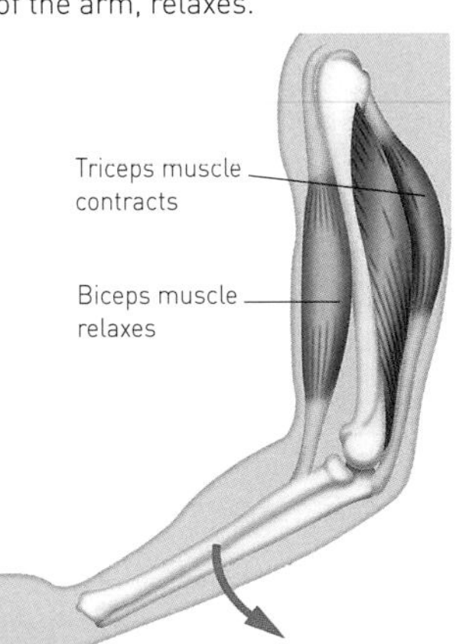

Bending the arm
The biceps muscle, at the front of the arm, shortens (contracts), pulling the bones of the forearm upwards to bend the arm. At the same time, the triceps muscle relaxes and lengthens.

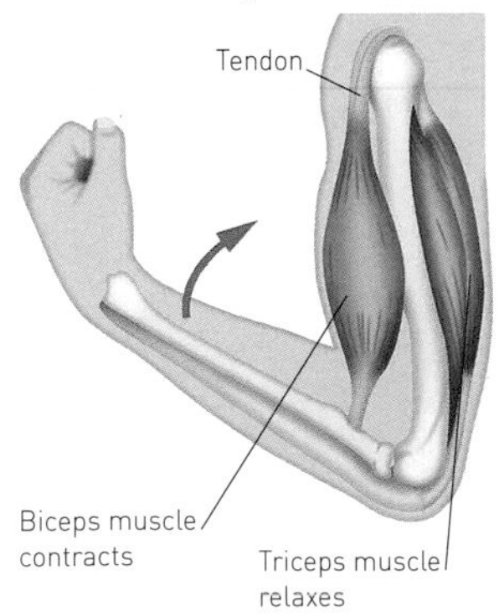

THE JOINTS

A joint is where one bone meets another. In a few joints (immovable joints), the bone edges fit together or are fused. Immovable joints are found in the skull and pelvis. Most joints are movable, and the bone ends are joined by fibrous tissue called ligaments, which form a capsule around the joint. The capsule lining (synovial membrane) produces fluid to lubricate the joint; the ends of the bones are also protected by smooth cartilage. Muscles that move the joint are attached to the bones by tendons. The degree and type of movement depends on the way the ends of the bones fit together, the strength of the ligaments and the arrangement of muscles.

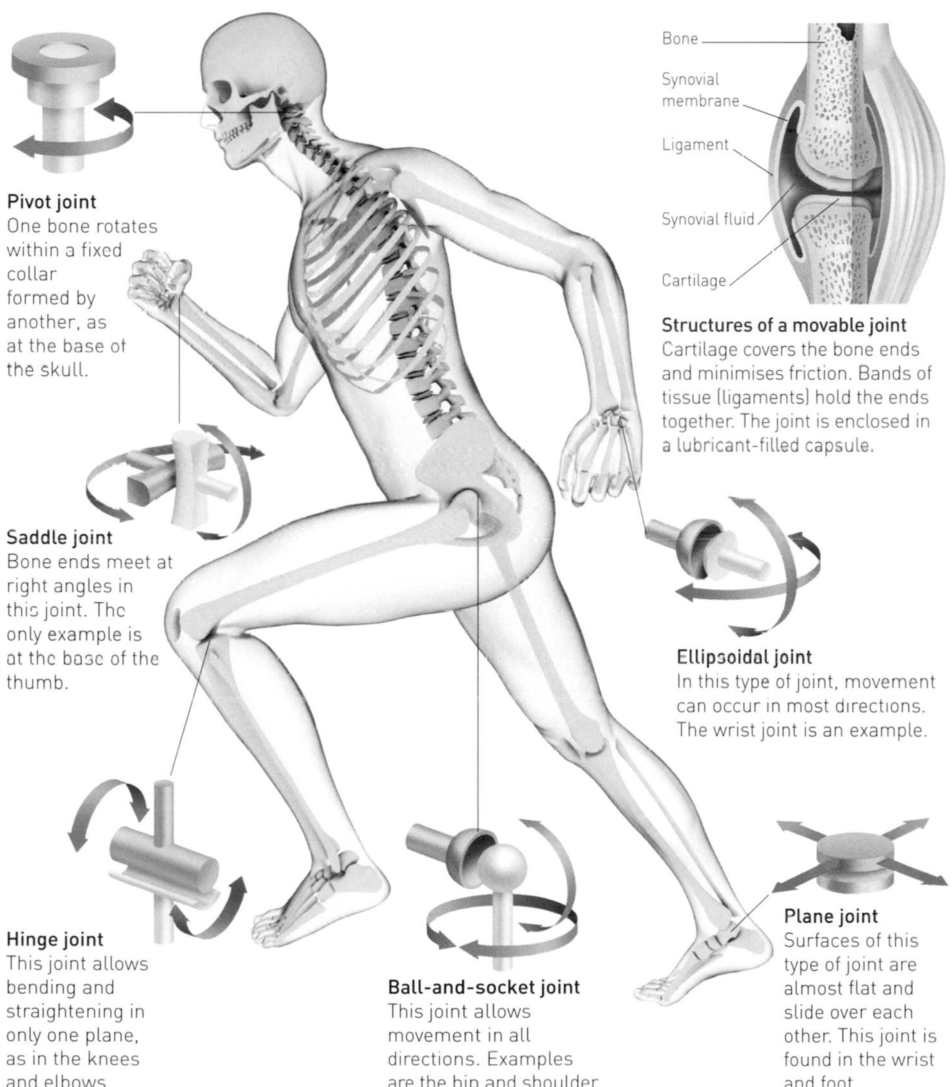

Structures of a movable joint
Cartilage covers the bone ends and minimises friction. Bands of tissue (ligaments) hold the ends together. The joint is enclosed in a lubricant-filled capsule.

Pivot joint
One bone rotates within a fixed collar formed by another, as at the base of the skull.

Saddle joint
Bone ends meet at right angles in this joint. The only example is at the base of the thumb.

Ellipsoidal joint
In this type of joint, movement can occur in most directions. The wrist joint is an example.

Hinge joint
This joint allows bending and straightening in only one plane, as in the knees and elbows.

Ball-and-socket joint
This joint allows movement in all directions. Examples are the hip and shoulder.

Plane joint
Surfaces of this type of joint are almost flat and slide over each other. This joint is found in the wrist and foot.

FRACTURES

RECOGNITION

There may be:
- Deformity, swelling and bruising at the fracture site;
- Pain and/or difficulty in moving the area;
- Shortening, bending or twisting of a limb;
- Coarse grating (crepitus) of the bone ends that can be heard or felt (by casualty). Do not try to seek this;
- Signs of shock, especially if the thigh bone or pelvis are fractured;
- Difficulty in moving a limb normally or at all (for example, inability to walk);
- A wound, possibly with bone ends protruding (Treating an open fracture p.138).

See also
Crush injury p.119
Internal bleeding p.113
Shock pp.116–17

A break or crack in a bone is called a fracture. Considerable force is needed to break a bone, unless it is diseased or old. However, bones that are still growing are supple and may split, bend or crack like a twig. A bone may break at the point where a heavy blow is received. Fractures may also result from a twist or a wrench (indirect force).

OPEN AND CLOSED FRACTURES

In an open fracture, one of the broken bone ends may pierce the skin surface, or there may be a wound at the fracture site. An open fracture carries a high risk of becoming infected.

In a closed fracture, the skin above the fracture is intact. However, bones may be displaced (unstable) causing internal bleeding and the casualty may develop shock (pp.116–17).

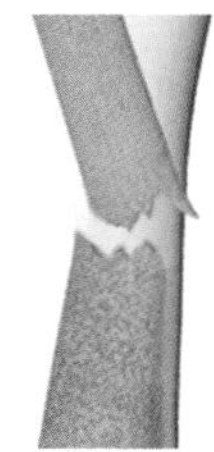

Open fracture
Bone is exposed at the surface where it breaks the skin. The casualty may suffer bleeding and shock. Infection is a risk.

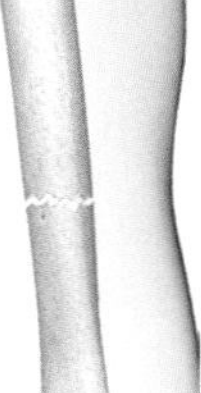

Closed fracture
The skin is not broken, although the bone ends may damage nearby tissues and blood vessels. Internal bleeding is a risk.

STABLE AND UNSTABLE FRACTURES

A stable fracture occurs when the broken bone ends do not move because they are not completely broken or they are impacted. Such injuries are common at the wrist, shoulder, ankle and hip. Usually, these fractures can be gently handled without further damage.

In an unstable fracture, the broken bone ends can easily move. There is a risk that they may damage blood vessels, nerves and organs around the injury. Unstable injuries can occur if the bone is broken or the ligaments are torn (ruptured). They should be handled carefully to prevent further damage.

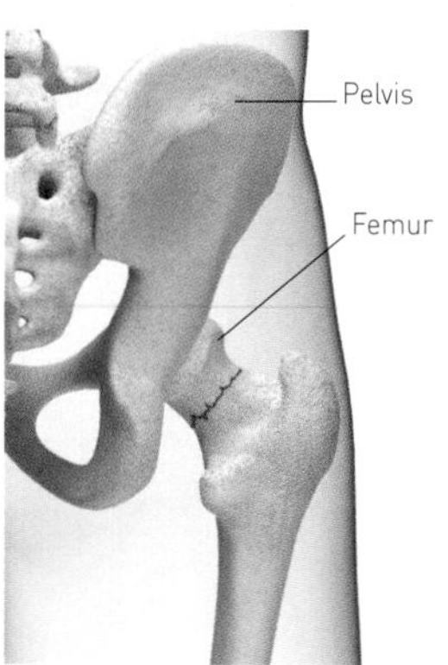

Stable fracture
Although the bone is fractured, the ends of the injury remain in place. The risk of bleeding or further damage is minimal.

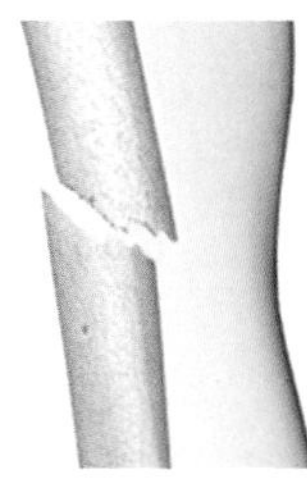

Unstable fracture
In this type of fracture, the broken bone ends can easily be displaced by movement or muscle contraction.

TREATING A CLOSED FRACTURE

YOUR AIMS

- To prevent movement at the injury site.
- To arrange removal to hospital, with comfortable support during transport.

CAUTION

- Do not move the casualty until the injured part is secured and supported, unless she is in immediate danger.
- Do not allow the casualty to eat or drink because an anaesthetic may be needed.

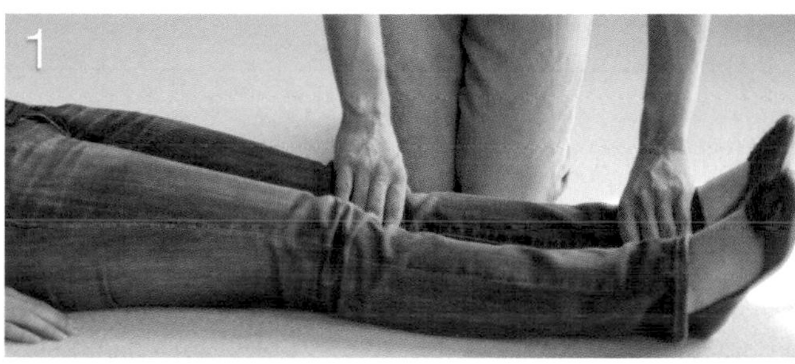

1 Advise the casualty to keep still. Support the joints above and below the injured area with your hands, or ask a helper to do this, until it is immobilized with a sling or bandages.

2 Place padding around the injury for extra support. Take or send the casualty to hospital; an arm injury may be transported by car; **call 999/112 for emergency help** for a leg injury.

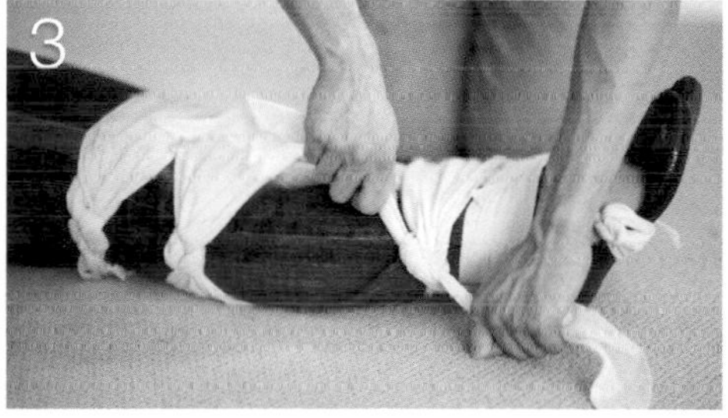

3 For firmer support and/or if removal to hospital is likely to be delayed, secure the injured part to an unaffected part of the body. For upper limb fractures, immobilise the arm with a sling (pp.251–52). For lower limb fractures, move the uninjured leg to the injured one and secure with broad-fold bandages (p.249). Always tie the knots on the uninjured side.

4 Treat for shock if necessary (pp.116–17) . Do not raise an injured leg. Elevate an uninjured limb if shock is present. Monitor and record vital signs (pp.52–53) while waiting for help. Check the circulation beyond a sling or bandage (p.243) every ten minutes. If the circulation is impaired, loosen the bandages.

SPECIAL CASE REALIGNING A LIMB

If a fractured limb is bent and you need to immobilise it because removal to hospital will be delayed, it may be gently realigned to restore it to a suitable position.

Pull gently in the line of the bone until the limb is straight. Pull only in a straight line and maintain in this position until the limb is immobilised with bandages. Stop immediately if your action increases the casualty's pain.

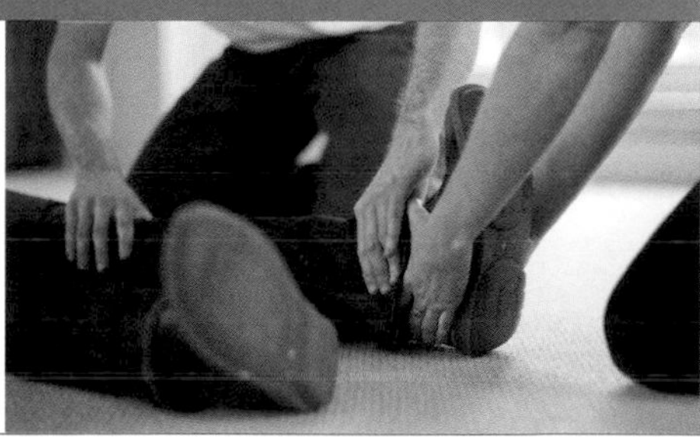

FRACTURES (continued)

TREATING AN OPEN FRACTURE

YOUR AIMS

- To prevent blood loss, movement and infection at the site of injury.
- To arrange removal to hospital, with comfortable support during transport.

CAUTION

- Do not move the casualty until the injured part is secured and supported, unless he is in immediate danger.
- Do not allow the casualty to eat or drink because an anaesthetic may be needed.
- Do not press directly on a protruding bone end.

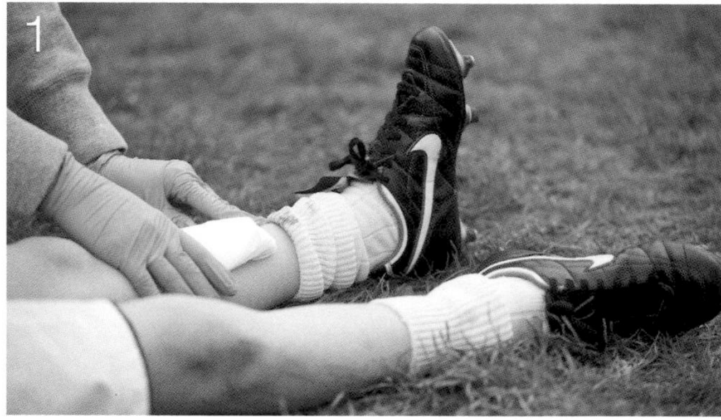

1 Cover the wound with a sterile dressing or large, clean, non-fluffy pad. Apply pressure around the injury to control bleeding (pp.114–15); be careful not to press on a protruding bone.

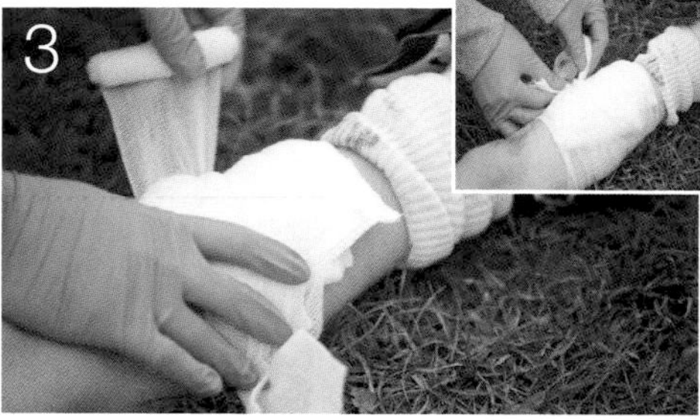

2 Carefully place a sterile wound dressing or more clean padding over and around the dressing.

3 Secure the dressing and padding with a bandage. Bandage firmly, but not so tightly that it impairs the circulation beyond the bandage.

4 Immobilise the injured part as for a closed fracture (p.137), and arrange to transport the casualty to hospital.

5 Treat the casualty for shock (pp.116–17) if necessary. Do not raise the injured leg. Monitor and record vital signs – level of response, breathing and pulse (pp.52–53) – while waiting for help to arrive. Check the circulation beyond the bandage (p.243) every ten minutes. If the circulation is impaired, loosen the bandages.

SPECIAL CASE PROTRUDING BONE

If a bone end is protruding, build up pads of clean, soft, non-fluffy material around the bone, until you can bandage over it without pressing on the injury.

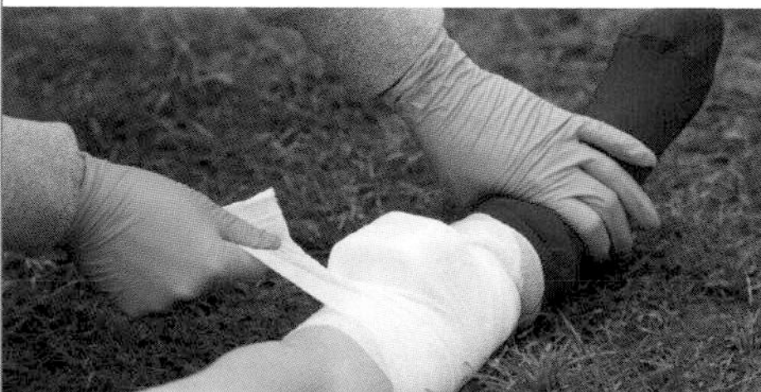

DISLOCATED JOINT

RECOGNITION

There may be:

- "Sickening", severe pain;
- Inability to move the joint;
- Swelling and bruising around the affected joint;
- Shortening, bending or deformity of the area.

YOUR AIMS

- To prevent movement at the injury site.
- To arrange removal to hospital, with comfortable support during transport.

CAUTION

- Do not try to replace a dislocated bone into its socket as this may cause further injury.
- Do not move the casualty until the injured part is secured and supported, unless she is in immediate danger.
- For a hand or arm injury remove bracelets, rings and watches in case of swelling.
- Do not allow the casualty to eat or drink because an anaesthetic may be needed.

See also
Fractures **pp.136–37**
Shock **pp.116–17**
Strains and sprains **pp.140–41**

This is a joint injury in which the bones are partially or completely pulled out of their normal position. Dislocation can be caused by a strong force wrenching the bone into an abnormal position, or by violent muscle contraction. This very painful injury most often affects the shoulder, knee, jaw or joints in the thumbs or fingers. Dislocations may be associated with torn ligaments (pp.140–41), or with damage to the synovial membrane that lines the joint capsule (p.135).

Joint dislocation can have serious consequences. If vertebrae are dislocated, the spinal cord can be damaged. Dislocation of the shoulder or hip may damage the large nerves that supply the limbs and result in paralysis. A dislocation of any joint may also fracture the bones involved. It is difficult to distinguish a dislocation from a closed fracture (p.136). If you are in any doubt, treat the injury as a fracture.

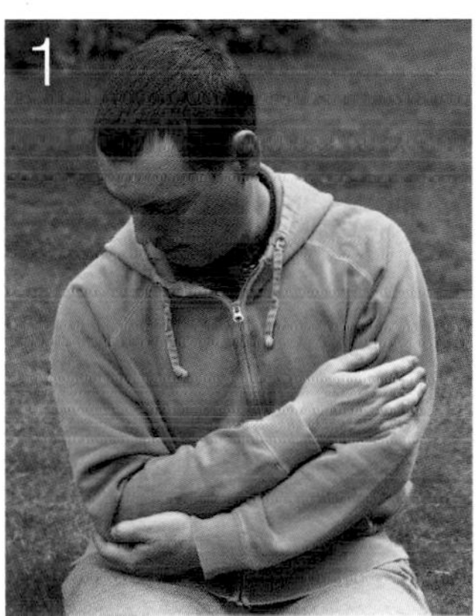

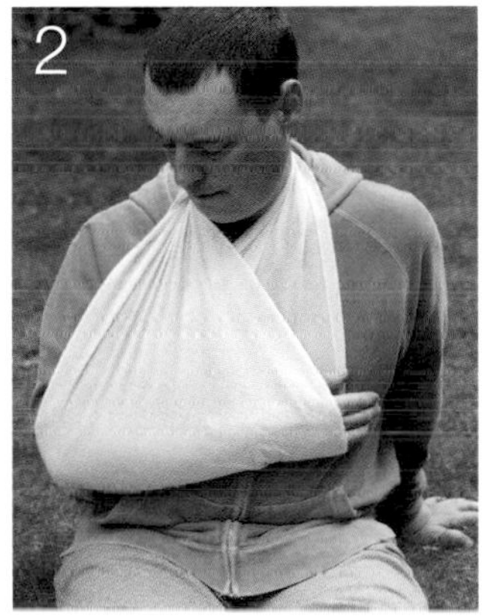

1 If, for example, the casualty has a dislocated shoulder, advise the casualty to keep still. Help him to support the injured arm in the position he finds most comfortable.

2 Immobilise the injured arm with a sling (p.251) or use padding and/or broad-fold bandages (p.249) for a leg injury, whichever is most comfortable.

3 For extra support for an injured arm, secure the limb to the chest by tying a broad-fold bandage (p.249) right around the chest and the sling.

4 Arrange to take or send the casualty to hospital. Treat for shock if necessary. Monitor and record vital signs (pp.52–53) while waiting for help to arrive.

5 Check the circulation beyond the bandages (p.243) every ten minutes.

STRAINS AND SPRAINS

The softer structures around bones and joints – the ligaments, muscles and tendons – can be injured in several ways. Injuries to these soft tissues are commonly called strains and sprains. They occur when the tissues are overstretched and partially or completely torn (ruptured) by violent or sudden movements. For this reason, strains and sprains are frequently associated with sporting activities.

Strains and sprains should be treated initially by the "RICE" procedure:

R – Rest the injured part;
I – Apply Ice pack or a cold pad;
C – Provide Comfortable support;
E – Elevate the injured part.

This procedure may be sufficient to relieve the symptoms, but if you are in any doubt as to the severity of the injury, treat it as a fracture (pp.136–37).

MUSCLE AND TENDON INJURY

Muscles and tendons may be strained, ruptured or bruised. A strain occurs when the muscle is overstretched; it may be partially torn, often at the junction between the muscle and the tendon that joins it to a bone. In a rupture, a muscle or tendon is torn completely; this may occur in the main bulk of the muscle or in the tendon. Deep bruising can be extensive in parts of the body where there is a large bulk of muscle. Injuries in these areas are usually accompanied by bleeding into the surrounding tissues, which can lead to pain, swelling and bruising.

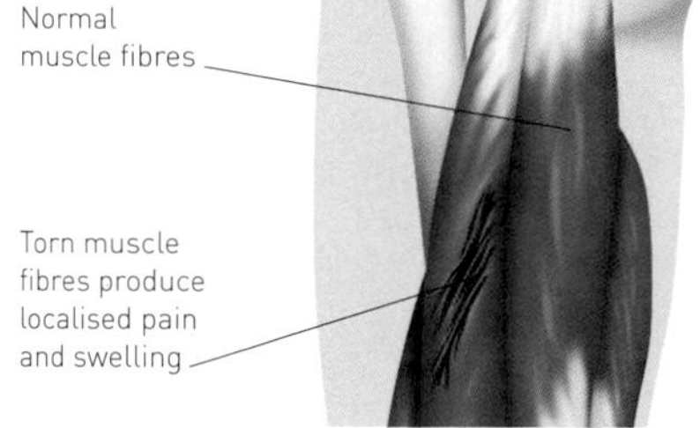

Muscle tears
Vigorous movements may cause muscle fibres, such as the hamstring in the leg, to tear. Muscle tears can cause severe pain and swelling.

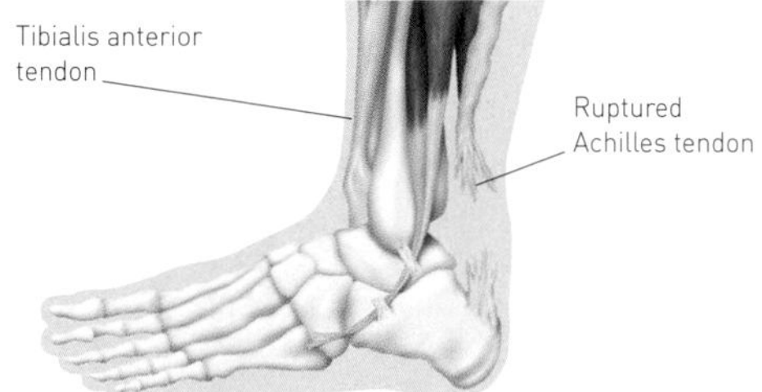

Ruptured tendon
The Achilles heel tendon attaches the calf muscle to the heel bone. It can snap after sudden exertion and may need surgery and immobilisation.

LIGAMENT INJURY

One common form of ligament injury is a sprain. This is the tearing of a ligament at or near a joint. It is often due to a sudden or unexpected wrenching motion that pulls the bones in the joint too far apart and tears the surrounding tissues.

Fibula
Sprained ligament
Heel bone

Sprained ankle
This is due to overstretching or tearing of a ligament – the fibrous cords that connect bones at a joint. In this example, one of the ligaments in the ankle is partially torn.

RECOGNITION

There may be:

- Pain and tenderness;
- Difficulty in moving the injured part, especially if it is a joint;
- Swelling and bruising in the area.

YOUR AIMS

- To reduce swelling and pain.
- To obtain medical help if necessary.

See also
Cold compresses **p.241**
Fractures **pp.136–37**

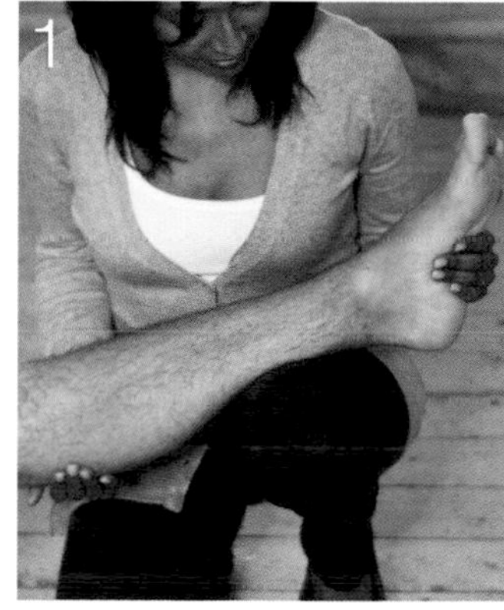

1 Help the casualty to sit or lie down. Support the injured part in a comfortable position, preferably raised.

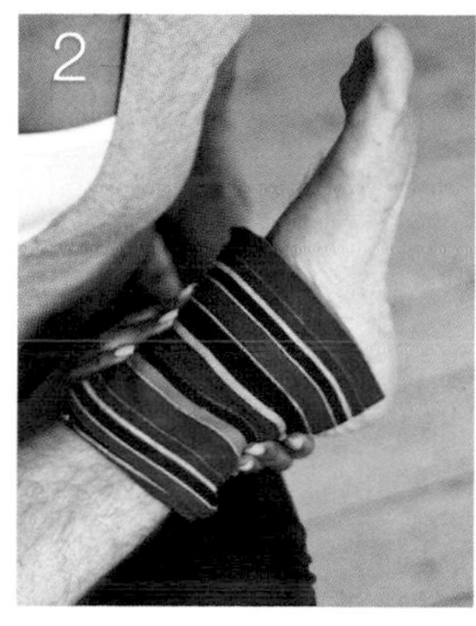

2 Cool the area by applying a cold compress, such as an ice pack or cold pad (p.241), to the injury. This helps to reduce swelling, bruising and pain.

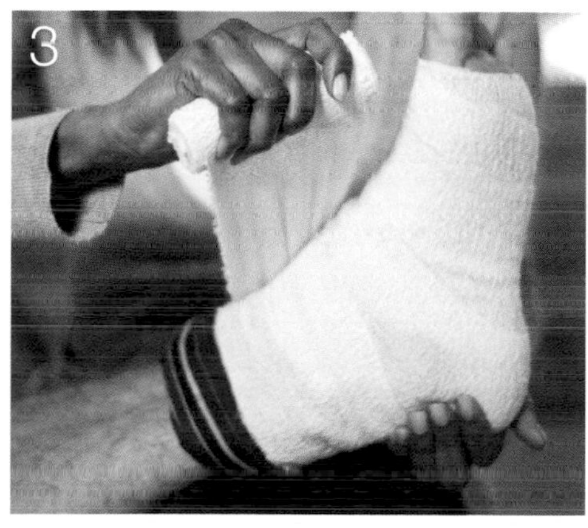

3 Apply comfortable support to the injured part. Leave the cold compress in place or wrap a layer of soft padding, such as cotton wool, around the area. Secure it with a support bandage that extends to the next joint; for an ankle injury, the bandage should extend from the base of the toes to the knees.

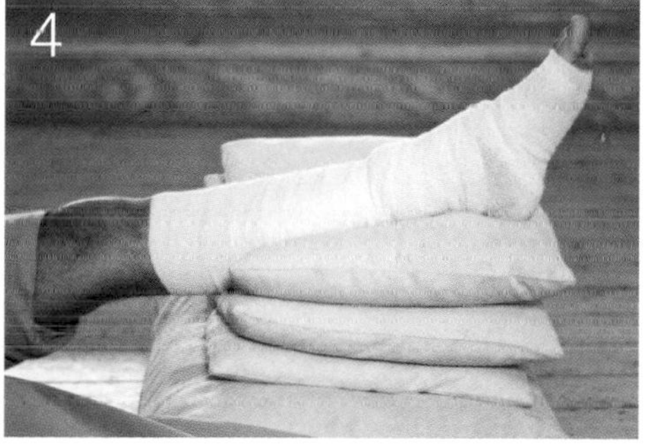

4 Support the injured part in a raised position to help minimise bruising and swelling in the area. Check the circulation beyond the bandages (p.243) every ten minutes. If the circulation is impaired, loosen the bandages.

5 If the pain is severe, or the casualty is unable to use the injured part, arrange to take or send him to hospital. Otherwise, advise the casualty to rest the injury and to seek medical advice if necessary.

FACIAL INJURY

RECOGNITION

There may be:

- Pain around affected area; if the jaw is affected, difficulty speaking, chewing or swallowing;
- Difficulty breathing;
- Swelling and distortion of the face;
- Bruising and/or a black eye;
- Clear fluid or watery blood from the nose or ear.

YOUR AIMS

- To keep the airway open.
- To minimise pain and swelling.
- To arrange urgent removal to hospital.

CAUTION

- Never place a bandage around the lower part of the face or lower jaw in case the casualty vomits or has difficulty breathing.
- Do not allow the casualty to eat or drink because an anaesthetic may be needed.
- If the casualty loses consciousness, open the airway and check breathing (The unconscious casualty pp.54–85).
- If an unconscious casualty is breathing, place him in the recovery position (pp.64–65) with his injured side downwards so that blood or other body fluids can drain away. Place soft padding under his head. Be aware of the risk of neck (spinal) injury.

Fractures of facial bones are usually due to hard impacts. Serious facial fractures may appear frightening. There may be distortion of the eye sockets, general swelling and bruising, as well as bleeding from displaced tissues or from the nose and mouth. The main danger with any facial fracture is that blood, saliva or swollen tissue may obstruct the airway and cause breathing difficulties.

When you are examining a casualty with a facial injury, assume that there is damage to the skull, brain or neck. There is also a danger that you may misinterpret the symptoms of a facial fracture as a black eye.

See also
Head injury **p.165**
Knocked-out adult tooth **p.126**
Shock **pp.116–17**
Spinal injury **pp.171–73**
The unconscious casualty **pp.54–85**

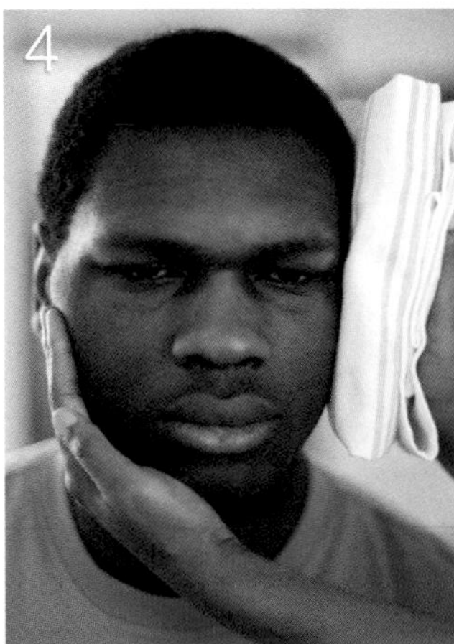

1 **Call 999/112 for emergency help.**

2 Help the casualty to sit down and make sure the airway is open and clear.

3 Ask the casualty to spit out any blood, displaced teeth or dentures from his mouth. Keep any teeth to send to hospital with him.

4 Gently place a cold compress (p.241) against the casualty's face to help reduce pain and minimise swelling. Treat for shock (pp.116–17) if necessary.

5 Monitor and record vital signs – level of response, breathing and pulse (pp.52–53) – while waiting for help to arrive.

CHEEKBONE AND NOSE INJURY

RECOGNITION

There may be:

- Pain, swelling and bruising;
- Obvious wound or bleeding from the nose or mouth.

YOUR AIMS

- To minimise pain and swelling.
- To arrange transport to hospital.

CAUTION

- If there is clear fluid or watery blood leaking from the casualty's nose, treat the casualty as for a head injury (p.165).
- Do not allow the casualty to eat or drink because an anaesthetic may be needed.

Fractures of the cheekbone and nose are usually the result of direct blows to the face. Swollen facial tissues are likely to cause discomfort, and the air passages in the nose may become blocked, making breathing difficult. These injuries should always be examined in hospital.

See also
Head injury **p.165**
Nosebleed **p.125**

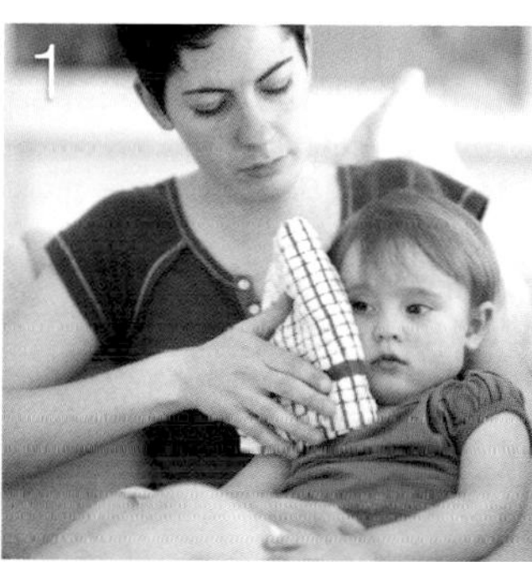

1 **Gently place a cold compress, such as a cold pad or ice pack (p.241), against the injured area to help reduce pain and minimise swelling.**

2 **If the casualty has a nosebleed, try to pinch the nose to stop the bleeding (p.125). Arrange to take or send the casualty to hospital.**

LOWER JAW INJURY

RECOGNITION

There may be:

- Difficulty speaking, swallowing and moving the jaw;
- Pain and nausea when moving the jaw;
- Displaced or loose teeth and dribbling;
- Swelling and bruising inside and outside the mouth.

YOUR AIMS

- To protect the airway.
- To arrange transport to hospital.

See also
Facial injury **opposite**
Head injury **p.165**
Knocked-out adult tooth **p.126**

Jaw fractures are usually the result of direct force, such as a heavy blow to the chin. In some situations, a blow to one side of the jaw produces indirect force, which causes a fracture on the other side of the face. A fall on to the point of the chin can fracture the jaw on both sides. The lower jaw may also be dislocated by a blow to the face, or is sometimes dislocated by yawning.

If the face is seriously injured, with the jaw fractured in more than one place, treat as for a facial injury (opposite).

1 **If the casualty is not seriously injured, help him to sit with his head forward to allow fluids to drain from his mouth. Encourage the casualty to spit out loose teeth, and keep them to send to hospital with him.**

2 **Give the casualty a soft pad to hold firmly against his jaw in order to support it.**

3 **Arrange to take or send the casualty to hospital. Keep his jaw supported throughout.**

UPPER ARM INJURY

RECOGNITION

There may be:

- Pain, increased by movement;
- Tenderness and deformity over the site of a fracture;
- Rapid swelling;
- Bruising, which may develop more slowly.

YOUR AIMS

- To immobilise the arm.
- To arrange transport to hospital.

CAUTION

- Do not allow the casualty to eat or drink because an anaesthetic may be needed.

The most serious form of upper arm injury is a fracture of the long bone in the upper arm (humerus). The bone may be fractured across the centre by a direct blow. However, it is much more common, especially in elderly people, for the arm bone to break at the shoulder end, usually in a fall.

A fracture at the top of the bone is usually a stable injury (p.136), as the broken bone ends stay in place. For this reason, it may not be immediately apparent that the bone is broken, although the arm is likely to be painful. There is a possibility that the casualty will cope with the pain and leave the fracture untreated for some time.

See also
Fractures **pp.136–38**

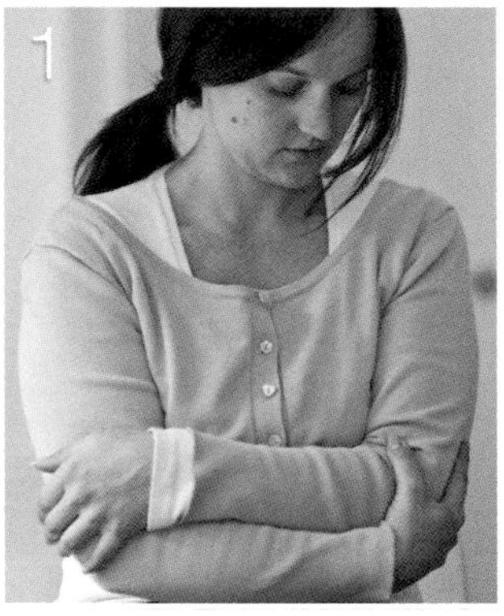

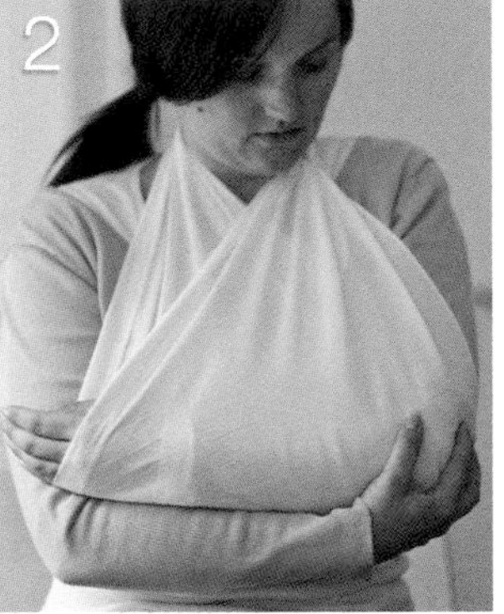

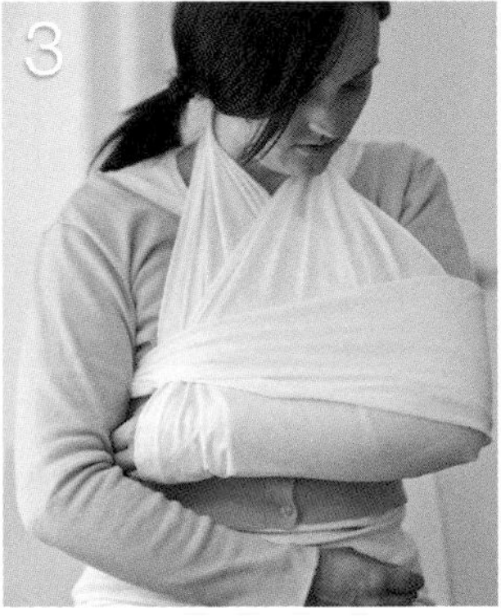

1 Help the casualty to sit down. Remove all jewellery such as bracelets, rings and watches. Gently place the forearm horizontally across her body in the position that is most comfortable. Ask her to support her elbow if possible.

2 Slide a triangular bandage in position between the arm and the chest, ready to make an arm sling (p.251). Place soft padding between the injured arm and the body, then support the arm and its padding in an arm sling.

3 For extra support, or if the journey to hospital is prolonged, secure the arm by tying a broad-fold bandage (p.249) around the chest and over the sling; make sure that the broad-fold bandage is below the fracture site.

4 Arrange to take or send the casualty to hospital.

ELBOW INJURY

RECOGNITION

There may be:
- Pain, increased by movement;
- Tenderness over the site of a fracture;
- Swelling, bruising and deformity;
- Fixed elbow.

YOUR AIMS

- To immobilise the arm without further injury to the joint.
- To arrange transport to hospital

CAUTION

- If the casualty feels faint, help her to lie down.
- Do not allow the casualty to eat or drink because an anaesthetic may be needed.
- Do not try to move the injured arm.

Fractures or dislocations at the elbow usually result from a fall onto the hand. Children often fracture the upper arm bone just above the elbow. This is an unstable fracture (p.136), and the bone ends may damage blood vessels. Circulation in the arm needs to be checked regularly. In any elbow injury, the elbow will be stiff and difficult to straighten. Never try to force a casualty to bend it.

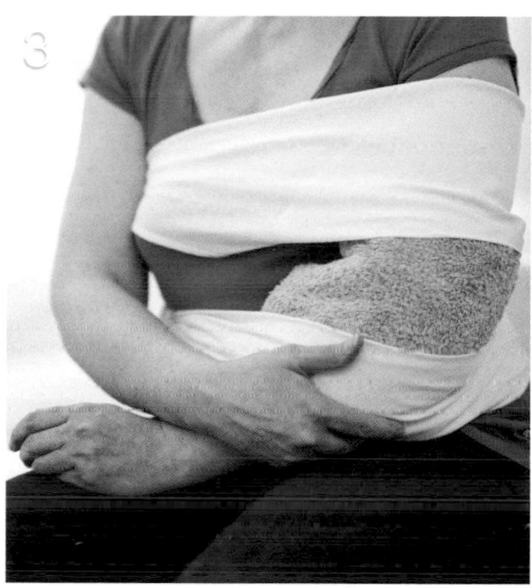

1 If the elbow can be bent, treat as for upper arm injury opposite. Remove all jewellery such as bracelets, rings and watches.

2 If the casualty cannot bend her arm, help her to sit down. Place padding, such as a towel, around the elbow for comfort and support.

3 Secure the arm in the most comfortable position for the casualty using broad-fold bandages. Keep the bandages clear of the fracture site.

4 Arrange to take or send the casualty to hospital.

5 Check the wrist pulse (p.53) in the injured arm every ten minutes until medical help arrives. If you cannot feel a pulse, gently undo the bandages and straighten the arm until the pulse returns. Support the arm in this position.

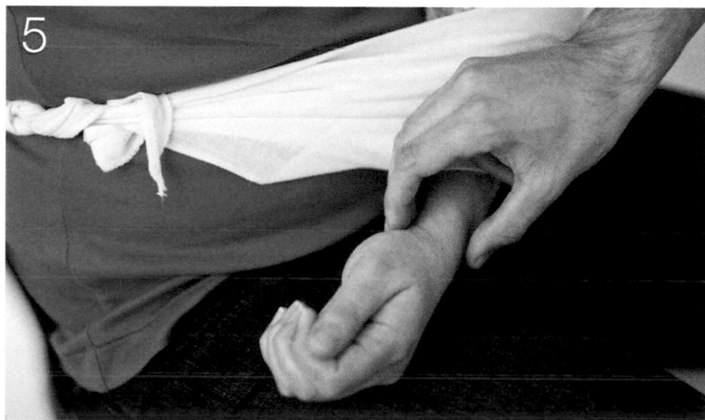

FOREARM AND WRIST INJURIES

RECOGNITION

There may be:

- Pain, increased by movement;
- Swelling, bruising and deformity;
- Possible bleeding with an open fracture.

YOUR AIMS

- To immobilise the arm.
- To arrange transport to hospital.

CAUTION

- Do not allow the casualty to eat or drink because an anaesthetic may be needed.

See also
Fractures **pp.136–38**
Severe external bleeding **pp.114–15**

The bones of the forearm (radius and ulna) can be fractured by an impact such as a heavy blow or a fall. As the bones have little fleshy covering, the broken ends may pierce the skin, producing an open fracture (p.138).

A fall onto an outstretched hand can result in a fracture of the wrist. This is called a Colles fracture and commonly occurs in elderly people.

The wrist joint is rarely dislocated, but is often sprained. It can be difficult to distinguish between a sprain and a fracture, especially if the tiny scaphoid bone (at the base of the thumb) is injured. If you are in any doubt about the injury treat as a fracture.

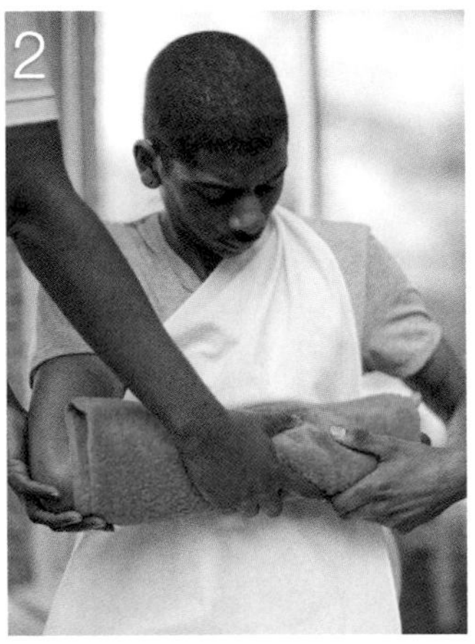

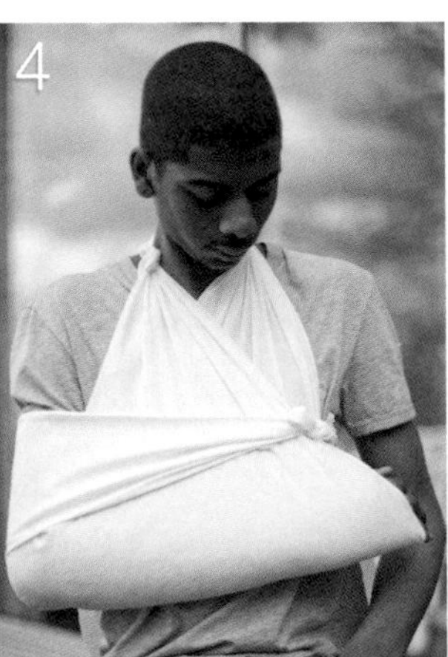

1 Ask the casualty to sit down. Steady and support the injured forearm and place it across his body; ask the casualty to support it if he can. Expose and treat any wound.

2 Slide a triangular bandage in position between the arm and the chest, ready to make an arm sling (p.251). Surround the forearm in soft padding, such as a small towel.

3 Support the arm and the padding with an arm sling; make sure the knot is tied on the injured side.

4 For extra support, or if the journey to hospital is likely to be prolonged, secure the arm to the body by tying a broad-fold bandage (p.249) over the sling and body. Position the bandage as close to the elbow as you can. Arrange to take or send the casualty to hospital.

HAND AND FINGER INJURIES

RECOGNITION

There may be:

- Pain, increased by movement;
- Swelling, bruising and deformity;
- Possible bleeding with an open fracture.

YOUR AIMS

- To elevate the hand and immobilise it.
- To arrange transport to hospital.

CAUTION

- Do not allow the casualty to eat or drink because an anaesthetic may be needed.

See also
Crush injury **p.119**
Dislocated joint **p.139**
Fractures **pp.136–38**
Wound to the palm **p.127**

The bones and joints in the hand can suffer various types of injury, such as fractures, cuts and bruising. Minor fractures are usually caused by direct force. A fracture of the knuckle often results from a punch.

Multiple fractures, affecting many or all of the bones in the hand, are usually caused by crushing injuries. The fractures may be open, with severe bleeding and swelling, needing immediate first aid treatment.

The joints in the fingers or thumb are sometimes dislocated or sprained as a result of a fall onto the hand (for example, while someone is skiing or ice skating).

Always compare the suspected fractured hand with the uninjured hand because finger fractures result in deformities that may not be immediately obvious.

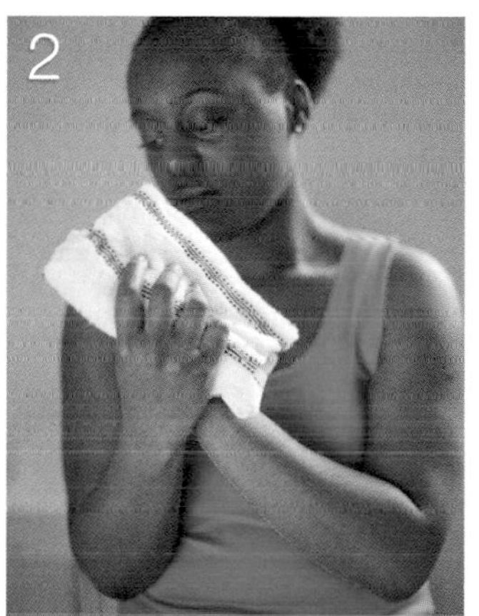

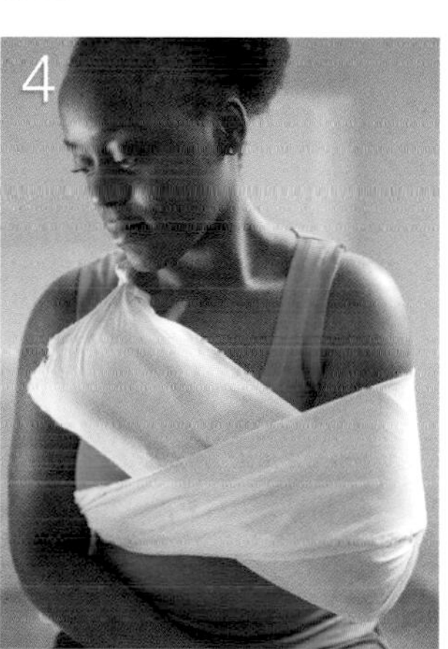

1 Help the casualty to sit down and ask her to raise and support the affected wrist and hand; help her if necessary. Treat any bleeding and losely cover the wound with a sterile dressing or large clean, non-fluffy pad.

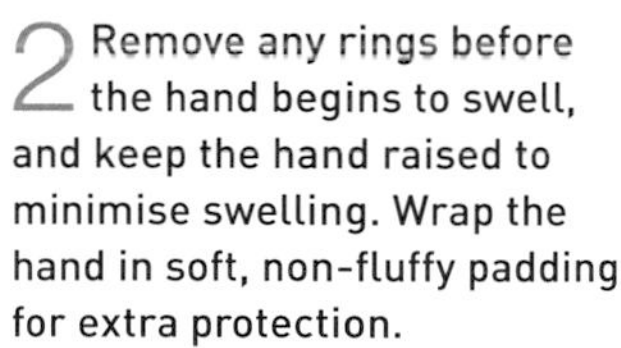

2 Remove any rings before the hand begins to swell, and keep the hand raised to minimise swelling. Wrap the hand in soft, non-fluffy padding for extra protection.

3 Gently support the affected arm across the casualty's body by placing it in an elevation sling (p.252).

4 For extra support, or if the journey to hospital is likely to be prolonged, secure the arm by tying a broad-fold bandage (p.249) around the chest and over the sling; keep it away from the injury. Arrange to take or send the casualty to hospital.

RIB INJURY

RECOGNITION

- Bruising, swelling or a wound at the fracture site.
- Pain at the site of injury.
- Pain on taking a deep breath.
- Shallow breathing.
- A wound over the fracture; you may hear air being "sucked" into chest cavity.
- Paradoxical breathing.
- Signs of internal bleeding (p.113) and shock (pp.116–17).

YOUR AIMS

- To support the chest wall.
- To arrange transport to hospital.

CAUTION

- Do not allow the casualty to eat or drink because an anaesthetic may be needed.
- If the casualty loses consciousness, open the airway and check breathing (The unconscious casualty pp.54–85). If he needs to be placed in the recovery position, lay him on his injured side to allow the lung on the uninjured side to work to its full capacity.

One or more ribs can be fractured by direct force to the chest from a blow or a fall, or by a crush injury (p.119). If there is a wound over the fracture, or if a broken rib pierces a lung, the casualty's breathing may be seriously impaired.

An injury to the chest can cause an area of fractured ribs to become detached from the rest of the chest wall, producing what is called a "flail-chest" injury. The detached area moves inwards when the casualty breathes in, and outwards as he breathes out. This "paradoxical" breathing causes severe breathing difficulties.

Fractures of the lower ribs may injure internal organs such as the liver and spleen, and may cause internal bleeding.

See also
Abdominal wound **p.128**
Penetrating chest wound **pp.102–03**
Shock **pp.116–17**

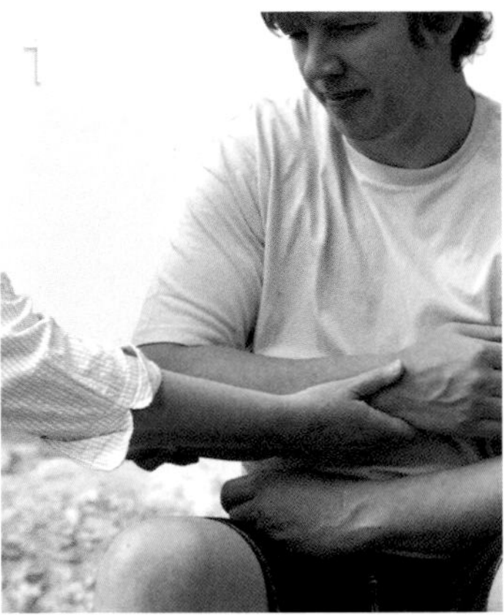

1 **Help the casualty to sit down and ask him to support the arm on the injured side; help him if necessary. For extra support place the arm on the injured side in a sling (pp.251–52).**

2 **Arrange to take or send the casualty to hospital.**

SPECIAL CASE A PENETRATING CHEST WOUND

If there is a penetrating wound, help the casualty to sit down on the floor, leaning towards the injured side. Cover and seal the wound along three edges (pp.102–03). Support the casualty with cushions and place the arm on the injured side in an elevation sling (p.252). **Call 999/112 for emergency help.** Monitor and record vital signs – level of response, breathing and pulse (pp.52–53) – while waiting for help to arrive.

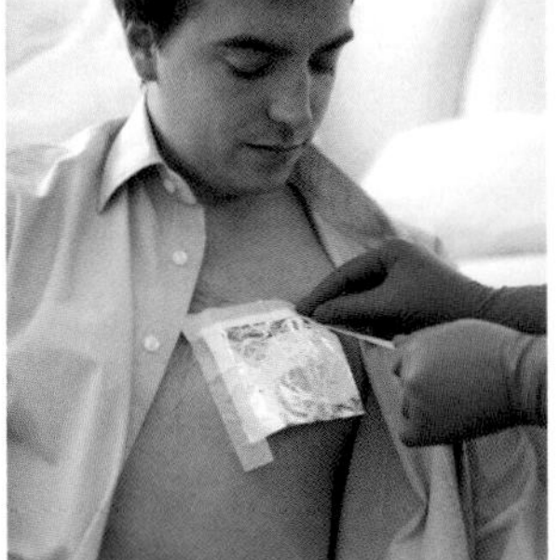

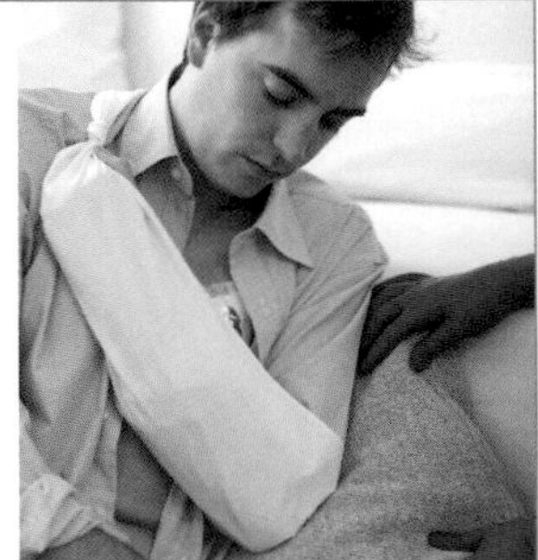

BACK PAIN

RECOGNITION

- Pain in the lower back following lifting or manual work.
- Possible pain radiating down the back of one leg with numbness or tingling in the affected leg – sciatica.

YOUR AIMS

- To relieve pain.

CAUTION

If any of the following symptoms or signs are present, **call 999/112 for emergency help**:

- Acute back pain in a casualty under 20 or over 55;
- Recent history of injury, such as a road traffic accident or fall from a height;
- Other symptoms of illness, such as fever, as well as back pain;
- Numbness and tingling down the back of both legs;
- Swelling or deformity along the spine;
- Difficulty with bladder and/or bowel function.

See also
Crush injury p.119
Dislocated joint p.139
Fractures pp.136–38
Spinal injury pp.171–73
Wound to the palm p.127

Lower back pain is common and most adults may experience it at some point in their lives. It may be acute (sudden onset) or chronic (long term). It is usually caused by age-related degenerative changes or results from minor injury affecting muscles, ligaments, vertebrae, discs or nerves. It may be the result of heavy manual work, a fall or a turning or twisting movement. Serious conditions causing back pain are rare and beyond the scope of first aid.

Most cases are simple backache, often in the lower back, in people aged 20–55 who are otherwise well. In a small number of casualties, the pain may extend down one leg. This is called sciatica and is caused by pressure on the nerve root (a so-called "trapped nerve").

Spine injuries in those under 20 or over 55, or that result from a more serious injury, require investigation and treatment and are dealt with in Nervous System Problems pp.160–75.

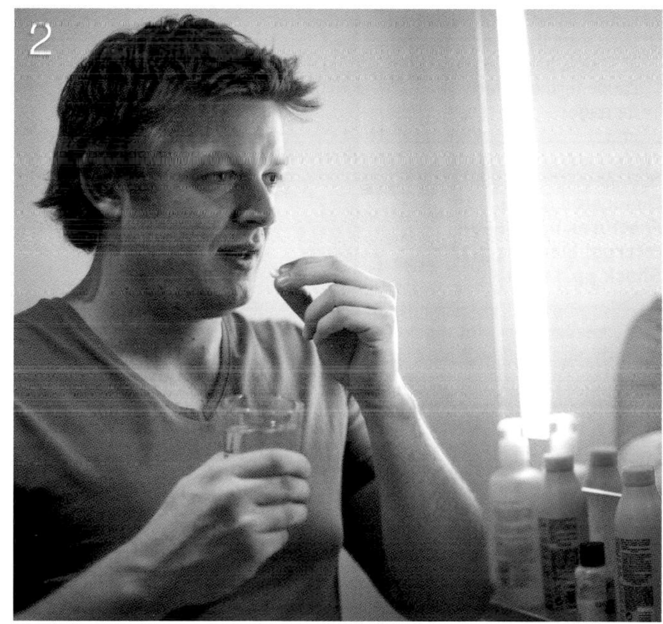

1 Advise the casualty to stay active to mobilise the injured area. Encourage him to return to normal activity as soon as possible.

2 An adult casualty may take the recommended dose of paracetamol tablets, or his own painkillers.

3 Advise the casualty to seek medical advice if necessary.

FRACTURED PELVIS

RECOGNITION

There may be:

- An inability to walk or even stand, although the legs appear uninjured;
- Pain and tenderness in the region of the hip, groin or back, which increases with movement;
- Difficulty or pain passing urine, and bloodstained clothing;
- Signs of shock and internal bleeding.

YOUR AIMS

- To minimise the risk of shock.
- To arrange urgent removal to hospital.

CAUTION

- Do not bandage the casualty's legs together if this increases the pain. In such cases, surround the injured area with soft padding, such as clothing or towels.
- Do not allow the casualty to eat or drink because an anaesthetic may be needed.

See also
Fractures **pp.136–38**
Internal bleeding **p.113**
Shock **pp.116–17**

Injuries to the pelvis are usually caused by indirect force, such as a car crash, a fall from a height or by crushing. These incidents can force the head of the thigh bone (femur) through the hip socket in the pelvis.

A fracture of the pelvic bones may also be complicated by injury to tissues and organs inside the pelvis, such as the bladder and the urinary passages. The bleeding from large organs and blood vessels in the pelvis may be severe and lead to shock.

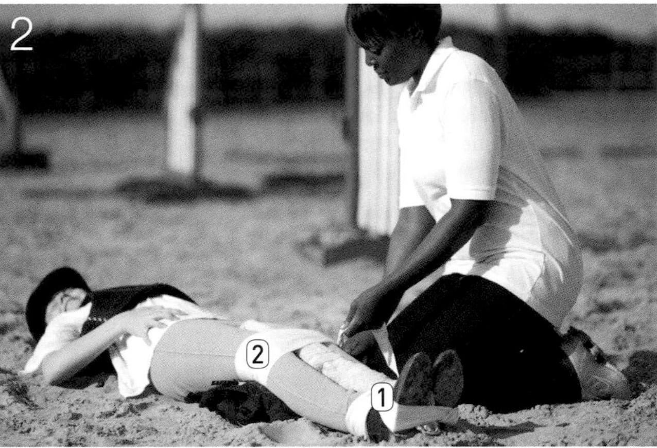

1 Help the casualty to lie down on her back with her head flat/low to minimise shock. Keep her legs straight and flat or, if it is more comfortable, help her to bend her knees slightly and support them with padding, such as a cushion or folded clothing.

2 Place padding between the bony points of the knees and the ankles. Immobilise the legs by bandaging them together with folded triangular bandages (p.249); secure the feet and ankles with a narrow-fold bandage (1), and the knees with a broad-fold bandage (2).

3 **Call 999/112 for emergency help.** Treat the casualty for shock (pp.116–17). Do not raise the legs.

4 Monitor and record vital signs – level of response, breathing and pulse (pp.52–53) – until help arrives.

KNEE INJURY

RECOGNITION

There may be:

- Pain on attempting to move the knee;
- Swelling at the knee joint.

YOUR AIMS

- To protect the knee in the most comfortable position.
- To arrange urgent removal to hospital.

CAUTION

- Do not attempt to straighten the knee forcibly. Displaced cartilage or internal bleeding may make it impossible to straighten the knee joint safely.
- Do not allow the casualty to eat or drink because an anaesthetic may be needed.
- Do not allow the casualty to walk.

See also
Strains and sprains **pp.140–41**

The knee is the hinge joint between the thigh bone (femur) and shin bone (tibia). It is capable of bending, straightening and, in the bent position, slight rotation.

The knee joint is supported by strong muscles and ligaments and is protected at the front by a disc of bone called the kneecap (patella). Discs of cartilage protect the end surfaces of the major bones. Direct blows, violent twists or sprains can damage these structures. Possible knee injuries include fracture of the patella, sprains and damage to the cartilage.

A knee injury may make it impossible for the casualty to bend the joint, and you should ensure that the casualty does not try to walk on the injured leg. Bleeding or fluid in the knee joint may cause marked swelling around the knee.

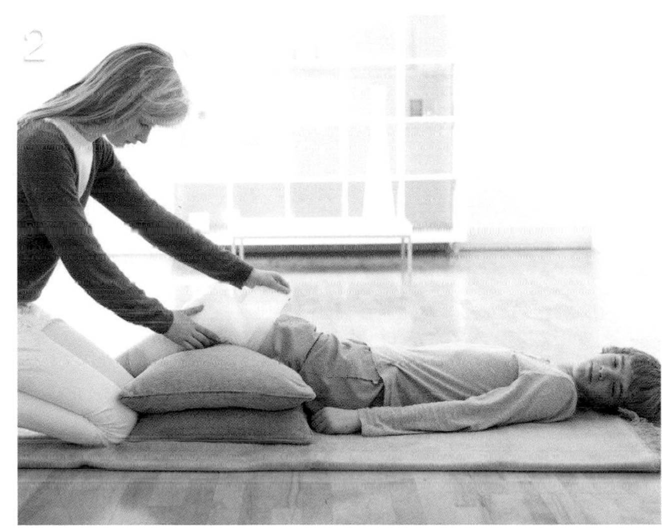

1 Help the casualty to lie down, preferably on a blanket to insulate him from the floor or ground. Place soft padding, such as pillows, blankets or coats, under his injured knee to support it in the most comfortable position.

2 Wrap soft padding around the joint. Secure padding with a roller bandage that extends from the middle of the lower leg to mid-thigh.

3 **Call 999/112 for emergency help.** The casualty needs to remain in the treatment position and so should be transported to hospital by ambulance.

LOWER LEG INJURY

RECOGNITION

There may be:

- Localised pain;
- Swelling, bruising and deformity of the leg;
- An open wound;
- Inability to stand on the injured leg.

YOUR AIMS

- To immobilise the leg.
- To arrange transport to hospital.

Injuries to the lower leg include fractures of the shin bone (tibia) and the splint bone (fibula), as well as damage to the soft tissues (muscles, ligaments and tendons).

Fractures of the tibia are usually due to a heavy blow (for example, from the bumper of a moving vehicle). As there is little flesh over the tibia, a fracture is more likely to produce a wound. The fibula can be broken by the twisting forces that sprain an ankle.

See also
Fractures **pp.136–38**
Severe external bleeding **pp.114–15**
Strains and sprains **pp.140–41**

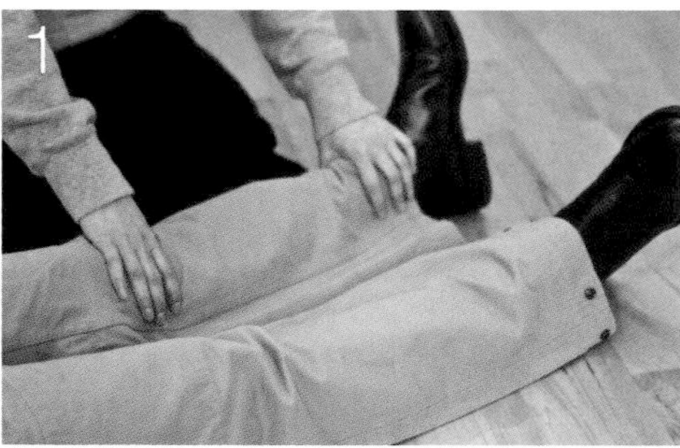

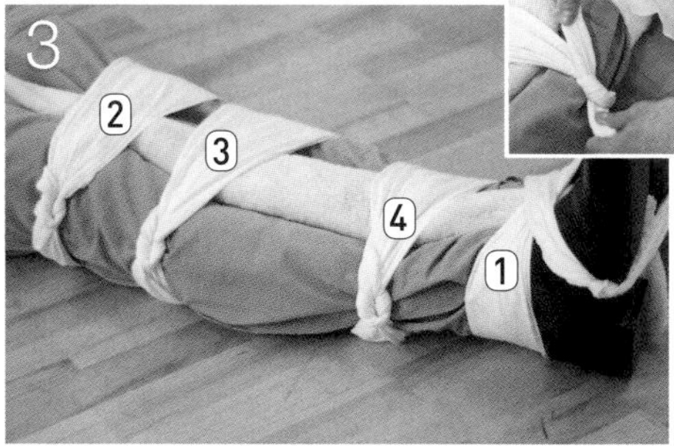

1 Help the casualty to lie down, and gently steady and support the injured leg. If there is a wound, carefully expose it and treat the bleeding. Place a dressing over the wound to protect it.

2 **Call 999/112 for emergency help.** Support the injured leg with your hands; hold the joints above and below the fracture site to prevent any movement. Maintain support until the ambulance arrives.

3 If the ambulance is delayed, support the injured leg by splinting it to the other leg. Bring the uninjured leg alongside the injured one and slide bandages under both legs. Position a narrow-fold bandage (p.249) at the feet and ankles (1), then broad-fold bandages at the knees (2) and above and below the fracture site (3 and 4). Insert padding between the lower legs. Tie a figure-of-eight bandage around the feet and ankles, then secure the other bandages, knotting them on the uninjured side.

4 If the casualty's journey to hospital is likely to be long and rough, place soft padding on the outside of the injured leg, from the knee to the foot. Secure the legs with broad-fold bandages as described above.

SPECIAL CASE
IF FRACTURE IS NEAR THE ANKLE

If the injury is very near the ankle, instead of tying the figure of eight bandage (above), place separate narrow-fold bandages above the ankle and around the feet.

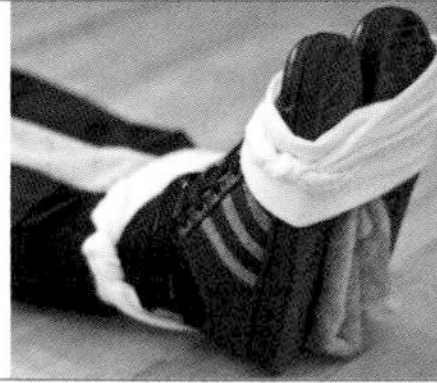

ANKLE INJURY

RECOGNITION

- Pain, increased either by movement or by putting weight on the foot.
- Swelling at the site of injury.

YOUR AIMS

- To relieve pain and swelling.
- To obtain medical aid if necessary.

CAUTION

- If you suspect a broken bone, tell the casualty not to put weight on the leg. Secure and support the lower leg (special case, opposite), and arrange to take or send the casualty to hospital.
- Do not allow the casualty to eat or drink because an anaesthetic may be needed.

If the ankle is broken, treat it as a fracture of the lower leg (opposite). A more common injury is a sprain (p.141), usually caused by a twist to the ankle. This problem can be treated by the RICE procedure: Rest the affected part, cool the injury with Ice, provide Comfortable support with bandaging, and Elevate the injury (p.140).

See also
Strains and sprains **pp.140–41**

1 Rest and support the ankle in the most comfortable position for the casualty, preferably raised.

2 Apply a cold compress, such as an ice pack or a cold pad (p.241), to the site to reduce swelling and bruising.

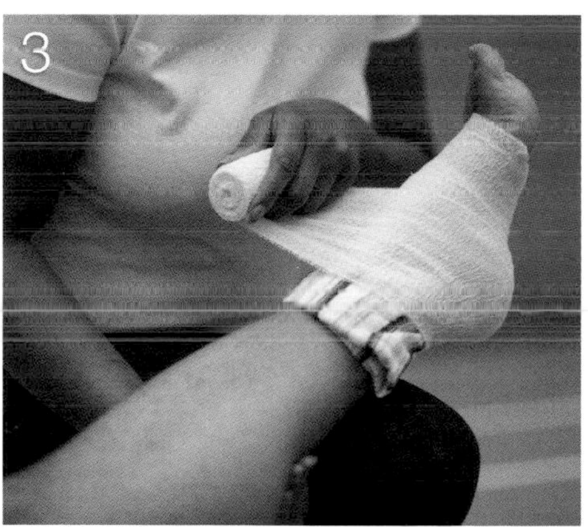

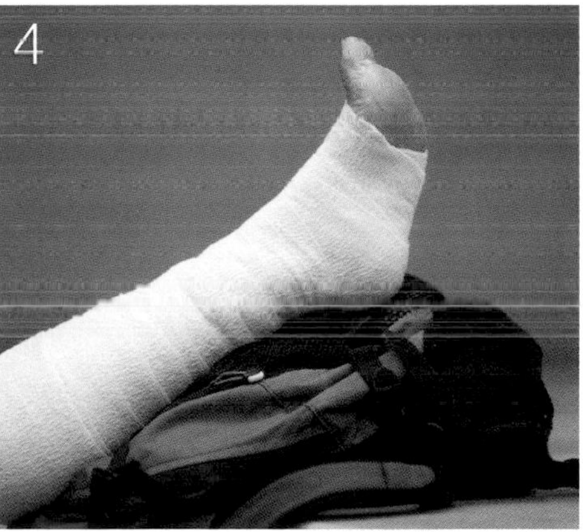

3 Apply comfortable support to the ankle. Leave the cold compress in place or wrap a layer of soft padding around the area. Bandage the ankle with a support bandage that extends from the base of the foot to the knee.

4 Raise and support the injured limb. Check the circulation beyond the bandaging (p.243) every ten minutes. If the circulation is impaired, loosen the bandage. Advise the casualty to rest the ankle and to seek medical advice if necessary.

FOOT AND TOE INJURIES

RECOGNITION

- Difficulty in walking.
- Stiffness of movement.
- Bruising and swelling.
- Deformity.

YOUR AIMS

- To minimise swelling.
- To arrange transport to hospital.

CAUTION

- Do not allow the casualty to eat or drink because an anaesthetic may be needed.

The bones and joints in the foot can suffer various types of injury, such as fractures, cuts and bruising. Minor fractures are usually caused by direct force. Always compare the injured foot with the uninjured foot, especially toes, because fractures can result in deformities that may not be immediately obvious. Multiple fractures, affecting many or all of the bones in the foot, are usually caused by crushing injuries. These fractures may be open, with severe bleeding and swelling, needing immediate first aid treatment. Foot and toe injures must be treated in hospital.

See also
Crush injury **p.119**

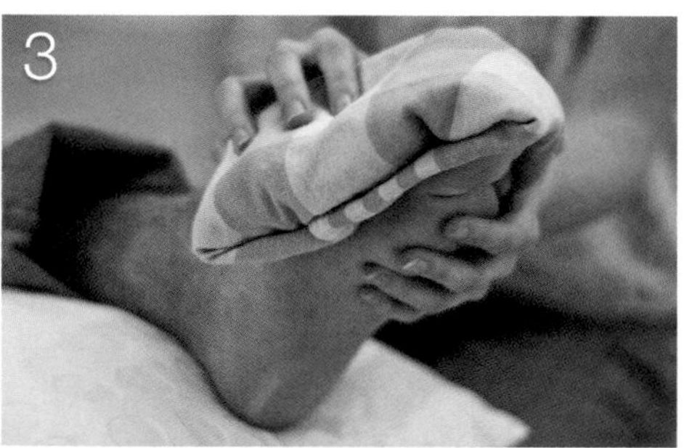

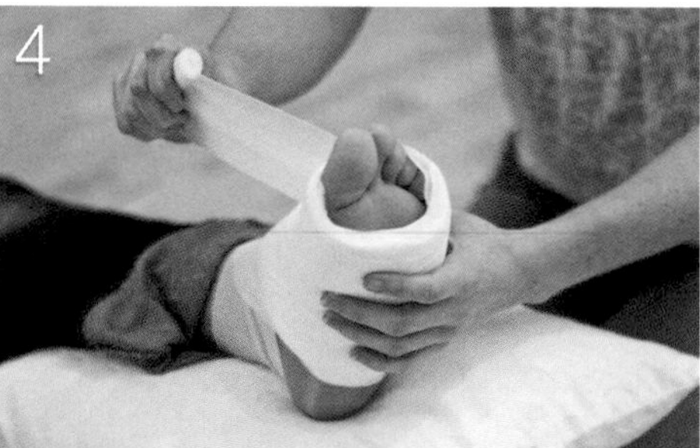

1 Help the casualty to lie down, and carefully steady and support the injured leg. If there is a wound, carefully expose it and treat the bleeding. Place a dressing over the wound to protect it.

2 Remove any foot jewellery before the area begins to swell.

3 Apply a cold compress, such as an ice pack or a cold pad (p.241). This will also help to relieve swelling and reduce pain.

4 Place padding around the casualty's foot and bandage firmly in place.

5 Arrange to take or send the casualty to hospital. If he is not being transported by ambulance, try to ensure that the injured foot remains elevated during travel.

CRAMP

YOUR AIMS

- To relieve the spasm and pain.

See also
Dehydration p.190
Heat exhaustion p.192

This condition is a sudden painful spasm in one or more muscles. Cramp commonly occurs during sleep. It can also develop after strenuous exercise, due to a build-up of chemical waste products in the muscles, or to excessive loss of salts and fluids from the body through sweating or dehydration. Cramp can often be relieved by stretching and massaging the affected muscles.

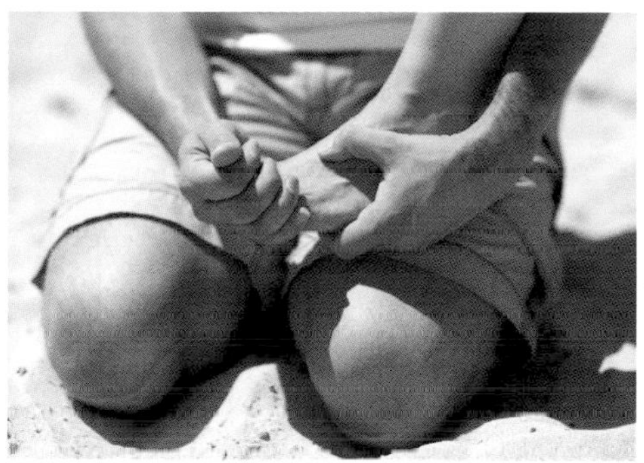

CRAMP IN THE FOOT

Help the casualty stand with his weight on the front of his foot; you can rest the foot on your knee to stretch the affected muscles. Once the spasm has passed, massage the affected part of the foot with your fingers.

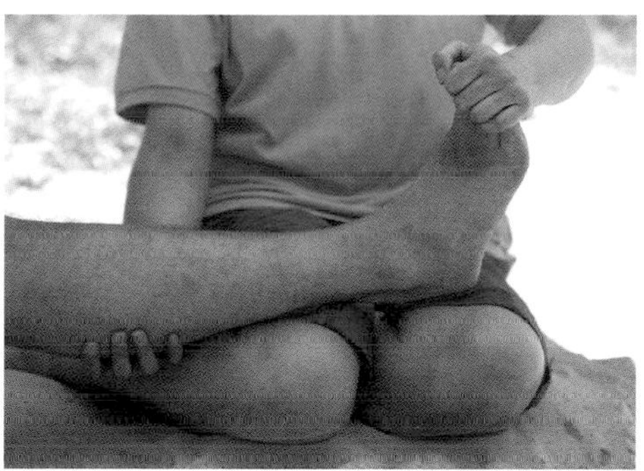

CRAMP IN THE CALF MUSCLES

Help the casualty straighten his knee, and support his foot. Flex his foot upwards towards his shin to stretch the calf muscles, then massage the affected area on the back of the calf.

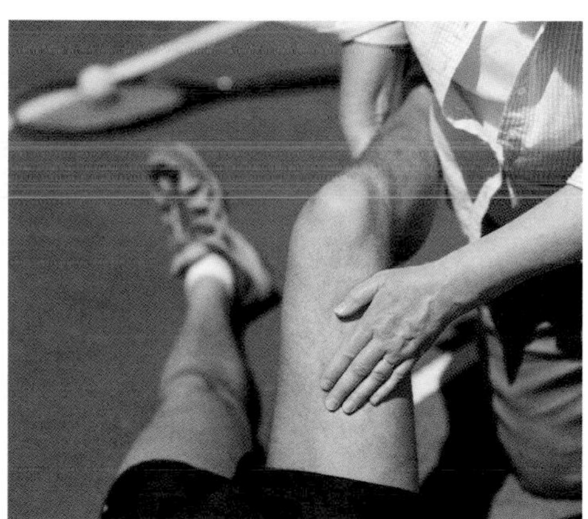

CRAMP IN THE FRONT OF THE THIGH

Help the casualty to lie down. Raise the leg and bend the knee to stretch the muscles. Massage the affected muscles once the spasm has passed.

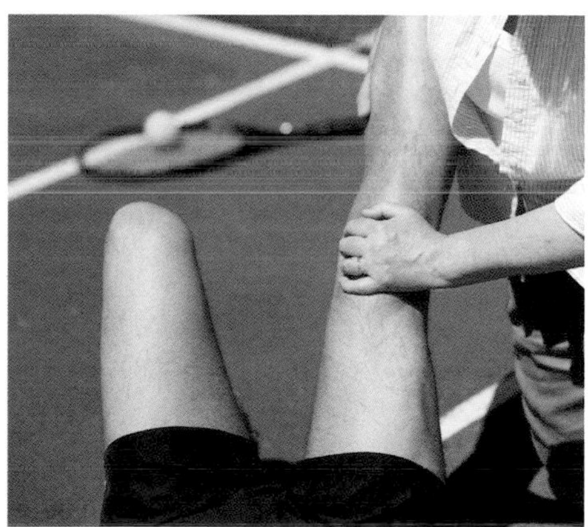

CRAMP IN THE BACK OF THE THIGH

Help the casualty to lie down. Raise the leg and straighten the knee to stretch the muscles. Massage the area once the spasm has passed.

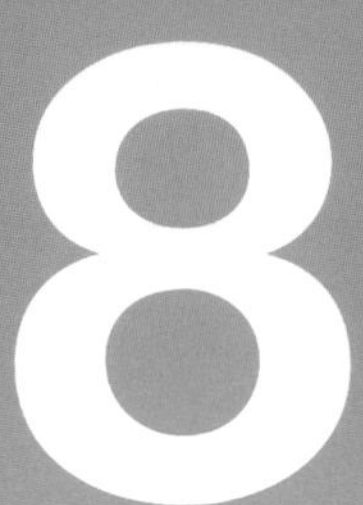

The nervous system is the most complex system in the body. Its control centre, the brain, is the source of consciousness, thought, speech and memory. It also receives and interprets sensory information and controls other body systems via the nerves.

When we are fully conscious we are alert and aware of our surroundings. However, if consciousness is impaired, even survival mechanisms such as the cough reflex, which normally keeps the airway clear, may not function.

Many of the injuries or conditions affecting the nervous system can result in impaired consciousness, so need immediate attention. In addition, damage to any part of the spinal cord can result in permanent injury so a casualty should be treated in the position you find him. Any casualty with a head injury may also have a spine injury, and vice versa.

AIMS AND OBJECTIVES

- To assess the casualty's condition quickly and calmly.
- To carry out any treatment necessary to improve the casualty's condition.
- To comfort and reassure the casualty.
- To protect the casualty from further injury.
- To look for and treat any injuries associated with the condition.
- To call 999/112 for emergency help if you suspect a serious illness or injury.
- To be aware of your own needs.

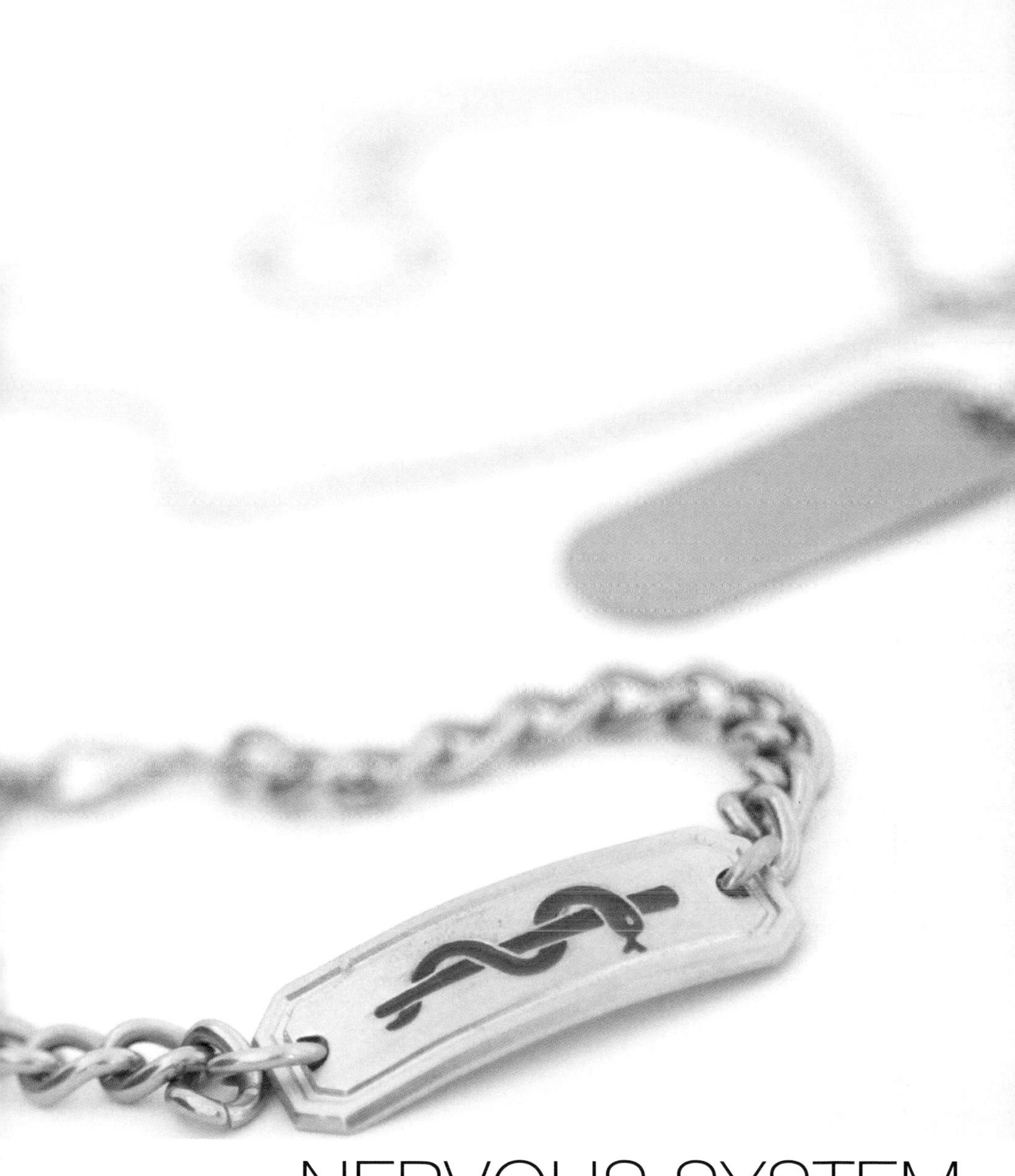

NERVOUS SYSTEM PROBLEMS

THE NERVOUS SYSTEM

This is the body's information-gathering, storage and control system. It consists of a central processing unit – the brain – and a network of nerve cells and fibres.

There are two main parts to the nervous system: the central nervous system, consisting of the brain and spinal cord, and the peripheral nervous system, which consists of all the nerves that connect the brain and the spinal cord to the rest of the body. In addition, the autonomic (involuntary) nervous system controls body functions such as digestion, heart rate and breathing. The central nervous system receives and analyses information from all parts of the body. The nerves carry messages, in the form of high-speed electrical impulses, between the brain and the rest of the nervous system.

Brain

Cranial nerves (12 pairs) extend directly from the underside of the brain; most serve the head, face, neck and shoulders

Vagus nerve, longest of the cranial nerves, serves organs in chest and abdomen; it controls the heart rate

Radial nerve controls muscles that straighten elbow and fingers

Sciatic nerve serves hip and hamstring muscles

Tibial nerve serves calf muscles

Structure of the nervous system
The system consists of the brain, spinal cord and a network of nerves that carry electrical impulses between the brain and the body.

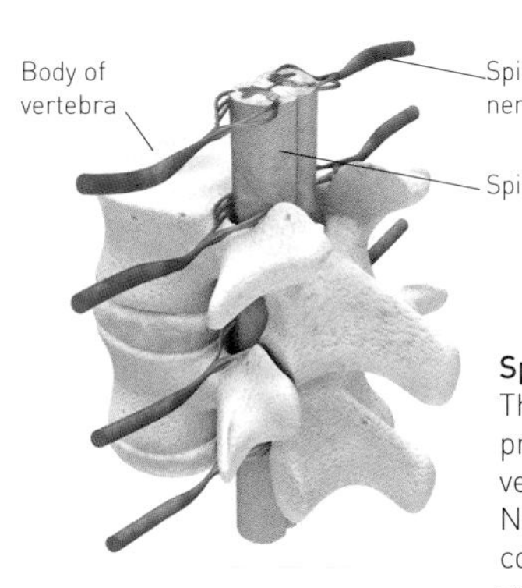

Spinal cord protection
The spinal cord is protected by the vertebral column. Nerves from the spinal cord emerge between vertebrae.

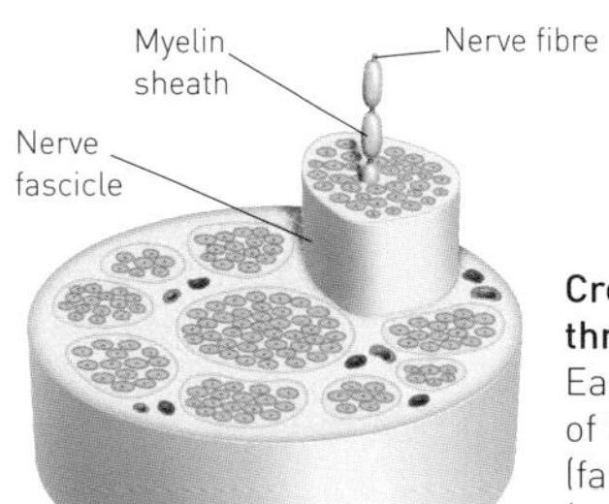

Cross-section through a nerve
Each nerve is made up of bundles of nerve fibres (fascicles). A fatty substance (myelin) surrounds and insulates larger nerve fibres.

CENTRAL NERVOUS SYSTEM

The brain and the spinal cord make up the central nervous system (CNS). This system contains billions of interconnected nerve cells (neurons) and is enclosed by three membranes called meninges. A clear fluid called cerebrospinal fluid flows around the brain and spinal cord. It functions as a shock absorber, provides oxygen and nutrients and removes waste products. The brain has three main structures: the cerebrum, which is concerned with thought, sensation and conscious movement; the cerebellum, which coordinates movement, balance and posture; and the brain stem, which controls basic functions such as breathing. The main function of the spinal cord is to convey signals between the brain and the peripheral nervous system (below).

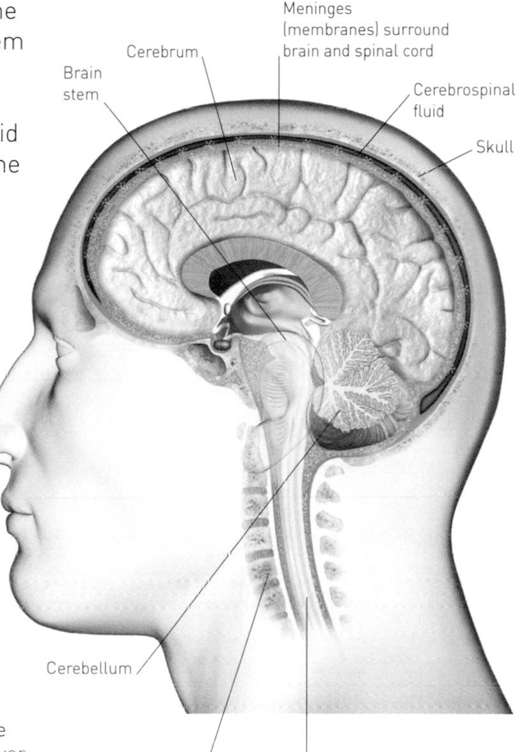

Structure of the brain
The brain is enclosed within the skull. It has three main parts: the cerebrum, which has an outer layer called the cortex; the cerebellum; and the brain stem.

PERIPHERAL NERVOUS SYSTEM

This part of the nervous system consists of two sets of paired nerves – the cranial and spinal nerves – connecting the CNS to the body. The cranial nerves emerge in 12 pairs from the underside of the brain. The 31 pairs of spinal nerves branch off at intervals from the spinal cord, passing into the rest of the body. Nerves comprise bundles of nerve fibres that can relay both incoming (sensory) and outgoing (motor) signals.

AUTONOMIC NERVOUS SYSTEM

Some of the cranial nerves, and several small spinal nerves, work as the autonomic nervous system. This system is concerned with vital body functions such as heart rate and breathing. The system's two parts, the sympathetic and parasympathetic systems, counterbalance each other. The sympathetic system prepares the body for action by releasing hormones that raise the heart rate and reduce the blood flow to the skin and intestines. The parasympathetic system releases hormones with a calming effect.

IMPAIRED CONSCIOUSNESS

YOUR AIMS

- To maintain an open airway.
- To assess and record level of response.
- To arrange urgent removal to hospital if necessary.

CAUTION

- Do not move the casualty unnecessarily.
- If you suspect that a casualty may have a neck (spinal) injury, support his head at all times. If he is unconscious, open the airway using the jaw-thrust method (p.173). Kneel behind the casualty's head and place your hands on each side of his face, with your fingertips at the angles of his jaw, then gently lift the jaw to open the airway.

See also
Diabetes mellitus p.218
Head injury opposite
Hypoxia p.90
Spinal injury pp.171–73
The unconscious casualty pp.54–85

There is no absolute dividing line between consciousness and unconsciousness. A person may be fully aware and awake (conscious), completely unresponsive to any stimulus (unconscious) or at any level between these two extremes. For example, a casualty may be "groggy" or respond only to loud sounds or to pain. Impaired consciousness is the term used to describe the condition of a casualty who is anything less than fully conscious.

AVPU SCALE

You can assess conscious levels by checking the casualty's level of response to stimuli using the AVPU code.

A – Is the casualty Alert? Are his eyes open and does he respond to questions?
V – Does the casualty respond to Voice? Does he answer simple questions and obey commands?
P – Does the casualty respond to Pain? Does he open his eyes or move if pinched?
U – Is the casualty Unresponsive to any stimulus?

Make a note of your findings at each assessment since a casualty's condition may change while you are attending him.

CAUSES OF IMPAIRED CONSCIOUSNESS

The main causes of impaired consciousness are structural damage to the brain or a lack of nutrients – oxygen and glucose (sugar) – reaching the brain. Structural damage may occur with a head injury or a brain tumour. Low oxygen (hypoxia) or low blood sugar (hypoglycaemia) may occur with any condition that reduces blood flow to the brain, such as a stroke, shock, fainting or a heart attack. It can also occur if blood flow is normal but there is insufficient oxygen or glucose in the blood – for example, due to poisoning, or a chemical imbalance caused by diabetes mellitus. Epilepsy can produce impaired consciousness due to abnormal electrical activity in the brain.

1 Perform a quick check of consciousness by assessing the level of response using the AVPU code (above). If the person is "groggy", but responds to sound or pain, support him in a comfortable, resting position and watch for any change in his level of response. **Call 999/112 for emergency help.**

2 If the casualty is unconscious, open his airway and check breathing (The unconscious casualty pp.54–85). **Call 999/112 for emergency help.** Monitor and record vital signs – level of response, breathing and pulse (pp.52–53) – while waiting for emergency help to arrive. Treat any associated injuries.

HEAD INJURY

YOUR AIMS

- Assess and monitor the casualty and call appropriate medical help if necessary.

CAUTION

- Support the casualty's head because of the risk of neck (spinal) injury.
- If the casualty is unconscious, open the airway using the jaw-thrust method and check breathing (The unconscious casualty pp.54–85).

See also
Cerebral compression **p.167**
Concussion **p.166**
Facial injury **p.142**
Scalp and head wounds **p.123**
Spinal injury **pp.171–73**
The unconscious casualty **pp.54–85**

All head injuries are potentially serious since they can result in impaired consciousness (opposite). Injuries may be associated with brain tissue or blood vessel damage inside the skull, or with a skull fracture. Assume a casualty with an injury to the head may have a neck (spinal) injury.

A head injury may produce concussion, a brief period of loss of consciousness that is followed by recovery or compression of the brain, which is life-threatening (below).

A head wound should alert you to the risk of underlying brain injury, which may be serious. Bleeding inside the skull may occur, which can lead to compression. Clear fluid or watery blood leaking from the ear or nose, and bruising around the eyes or ears are signs of serious injury.

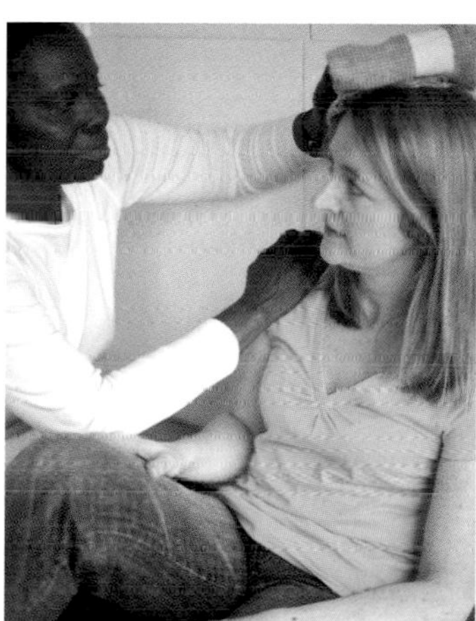

FOR A CONSCIOUS CASUALTY

If the casualty is fully conscious, help her to sit down in a comfortable position. Give her a cold compress to hold against her head. Monitor her condition. If she does not recover fully, or if she becomes drowsy or confused, complains of worsening headache, double vision or vomiting, **call 999/112 for emergency help**.

RECOGNISING A POTENTIALLY SERIOUS HEAD INJURY

Advise a casualty that if following a head injury he develops any of the following he should seek medical advice:

- Increasing drowsiness;
- Worsening headache;
- Confusion/strange behaviour or loss of memory or any vomiting episodes since the injury;
- Weakness in an arm or leg or speech difficulties;
- Dizziness, loss of balance or seizures;
- Any visual problems;
- Blood, or clear fluid, leaking from the nose or ear;
- Unusual breathing problems;

Advise the casualty not to take any alcohol or drugs (other than his prescribed medication) until fully recovered.

CONCUSSION

RECOGNITION

- Brief period of impaired consciousness following a blow to the head.

There may also be:

- Dizziness or nausea;
- Loss of memory of events at the time of, or immediately preceding, the injury;
- Mild, generalised headache;
- Confusion.

YOUR AIMS

- To ensure the casualty recovers fully and safely.
- To place the casualty in the care of a responsible person.
- To obtain medical aid if necessary.

CAUTION

- If the casualty does not recover fully, or if there is a deteriorating level of response after an initial recovery, **call 999/112 for emergency help**.

See also
Cerebral compression **opposite**
Spinal injury **pp.171–73**
The unconscious casualty **pp.54–85**

The brain is free to move a little within the skull, and can thus be "shaken" by a blow to the head. This shaking is called concussion. Among the more common causes of concussion are traffic incidents, sports injuries and falls.

Concussion produces temporary disturbance of normal brain activity but is not usually associated with any lasting damage to the brain. The casualty will suffer impaired consciousness and may be confused, but this lasts only a short time (usually only a few minutes) and is followed by a full recovery.

A casualty who has been concussed should be monitored and advised to obtain medical help if symptoms such as headache or blurred vision develop later. Always suspect a neck injury in any casualty who has a head injury (pp.171–73).

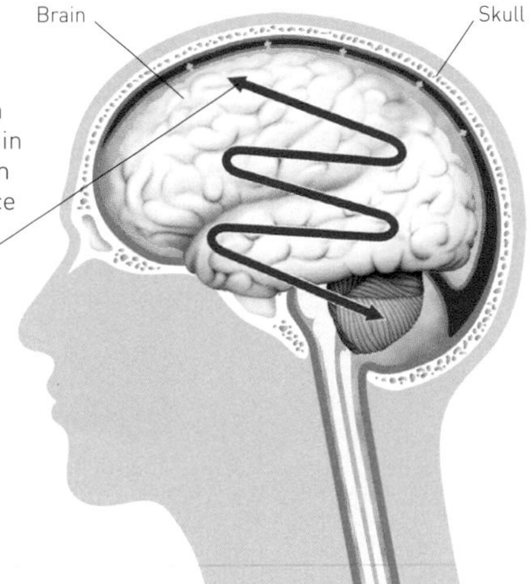

Mechanism of concussion
Concussion usually occurs as a result of a blow to the head, which "shakes" the brain within the skull. This results in a temporary disturbance of brain function.

1 Treat the casualty as for impaired consciousness (p.164).

2 Regularly monitor and record vital signs – level of response, breathing and pulse (pp.52–53). Even if the casualty appears to recover fully, watch him for subsequent deterioration in his level of response.

3 When the casualty has recovered, place him in the care of a responsible person. If a casualty has been injured on the sports field, never allow him to "play on" without first obtaining medical advice.

4 Advise the casualty to go to hospital if, following a blow to the head, he develops symptoms such as headache, vomiting, confusion, drowsiness or double vision.

CEREBRAL COMPRESSION

RECOGNITION

- Deteriorating level of response – casualty may lose consciousness.

There may also be:

- History of a recent head injury;
- Intense headache;
- Noisy breathing, becoming slow;
- Slow, yet full and strong pulse;
- Unequal pupil size;
- Weakness and/or paralysis down one side of the face or body;
- Drowsiness;
- Change in personality or behaviour, such as irritability or disorientation.

YOUR AIMS

- To arrange urgent removal of the casualty to hospital.

CAUTION

- Do not allow the casualty to eat or drink because an anaesthetic may be needed.
- If the casualty is unconscious, open the airway using the jaw-thrust method (p.173) and check breathing (The unconscious casualty pp.54–85). If the casualty is breathing, try to maintain the airway in the position the casualty was found because of the risk of spinal injury.

See also
Spinal injury **pp.171–73**
Stroke **pp.174–75**
The unconscious casualty **pp.54–85**

Compression of the brain – cerebral compression – is very serious and almost invariably requires surgery. Cerebral compression occurs when there is a build-up of pressure on the brain. This pressure may be due to one of several different causes, such as an accumulation of blood within the skull or swelling of injured brain tissues.

Cerebral compression is usually caused by a head injury. However, it can also be due to other causes, such as a stroke (pp.174–75), infection or a brain tumour. The condition may develop immediately after a head injury, or it may appear a few hours or even days later. For this reason, you should always try to find out whether a casualty has a recent history of a head injury.

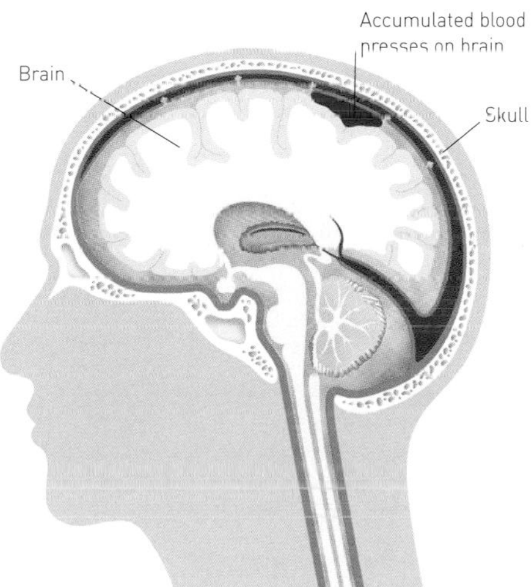

Compression caused by bleeding Bleeding may occur within the skull following a head injury or a disorder such as a stroke. The escaped blood may put pressure on tissues in the brain.

1 **Call 999/112 for emergency help.** If the casualty is conscious, steady and support his head.

2 Monitor and record the casualty's vital signs – level of response, breathing and pulse (pp.52–53) – while waiting for emergency help to arrive.

SEIZURES IN ADULTS

RECOGNITION

- Sudden unconsciousness.
- Rigidity and arching of the back.
- Convulsive movements.

In epilepsy, the following sequence is common:

- The casualty suddenly loses consciousness;
- He becomes rigid, arching his back;
- Breathing may become difficult. The lips may show a grey-blue tinge (cyanosis) and the face and neck may become red and puffy;
- Convulsive movements begin. The jaw may be clenched and breathing may be noisy. Saliva may appear at the mouth and may be bloodstained if the lips or tongue have been bitten;
- Possible loss of bladder or bowel control;
- Muscles relax and breathing becomes normal; the casualty recovers consciousness, usually within a few minutes. He may feel dazed, or act strangely. He may be unaware of his actions;
- After a seizure, the casualty may feel tired and fall into a deep sleep.

YOUR AIMS

- To protect the casualty from injury during the seizure.
- To care for the casualty when consciousness is regained and arrange removal to hospital if necessary.

See also
Impaired consciousness **p.164**
The unconscious casualty **pp.54–85**

A seizure – also called a convulsion or fit – consists of involuntary contractions of many of the muscles in the body. The condition is due to a disturbance in the electrical activity of the brain. Seizures usually result in loss or impairment of consciousness. The most common cause is epilepsy. Other causes include head injury, some brain-damaging diseases, shortage of oxygen or glucose in the brain and the intake of certain poisons, including alcohol or drugs.

Epileptic seizures result from recurrent, major disturbances of brain activity. These seizures can be sudden and dramatic. Just before a seizure, a casualty may have a brief warning period (aura) with, for example, a strange feeling or a special smell or taste.

No matter what the cause of the seizure, care must always include maintaining an open, clear airway and monitoring of the casualty's vital signs – level of response, breathing and pulse. You will also need to protect the casualty from further harm during a seizure and arrange appropriate aftercare once he has recovered.

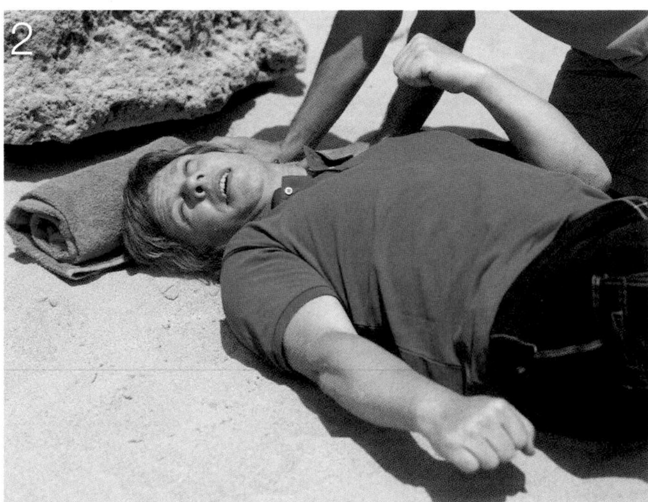

1 **Make space around the casualty; ask bystanders to move away. Remove potentially dangerous items, such as hot drinks and sharp objects. Note the time that the seizure started.**

2 **Protect the casualty's head from objects nearby; place soft padding such as rolled towels underneath or around his neck if possible. Loosen tight clothing around his neck if necessary.**

CAUTION

- Do not move the casualty unless he is in immediate danger.
- Do not put anything in his mouth or attempt to restrain him during a seizure.

Call 999/112 for emergency help if:

- The casualty is having repeated seizures or having his first seizure;
- The casualty is not aware of any reason for the seizure;
- The seizure continues for more than five minutes;
- The casualty is unconscious for more than ten minutes.

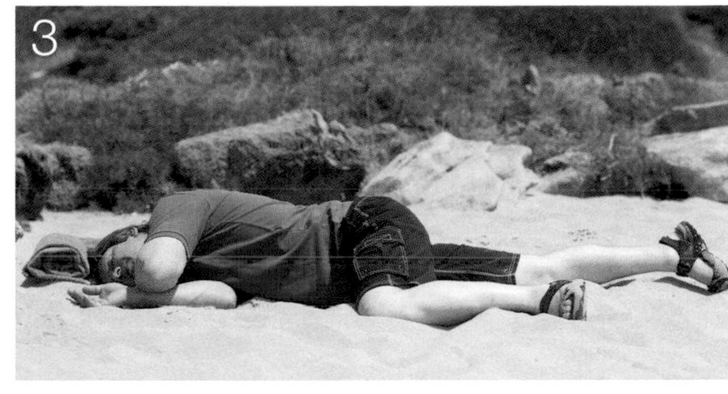

3 **When the convulsive movements have ceased, open the casualty's airway and check breathing. If he is breathing, place him in the recovery position.**

4 **Monitor and record vital signs – level of response, breathing and pulse (pp.52–53) – until he recovers. Note the duration of the seizure.**

ABSENCE SEIZURES

RECOGNITION

- Sudden "switching off"; the casualty may stare blankly ahead.
- Slight or localised twitching or jerking of the lips, eyelids, head or limbs.
- Odd "automatic" movements, such as lip-smacking, chewing or making noises.

YOUR AIMS

- To protect the casualty until he is fully recovered.

Some people experience a mild form of epilepsy, with small seizures during which they appear distant and unaware of their surroundings. These episodes, called "absence seizures", tend to affect children more than adults. There is unlikely to be any convulsive movement or loss of consciousness, but a full seizure may follow.

1 **Help the casualty to sit down in a quiet place. Make space around him; remove any potentially dangerous items, such as hot drinks and sharp objects.**

2 **Talk to the casualty in a calm and reassuring way. Do not pester him with questions. Stay with him until you are sure that he is fully recovered.**

3 **If the casualty does not recognise or have any awareness of his condition, advise him to seek medical advice as soon as possible.**

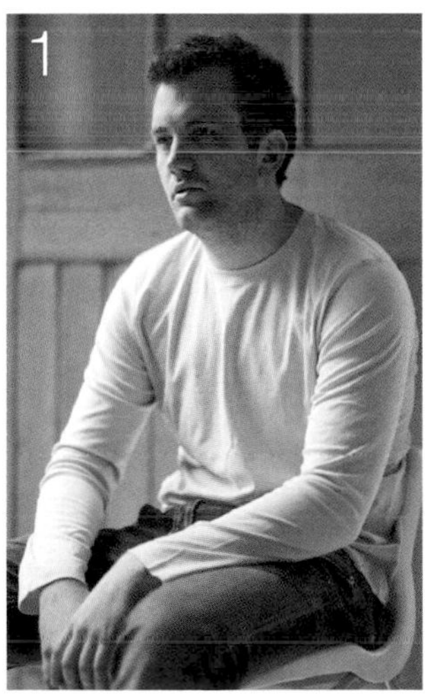

SEIZURES IN CHILDREN

RECOGNITION

- Violent twitching, with clenched fists and an arched back.

There may also be:

- Obvious signs of fever: hot, flushed skin and perhaps sweating;
- Twitching of the face and squinting, fixed or upturned eyes;
- Breath-holding, with red, "puffy" face and neck and drooling at the mouth;
- Loss of or impaired consciousness.

YOUR AIMS

- To protect the child from injury during the seizure.
- To cool the child.
- To reassure the parents.
- To arrange removal to hospital.

See also
The unconscious casualty **pp.54–85**

In young children, seizures – sometimes called fits or convulsions – are most often the result of a raised body temperature associated with a throat or ear infection or other infections. This type of seizure, also known as a febrile seizure, occurs because the electrical systems in the brain are not mature enough to deal with the body's high temperature.

Although seizures can be alarming, they are rarely dangerous if properly dealt with. However, you should always seek medical advice for the child to rule out any serious underlying condition.

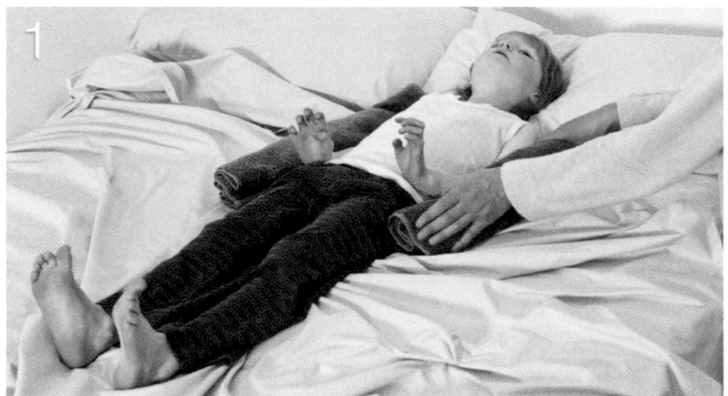

1 **Place pillows or soft padding around the child so that even violent movement will not result in injury. Do not restrain the child in any way.**

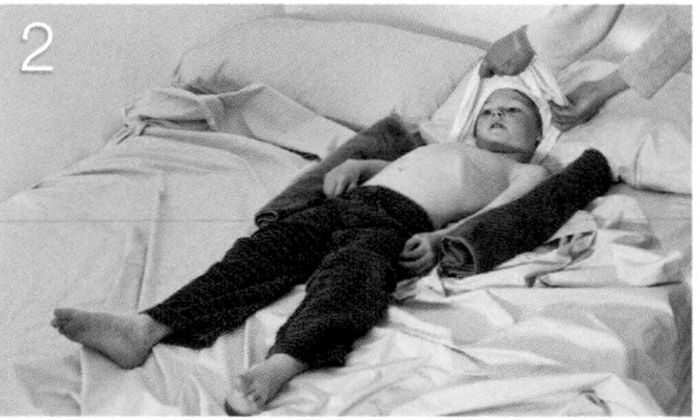

2 **Cool the child. Remove any bedding and clothes, for example T-shirt or pyjama top; you may have to wait until the seizure stops. Ensure a good supply of fresh air (but be careful not to overcool the child).**

3 **Once the seizures have stopped, maintain an open airway by placing the casualty in the recovery position. Call 999/112 for emergency help.**

4 **Reassure the child as well as the parents or carer. Monitor and record vital signs – level of response, breathing and pulse (pp.52–53) – until emergency help arrives.**

SPINAL INJURY

RECOGNITION

When the vertebrae are damaged, there may be:

- Pain in the neck or back at the injury site. This may be masked by other, more painful, injuries;
- Step, irregularity or twist in the normal curve of the spine;
- Tenderness and /or bruising in the skin over the spine.

When the spinal cord is damaged, there may be:

- Loss of control over limbs; movement may be weak or absent;
- Loss of sensation, or abnormal sensations such as burning or tingling; a casualty may tell you that his limbs feel stiff, heavy or clumsy;
- Loss of bladder and/or bowel control;
- Breathing difficulties.

See also
Head injury p.165
Impaired consciousness p.164
Mechanisms of injury p.42

Injuries to the spine can involve one or more parts of the back and/or neck: the bones (vertebrae), the discs of tissue that separate the vertebrae, the surrounding muscles and ligaments, or the spinal cord and the nerves that branch off from it.

The most serious risk associated with spinal injury is damage to the spinal cord. Such damage can cause loss of power and/or sensation below the injured area. The spinal cord or nerve roots can suffer temporary damage if they are pinched by displaced or dislocated discs, or by fragments of broken bone. If the cord is partly or completely severed, damage may be permanent.

The most important indicator is the mechanism of the injury. Suspect spinal injury if abnormal forces have been exerted on the back or neck, and particularly if a casualty complains of any changes in sensation or difficulties with movement. If the incident involved violent forward or backward bending, or twisting of the spine, you must assume that the casualty has a spinal injury. You must take particular care to avoid unnecessary movement of the head, neck and spine at all times.

Although spinal cord injury may occur without any damage to the vertebrae, spinal fracture greatly increases the risk. The areas that are most vulnerable are the bones in the neck and those in the lower back.

Any of the following incidents should alert you to a possible spinal injury:

- **Falling from a height,** such as a ladder;
- **Falling awkwardly,** for instance, while doing gymnastics or trampolining;
- **Diving into a shallow pool** and hitting the bottom;
- **Falling from a horse** or motorbike;
- **Collapsed rugby scrum;**
- **Sudden deceleration** in a motor vehicle;
- **A heavy object falling** across the back;
- **Injury to the head** or the face.

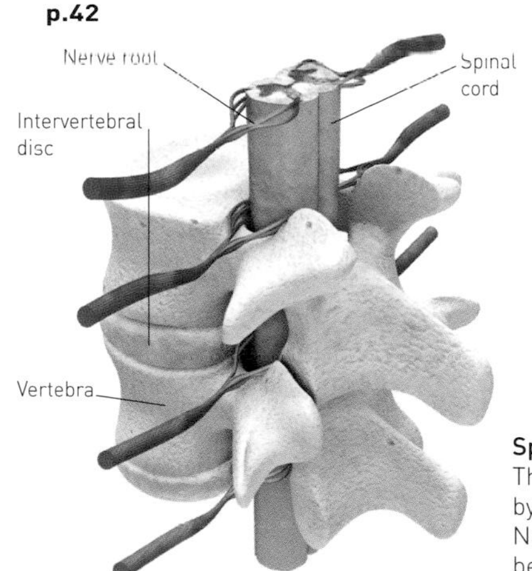

Spinal cord protection
The spinal cord is protected by the bony vertebral (spinal) column. Nerves branching from the cord emerge between adjacent vertebrae.

SPINAL INJURY (continued)

TREATING A CONSCIOUS CASUALTY WITH SPINAL INJURY

YOUR AIMS

- To prevent further injury.
- To arrange urgent removal to hospital.

CAUTION

- Do not move the casualty from the position in which you found her unless she is in immediate danger.
- If the casualty has to be moved, use the log-roll technique (opposite).

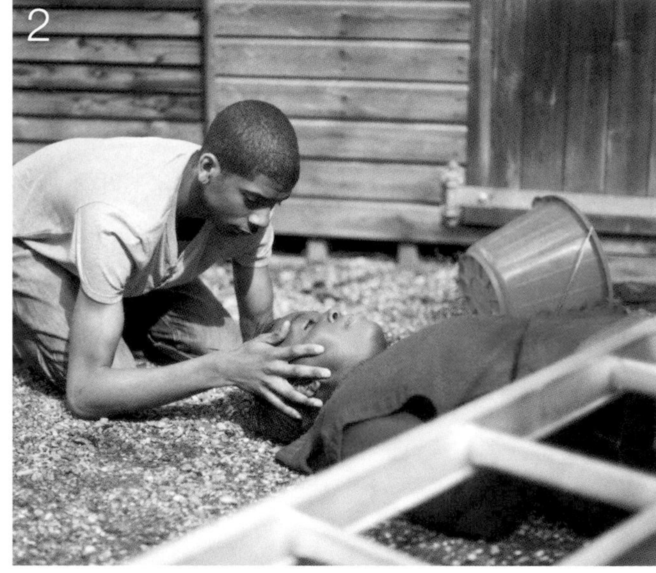
2

1 Reassure the casualty and advise her not to move. **Call 999/112 for emergency help**, or ask a helper to do this.

2 Kneel or lie behind the casualty's head. Rest your elbows on the ground or on your knees to keep your arms steady. Grasp the sides of the casualty's head. Spread your fingers so that you do not cover her ears – she needs to be able to hear you. Steady and support her head in this neutral position, in which the head, neck and spine are aligned.

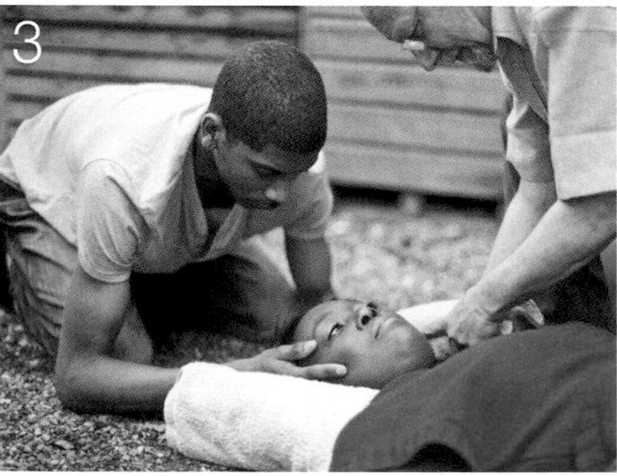
3

3 Ask a helper to place rolled-up blankets, towels or items of clothing on either side of the casualty's head and neck, while you keep her head in the neutral position. Continue to support the casualty's head until emergency services take over, no matter how long this may be.

4 Get your helper to monitor and record vital signs – level of response, breathing and pulse (pp.52–53) – while waiting for help.

TREATING AN UNCONSCIOUS CASUALTY WITH SPINAL INJURY

YOUR AIMS

- To maintain an open airway.
- To begin CPR if necessary.
- To prevent further spinal damage.
- To arrange urgent removal to hospital.

CAUTION

- If the casualty has to be moved and you have help, use the log roll technique (below).
- If you are alone and you need to leave the casualty to call for emergency help, and if the casualty is unable to maintain an open airway, you should place her in the recovery position (pp.64–65) before you leave her.

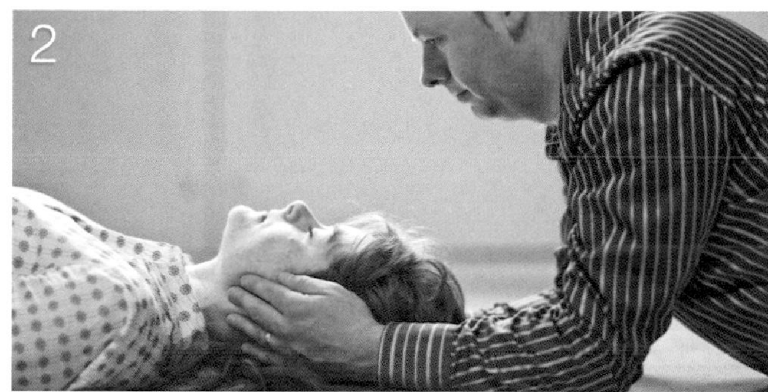

1 Kneel or lie behind the casualty's head. Rest your elbows on the ground or on your knees to keep your arms steady. Grasp the sides of her head. Support her head so that her head, trunk and legs are in a straight line.

2 Open the casualty's airway using the jaw-thrust technique. Place your fingertips at the angles of her jaw. Gently lift the jaw to open the airway. Take care not to tilt the casualty's neck.

3 Check the casualty's breathing. If she is breathing, continue to support her head. **Call 999/112 for emergency help** or ask a helper to do this.

4 If the casualty is not breathing, begin CPR (pp.66–67). If you need to turn the casualty, use the log-roll technique (below).

5 Monitor and record vital signs – level of response, breathing and pulse (pp.52–53) – while waiting for help.

SPECIAL CASE LOG-ROLL TECHNIQUE

1 This technique should be used to turn a casualty with a spinal injury. While you support the casualty's head and neck, ask your helpers to straighten her limbs gently. Position three people along one side to pull the casualty towards them, and two on the other to guide her forwards. The person at the legs should place her hands under the furthest leg. The middle helper supports the casualty's leg and hip.

2 Direct your helpers to roll the casualty. Keep the casualty's head, trunk and legs in a straight line at all times; the upper leg should be supported in a slightly raised position to keep the spine straight.

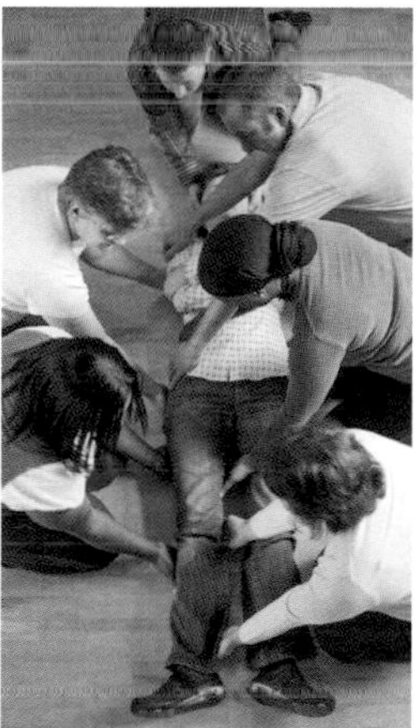

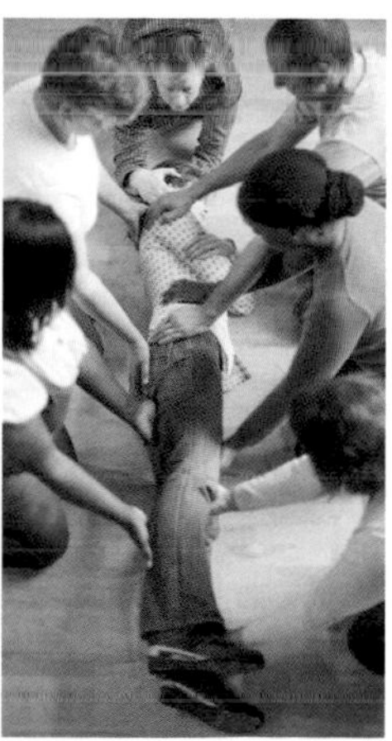

STROKE

RECOGNITION

- Facial weakness – the casualty is unable to smile evenly and the mouth or eye may be droopy.
- Arm weakness – the casualty is only able to raise one arm.
- Speech problems – the casualty is unable to speak clearly.

There may also be:

- Sudden weakness or numbness of the face, arm or leg on one or both sides of the body;
- Sudden loss or blurring of vision in one or both eyes;
- Sudden difficulty with speech or understanding the spoken word;
- Sudden confusion;
- Sudden severe headache with no apparent cause;
- Dizziness, unsteadiness or sudden fall.

YOUR AIMS

- To arrange urgent admission to hospital.
- To reassure and comfort the casualty.

CAUTION

- Be aware of signs of cerebral compression.
- If the person loses consciousness, open the airway and check breathing (The unconscious casualty pp.54–85).

A stroke or brain attack is a medical emergency that occurs when the blood supply to the brain is disrupted. Strokes are the third most common cause of death in the UK and many people live with long-term disability as a result of a stroke. This condition is more common later in life and is associated with disorders of the circulatory system, such as high blood pressure.

The majority of strokes are caused by a clot in a blood vessel that blocks the flow of blood to the brain. However, some strokes are the result of a ruptured blood vessel that causes bleeding into the brain. If a stroke is due to a blood clot, it may be possible to give drugs to limit the extent of damage to the brain and improve recovery. The earlier the casualty receives care in hospital, the better.

Use the FAST (Face-Arm-Speech-Time) guide if you suspect a casualty has had a stroke:

F – Facial weakness – the casualty is unable to smile evenly and the mouth or eye may be droopy;

A – Arm weakness – the casualty is only able to raise one of his arms;

S – Speech problems – the casualty is unable to speak clearly or may not understand the spoken word;

T – Time to call 999/112 for emergency help if you suspect that the casualty has had a stroke.

TRANSIENT ISCHAEMIC ATTACK (TIA)

A transient ischaemic attack, or TIA, is sometimes called a mini-stroke. It is similar to a full stroke, but the symptoms may only last a few minutes, will improve and eventually disappear. If you suspect a TIA, it is important to seek medical advice to confirm the casualty's condition. If there is any doubt assume that it is a stroke.

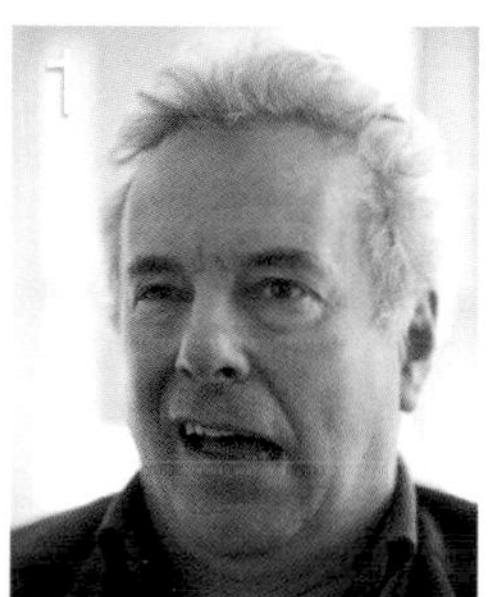

1 Look at the casualty's face. Ask him to smile: if he has had a stroke he may only be able to smile on one side – the other side of his mouth may droop.

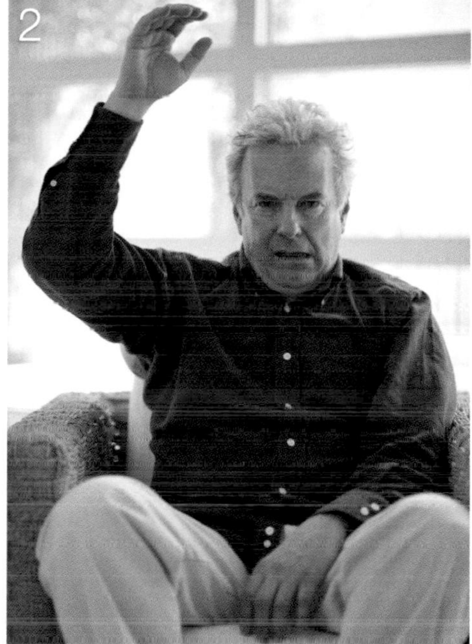

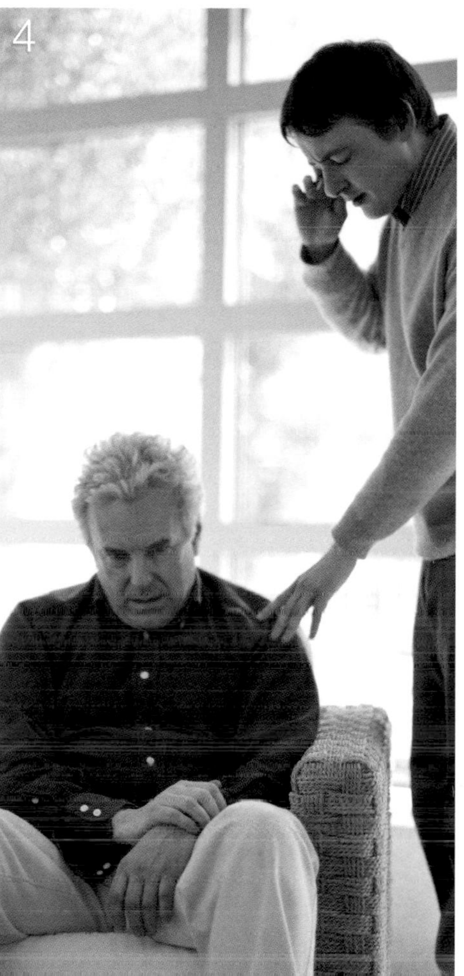

2 Ask the casualty to raise both his arms: if he has had a stroke, he may only be able to lift one arm.

3 Find out whether the person can speak clearly and understand what you say. When you ask a question does he respond appropriately?

4 **Call 999/112 for emergency help.** Tell ambulance control that you have used the FAST guide and you suspect a stroke.

5 Keep the casualty comfortable and supported. If the casualty is conscious, you can help him to lie down. Reassure him that help is on its way.

6 Regularly monitor and record vital signs – level of response, breathing and pulse (pp.52–53) – while waiting for help to arrive. Do not give the casualty anything to eat or drink since it may be difficult for him to swallow.

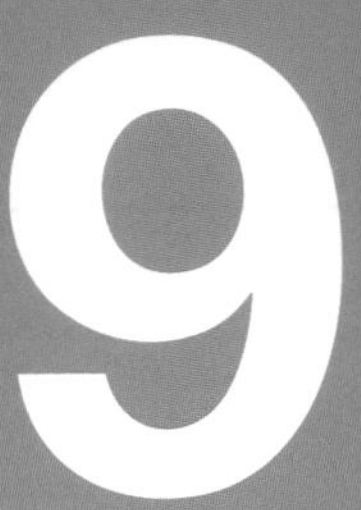

This chapter deals with the effects of injuries and illnesses caused by environmental factors such as extremes of heat and cold.

The skin protects the body and helps to maintain body temperature within a normal range. It can be damaged by fire, hot liquids or caustic substances. This chapter contains advice on how to assess burns, whether minor or severe.

The effects of temperature extremes can also impair skin and other body functions. Injuries may be localised – such as frostbite or sunburn – or generalised, as in heat exhaustion or hypothermia. Young children and the elderly are most susceptible to problems caused by extremes of temperature.

AIMS AND OBJECTIVES

- To assess the casualty's condition quickly and calmly.
- To comfort and reassure the casualty.
- To call 999/112 for emergency help if you suspect a serious illness or injury.
- To be aware of your own needs.

For burns:

- To protect yourself and the casualty from danger;
- To assess the burn, prevent further damage and relieve symptoms.

For extremes of temperature:

- To protect the casualty from heat or cold;
- To restore normal body temperature.

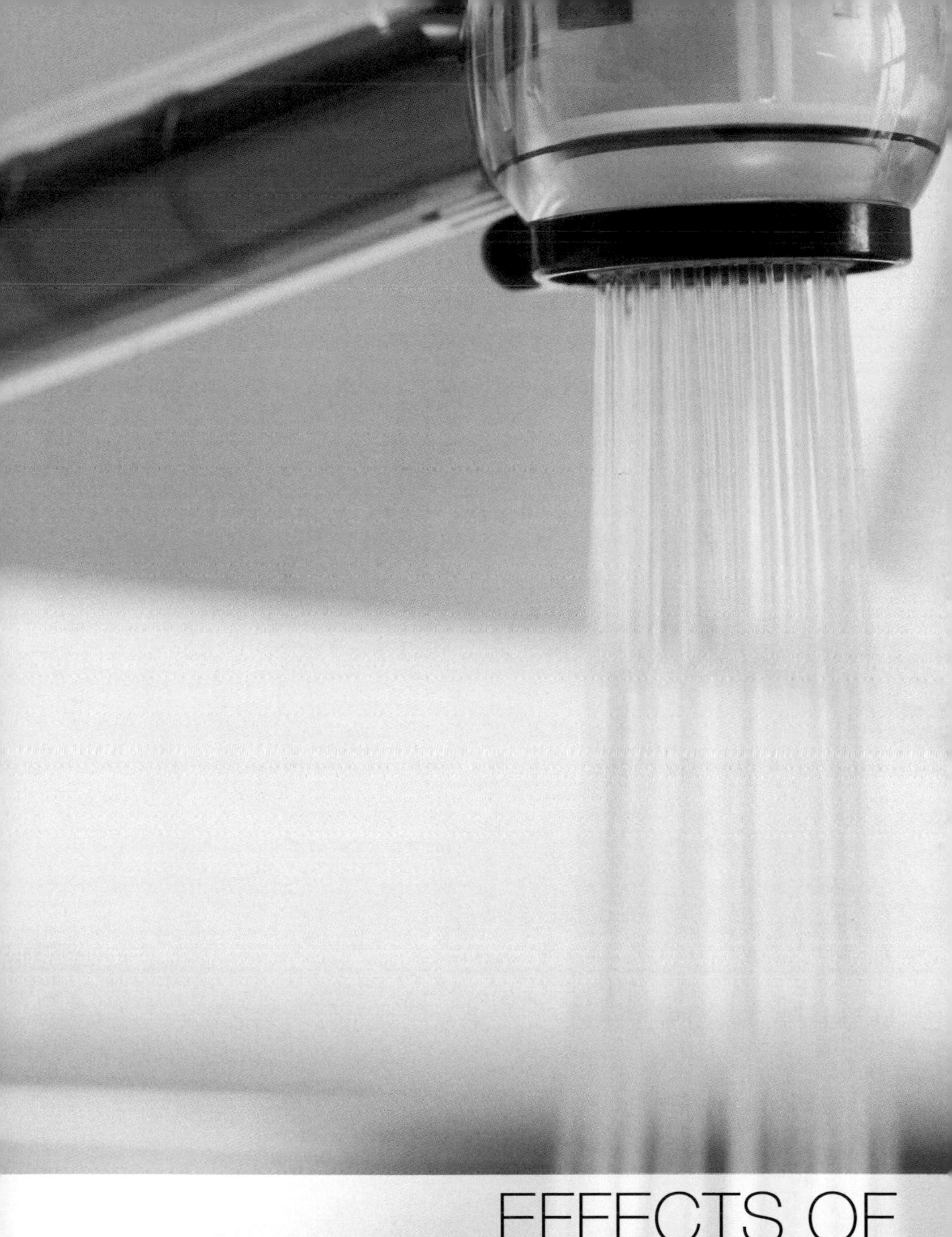

EFFECTS OF HEAT AND COLD

THE SKIN

One of the largest organs, the skin plays key roles in protecting the body from injury and infection and in maintaining the body at a constant temperature.

The skin consists of two layers of tissue – an outer layer (epidermis) and an inner layer (dermis) – which lie on a layer of fatty tissue (subcutaneous fat). The top part of the epidermis is made up of dead, flattened skin cells, which are constantly shed and replaced by new cells made in the lower part of this layer. The epidermis is protected by an oily substance called sebum – secreted from glands called sebaceous glands – which keeps the skin supple and waterproof.

The lower layer of the skin, the dermis, contains the blood vessels, nerves, muscles, sebaceous glands, sweat glands and hair roots (follicles). The ends of sensory nerves within the dermis register sensations from the body's surface, such as heat, cold, pain and even the slightest touch. Blood vessels supply the skin with nutrients and help to regulate body temperature by preserving or releasing heat (opposite).

Structure of the skin
The skin is made up of two layers: the thin, outer epidermis and the thicker dermis beneath it. Most of the structures of the skin, such as blood vessels, nerves and hair roots, are contained within the dermis.

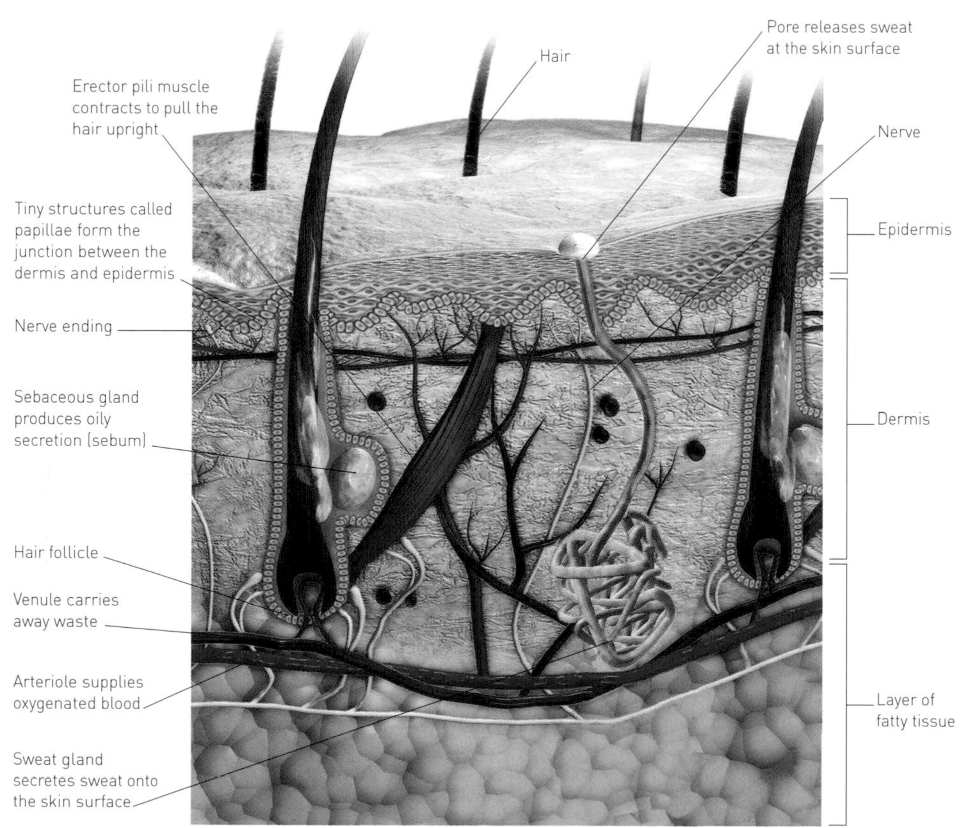

MAINTAINING BODY TEMPERATURE

One of the major functions of the skin is to help maintain the body temperature within its optimum range of 36–37°C (97–99°F). An organ in the brain called the hypothalamus regulates body temperature. If the temperature of blood passing through this thermostat falls or rises to a level outside the optimum range, various mechanisms are activated to either warm or cool the body as necessary.

HOW THE BODY KEEPS WARM

When the body becomes too cold, changes take place to prevent heat from escaping. Blood vessels at the body surface narrow (constrict) to keep warm blood in the main part (core) of the body. The activity of the sweat glands is reduced, and hairs stand on end to "trap" warm air close to the skin. In addition to the mechanisms that prevent heat loss, other body systems act to produce more warmth. The rate of metabolism is increased. Heat is also generated by muscle activity, which may be either voluntary (for example, during physical exercise) or, in cold conditions, involuntary (shivering).

HOW THE BODY LOSES HEAT

In hot conditions, the body activates a number of mechanisms to encourage heat loss and thus prevent the body temperature from becoming too high. Blood vessels that lie in or just under the skin widen (dilate). As a result, blood flow to the body surface increases and more heat is lost. In addition, the sweat glands become more active and secrete more sweat. This sweat then cools the skin as it evaporates.

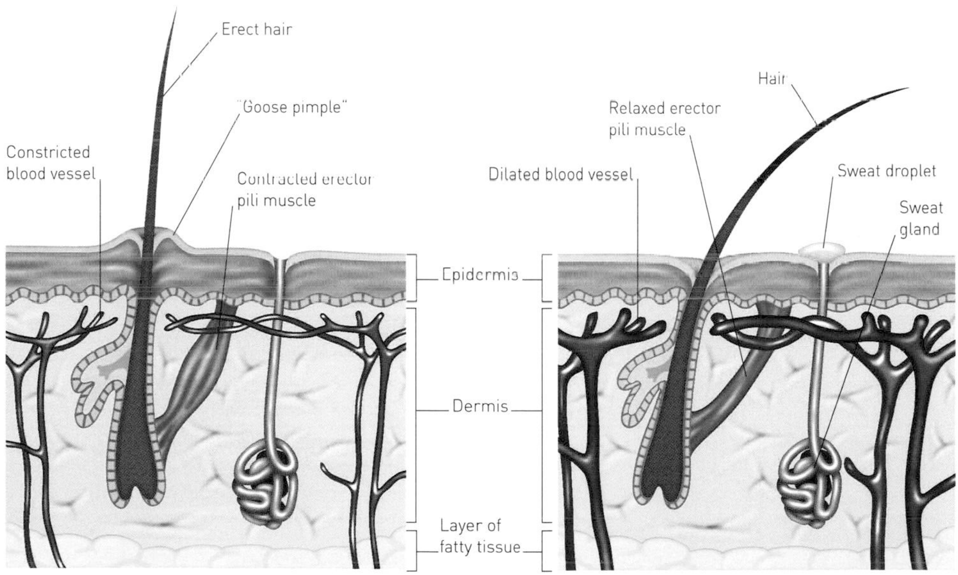

How skin responds to low body temperature
Blood vessels narrow (constrict) to reduce blood flow to the skin. The erector pili muscles contract, making the hairs stand upright and trap warm air close to the skin.

How skin responds to high body temperature
Blood vessels widen (dilate), making the skin appear flushed, and heat is lost. Sweat glands become active and produce sweat droplets, which evaporate to cool the skin.

ASSESSING A BURN

When skin is damaged by burning, it can no longer function effectively as a natural barrier against infection. In addition, body fluid may be lost because tiny blood vessels in the skin leak tissue fluid (serum). This fluid either collects under the skin to form blisters or leaks through the surface.

There may be related injuries, significant fluid loss and infection may develop later.

WHAT TO ASSESS

It is particularly important to consider the circumstances in which the burn has occurred; whether or not the airway is likely to have been affected; and the extent, location and depth of the burn.

There are many possible causes of burns (below). By establishing the cause of the burn, you may be able to identify any other potential problems that could result. For example, a fire in an enclosed space is likely to have produced poisonous carbon monoxide gas, or other toxic fumes may have been released if burning material was involved. If the casualty's airway has been affected, he may have difficulty breathing and will need urgent medical attention and admission to hospital.

The extent of the burn will also indicate whether or not shock is likely to develop. Shock is a life-threatening condition and occurs whenever there is a serious loss of body fluids (p.116). In a burn that covers a large area of the body, fluid loss will be significant and the risk of shock high.

If the burn is on a limb, fluid may collect in the tissues around it, causing swelling and pain. This build-up of fluid is particularly serious if the limb is being constricted, for example by clothing or footwear.

Burns allow germs to enter the skin and so carry a serious risk of infection. The risk of infection increases with the depth of the burn.

TYPES OF BURN AND POSSIBLE CAUSES

TYPE OF BURN	CAUSES
Dry burn	▪ Flames ▪ Contact with hot objects, such as domestic appliances or cigarettes ▪ Friction – for example, rope burns
Scald	▪ Steam ▪ Hot liquids, such as tea and coffee, or hot fat
Electrical burn	▪ Low-voltage current, as used by domestic appliances ▪ High-voltage currents, as carried in mains overhead cables ▪ Lightning strikes
Cold injury	▪ Frostbite ▪ Contact with freezing metals ▪ Contact with freezing vapours, such as liquid oxygen or liquid nitrogen
Chemical burn	▪ Industrial chemicals, including inhaled fumes and corrosive gases ▪ Domestic chemicals and agents, such as paint stripper, caustic soda, weed killers, bleach, oven cleaner or any other strong acid or alkali chemical
Radiation burn	▪ Sunburn ▪ Over-exposure to ultraviolet rays from a sunlamp ▪ Exposure to a radioactive source, such as an X-ray

DEPTH OF BURNS

Burns are classified according to the depth of skin damage. There are three depths: superficial, partial-thickness and full-thickness. A casualty may suffer one or more depths of burn in a single incident.

A superficial burn involves only the outermost layer of skin, the epidermis. This type of injury usually heals well if first aid is given promptly and if blisters do not form. Sunburn is one of the most common types of superficial burn. Other causes include minor domestic incidents. Partial-thickness burns are very painful, destroying the epidermis and causing the skin to become red and blistered. They usually heal well, but can be serious if they affect more than 20 per cent of the body in an adult and 10 per cent in a child.

In full-thickness burns, pain sensation can be lost, which masks the severity of the injury. The skin may look waxy, pale or charred and needs urgent medical attention.

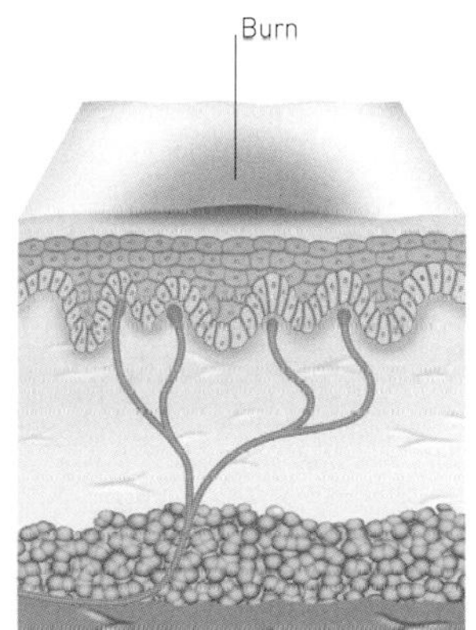

Superficial burn
This type of burn involves only the outermost layer of skin. Superficial burns are characterised by redness, swelling and tenderness.

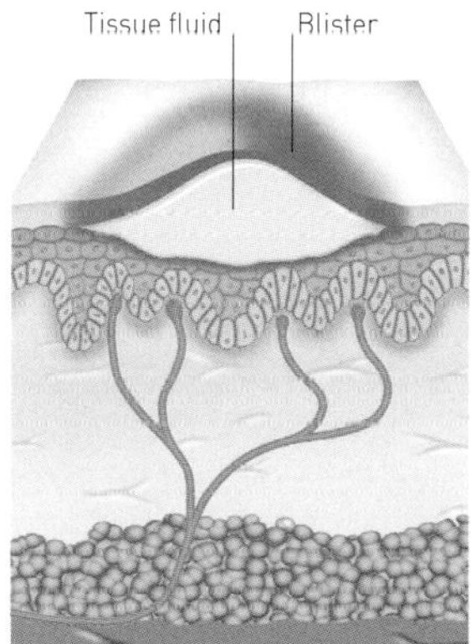

Partial-thickness burn
This affects the epidermis, and the skin becomes red and raw. Blisters form over the skin due to fluid released from the damaged tissues beneath.

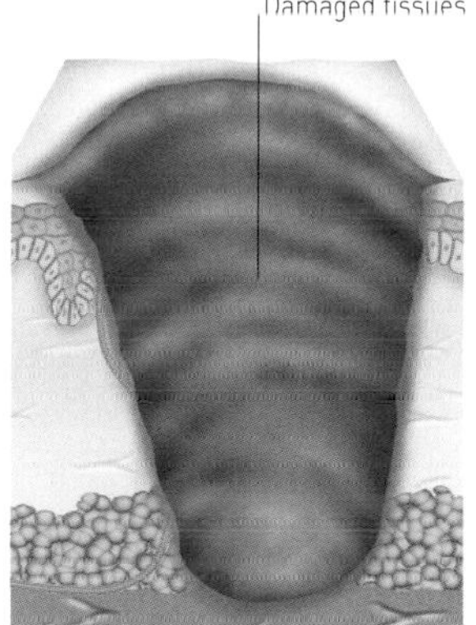

Full-thickness burn
With this type of burn, all the layers of the skin are affected; there may be some damage to nerves, fat tissue, muscles and blood vessels.

BURNS THAT NEED HOSPITAL TREATMENT

If the casualty is a child, seek medical advice or take the child to hospital, however small the burn appears. For adults, medical attention should be sought for any serious burn. Such burns include:

- All full-thickness burns;
- All burns involving the face, hands, feet or genital area;
- All burns that extend right around an arm or a leg;
- All partial-thickness burns larger than one per cent of the body surface (an area the size of the casualty's palm and fingers);
- All superficial burns larger than five per cent of the casualty's body surface (equivalent to five palm areas);
- Burns comprising a mixed pattern of varying depths.

If you are unsure about the severity of any burn, seek medical advice.

SEVERE BURNS AND SCALDS

RECOGNITION

There may be:

- Possible areas of superficial, partial thickness and/or full-thickness burns;
- Pain;
- Difficulty breathing;
- Features of shock (pp.116–17).

YOUR AIMS

- To stop the burning and relieve pain.
- To maintain an open airway.
- To treat associated injuries.
- To minimise the risk of infection.
- To minimise the risk of shock.
- To arrange urgent removal to hospital.
- To gather information for the emergency services.

See also
Burns to the airway **p.185**
Fires **pp.32–33**
Shock **pp.116–17**

Take great care when treating burns that are deep or extensive. The longer the burning continues, the more severe the injury will be. If the casualty has been injured in a fire, you should assume that smoke or hot air has also affected his breathing.

Your priorities are to cool the burn (which stops the burning process and relieves the pain) and to monitor his breathing. A casualty with a severe burn or scald injury will almost certainly be suffering from shock because of the fluid loss and will need urgent hospital treatment.

The possibility of non-accidental injury must always be considered, no matter what the age of the casualty. Keep an accurate record of what has happened and any treatment you have given. If you have to remove or cut away clothing, keep it in case of future investigation.

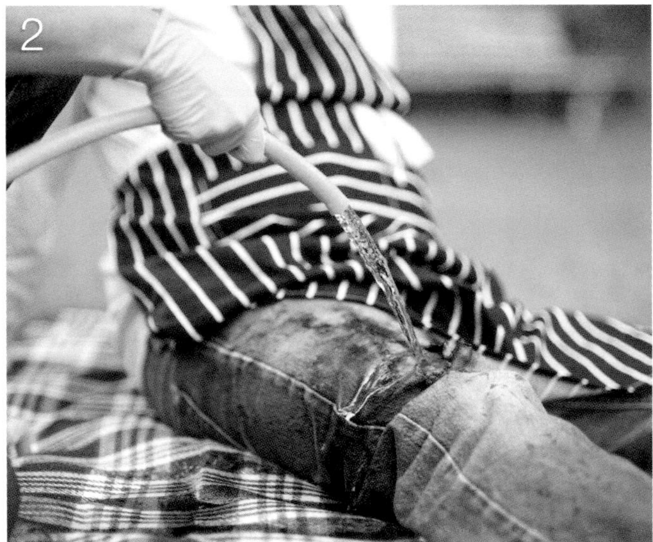

1 Help the casualty to sit or lie down. If possible, try to prevent the burnt area from coming into contact with the ground.

2 Start cooling the injury. Flood the burn with plenty of cold water, but do not delay the casualty's removal to hospital. **Call 999/112 for emergency help**; if possible, get someone to do this while you cool the burn.

3 Continue cooling the affected area for at least ten minutes, or until the pain is relieved. Watch for signs of breathing difficulty. Do not over-cool the casualty because you may lower the body temperature to a dangerous level. This is a particular hazard for babies and elderly people.

CAUTION

- Do not remove anything sticking to the burn; you may cause further damage and introduce infection into the burnt area.
- Do not burst any blisters.
- Do not apply any type of lotion or ointment to the burnt area; it may damage tissues and increase the risk of infection.
- The use of specialised dressings, sprays and gels to cool burns is not recommended.
- Do not use adhesive dressings or apply adhesive tape to the skin; a burn may be more extensive than it first appears.
- If the casualty has a burn on his face, do not cover the injury; you could cause the casualty distress and obstruct the airway.
- Do not allow the casualty to eat or drink because he may need an anaesthetic.

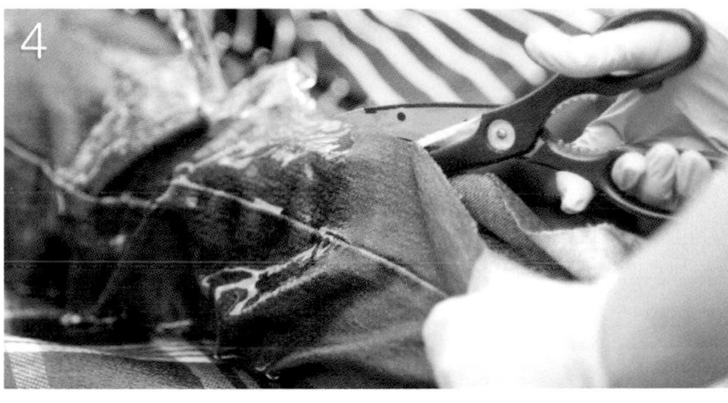

4 Do not touch or otherwise interfere with the burn. Gently remove any rings, watches, belts, shoes and burnt or smouldering clothing before the tissues begin to swell. A helper can do this while you are cooling the burn. Do not remove clothing that is stuck to the burn.

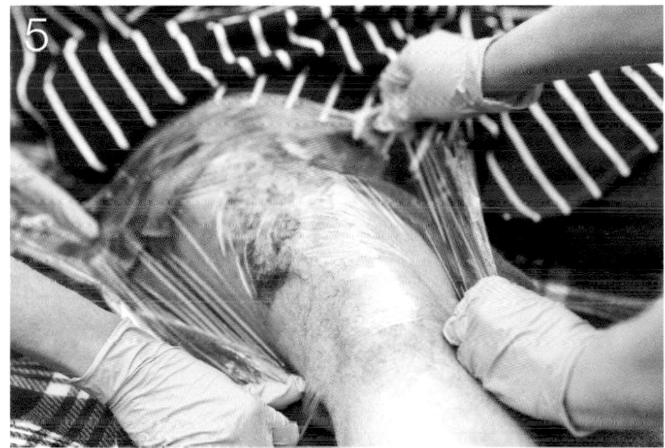

5 Cover the injured area with kitchen film to protect it from infection. Discard the first two turns from the roll and then apply it lengthways over the burn. A clean plastic bag can be used to cover a hand or foot; secure it with a bandage or adhesive tape applied over the plastic, not the damaged skin. If there is no plastic film available, use a sterile dressing, or improvise with non-fluffy material, such as a folded triangular bandage (p.249).

6 Reassure the casualty and treat him for shock (pp.116–17) if necessary. Record details of the casualty's injuries. Monitor and record his vital signs – level of response, breathing and pulse (pp.52–53) – while waiting for help.

MINOR BURNS AND SCALDS

RECOGNITION

- Reddened skin.
- Pain in the area of the burn.

Later there may be:

- Blistering of the affected skin.

YOUR AIMS

- To stop the burning.
- To relieve pain and swelling.
- To minimise the risk of infection.

CAUTION

- Do not break blisters or otherwise interfere with the injured area.
- Do not apply adhesive dressings or adhesive tape to the skin; removing them may tear damaged skin.
- Do not apply ointments or fats; they may damage tissues and increase the risk of infection.
- The use of specialised dressings, sprays and gels to cool burns is not recommended.
- Do not put blister plasters on blisters caused by a burn.

See also
Assessing a burn pp.180–81

SPECIAL CASE BLISTERS

Never burst a blister; they usually need no treatment. However, if a blister breaks or is likely to burst, cover it with a non-adhesive sterile dressing that extends well beyond the edges of the blister. Leave the dressing in place until the blister subsides.

Small, superficial burns and scalds are often due to domestic incidents, such as touching a hot iron or spilling boiling water on the skin. Most minor burns can be treated successfully by first aid and will heal naturally. However, you should advise the casualty to seek medical advice if you are at all concerned about the severity of the injury (Assessing a burn pp.180–81).

After a burn, blisters may form. These thin "bubbles" are caused by tissue fluid leaking into the burnt area just beneath the skin's surface. You should never break a blister caused by a burn because you may introduce infection into the wound.

1 **Flood the injured part with cold water for at least ten minutes or until the pain is relieved. If water is not available, any cold, harmless liquid, such as milk or canned drinks, can be used.**

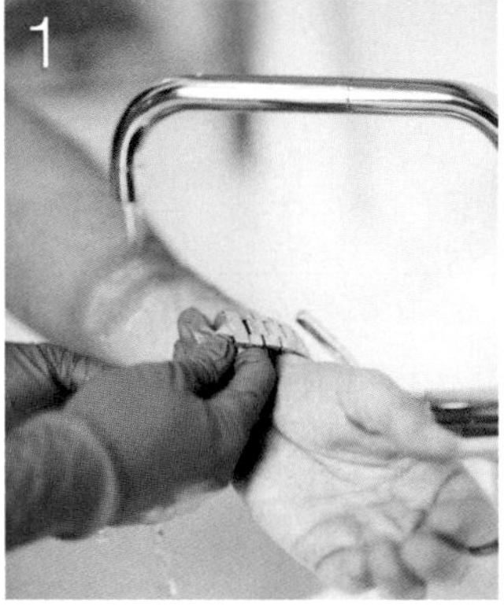

2 **Gently remove any jewellery, watches, belts or constricting clothing from the injured area before it begins to swell.**

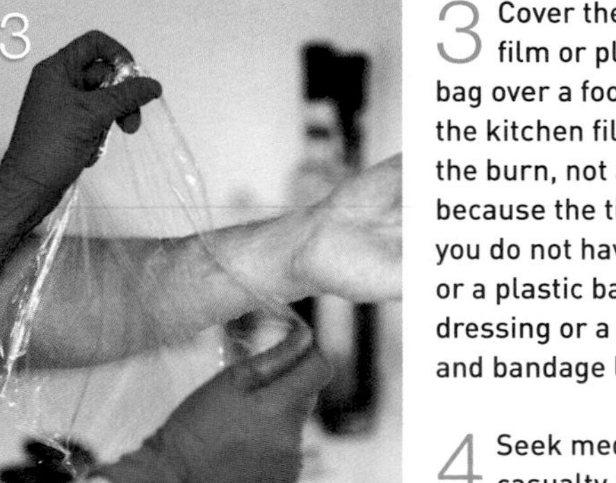

3 **Cover the burn with kitchen film or place a clean plastic bag over a foot or hand. Apply the kitchen film lengthways over the burn, not around the limb because the tissues swell. If you do not have kitchen film or a plastic bag, use a sterile dressing or a non-fluffy pad, and bandage loosely in place.**

4 **Seek medical advice if the casualty is a child, or if you are in any doubt about the casualty's condition.**

BURNS TO THE AIRWAY

RECOGNITION

There may be:

- Soot around the nose or mouth;
- Singeing of the nasal hairs;
- Redness, swelling or actual burning of the tongue;
- Damage to the skin around the mouth;
- Hoarseness of the voice;
- Breathing difficulties.

YOUR AIMS

- To maintain an open airway.
- To arrange urgent removal to hospital.

CAUTION

If the casualty loses consciousness, open the airway and check breathing (The unconscious casualty pp.54–85).

Any burn to the face and/or within the mouth or throat is very serious because the air passages rapidly become swollen. Usually, signs of burning will be evident. Always suspect damage to the airway if a casualty sustains burns in a confined space since he is likely to have inhaled hot air or gases.

There is no specific first aid treatment for an extreme case of burns to the airway; the swelling will rapidly block the airway, and there is a serious risk of hypoxia. Immediate and specialised medical help is required.

See also
Hypoxia **p.90**
Shock **pp.116–17**
The unconscious casualty **pp.54–85**

1 **Call 999/112 for emergency help.** Tell ambulance control that you suspect burns to the casualty's airway.

2 **Take any steps possible to improve the casualty's air supply, such as loosening clothing around his neck.**

3 **Offer the casualty ice or small sips of cold water to reduce swelling and pain.**

4 **Reassure the casualty. Monitor and record vital signs – level of response, breathing and pulse (pp.52–53) – while waiting for help to arrive.**

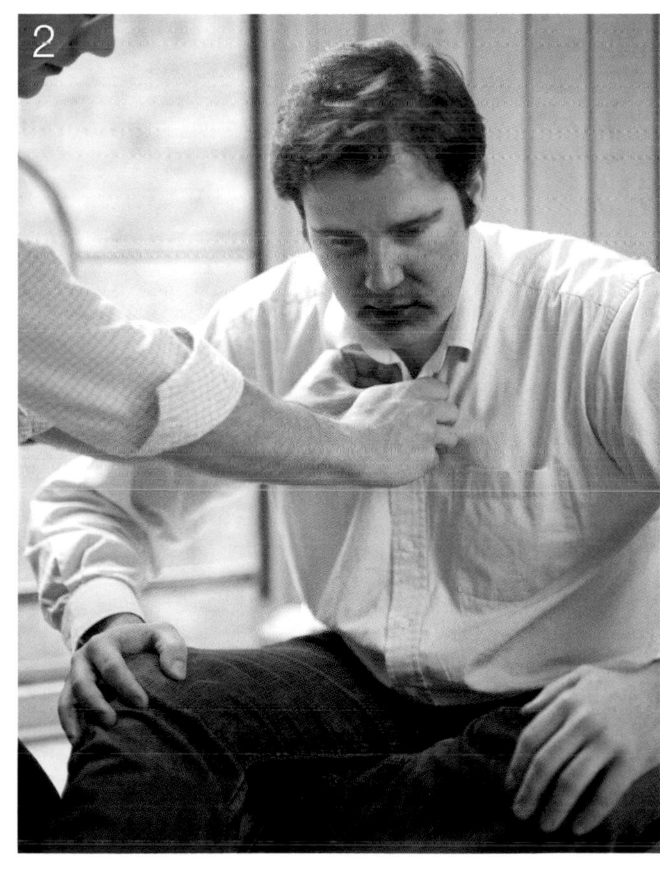
2

ELECTRICAL BURN

RECOGNITION

There may be:

- Unconsciousness;
- Full-thickness burns, with swelling, scorching and charring;
- Burns at points of entry and exit of electricity;
- Signs of shock.

YOUR AIMS

- To treat the burns and shock.
- To arrange urgent removal to hospital.

CAUTION

- Do not approach a victim of high-voltage electricity until you are officially told that the current has been switched off (pp.34–35).
- If the casualty is unconscious, open the airway and check his breathing (The unconscious casualty pp.54–85).

See also
Electrical injury **pp.34–35**
Severe burns and scalds **pp.182–83**
Shock **pp.116–17**
The unconscious casualty **pp.54–85**

Burns may occur when electricity passes through the body. There may be surface damage along the point of contact, or at the points of entry and exit of the current. In addition, there may also be internal damage between the entry and exit points; the position and direction of wounds will alert you to the likely site and extent of hidden injury, and to the degree of shock that the casualty may suffer.

Burns may be caused by a lightning strike or by a low- or high-voltage electric current. Electric shock can cause cardiac arrest. If the casualty is unconscious, your priority, once the area is safe, is to open his airway and check his breathing.

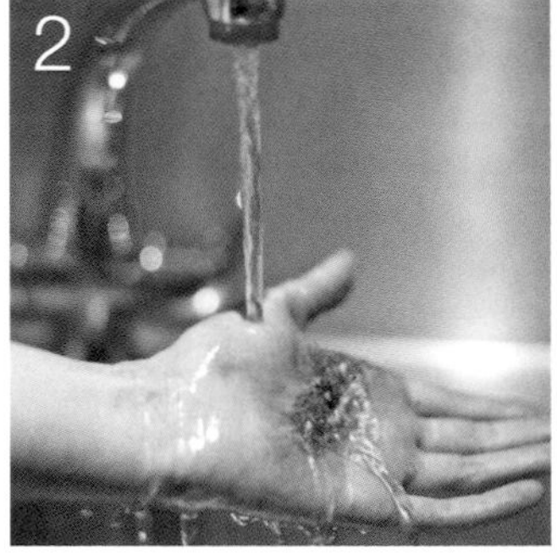

1 Make sure that contact with the electrical source is broken before you touch the casualty (pp.34–35).

2 Flood the injury with cold water (at the entry and exit points if both are present) for at least ten minutes or until pain is relieved. If water is not available, any cold, harmless liquid can be used.

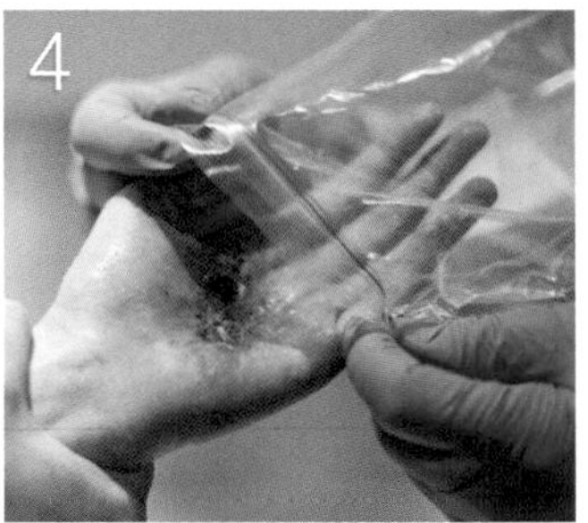

3 Gently remove any jewellery, watches, belts or constricting clothing from the injured area before it begins to swell. Do not touch the burn.

4 Place a clean plastic bag over a burn on a foot or hand, or cover the burn with kitchen film. The burnt tissues will swell. Apply the film along the length of the limb so that it does not become too hot. Tape the bag loosely in place (tape the bag not the skin), or use a sterile dressing or a clean, non-fluffy pad, and bandage loosely.

5 **Call 999/112 for emergency help.** Reassure the casualty and treat him for shock (pp.116–17). Monitor and record vital signs – level of response, breathing and pulse (pp.52–53) – while waiting for help to arrive.

CHEMICAL BURN

RECOGNITION

There may be:

- Evidence of chemicals in the vicinity;
- Intense, stinging pain.

Later:

- Discoloration, blistering and peeling;
- Swelling of the affected area.

YOUR AIMS

- To make the area safe and inform the relevant authority.
- To disperse the harmful chemical.
- To arrange transport to hospital.

CAUTION

- Never attempt to neutralise acid or alkali burns unless trained to do so.
- Do not delay starting treatment by searching for an antidote.
- If the incident occurs in the workplace, notify the safety officer and/or emergency services.

See also
Chemical burn to the eye p.188
Inhalation of fumes pp.96–97

Certain chemicals may irritate, burn or penetrate the skin, causing widespread and sometimes fatal damage. Most strong, corrosive chemicals are found in industry, but chemical burns can also occur in the home; for instance from dishwasher products (the most common cause of alkali burns in children), oven cleaners, pesticides and paint stripper.

Chemical burns are always serious, and the casualty may need urgent hospital treatment. If possible, note the name or brand of the burning substance. Before treating the casualty, ensure the safety of yourself and others because some chemicals give off poisonous fumes, causing breathing difficulties.

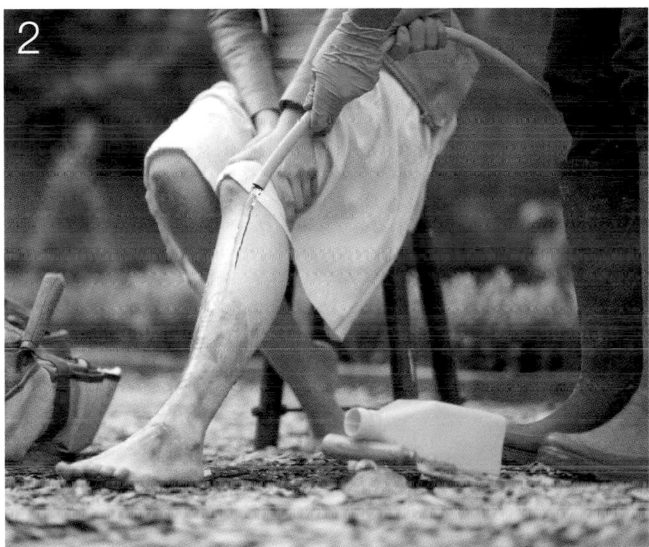

1 Make sure that the area around the casualty is safe. Ventilate the area to disperse fumes. Wear protective gloves to prevent you from coming into contact with the chemical. If it is safe to do so, seal the chemical container. Move the casualty if necessary. If the chemical is in powder form, it can be brushed off the skin.

2 Flood the burn with water for at least 20 minutes to disperse the chemical and stop the burning. If treating a casualty lying on the ground, ensure that the contaminated water does not collect underneath her. Pour water away from yourself to avoid splashes.

3 Gently remove any contaminated clothing while flooding the injury.

4 Arrange to take or send the casualty to hospital. Monitor vital signs – level of response, breathing and pulse (pp.52–53) – while waiting for medical help. Pass on details of the chemical to medical staff if you can identify it.

CHEMICAL BURN TO THE EYE

RECOGNITION

There may be:

- Intense pain in the eye;
- Inability to open the injured eye;
- Redness and swelling around the eye;
- Copious watering of the eye;
- Evidence of chemical substances or containers in the immediate area.

YOUR AIMS

- To disperse the harmful chemical.
- To arrange transport to hospital.

CAUTION

- Do not allow the casualty to touch the injured eye.
- Do not forcibly remove a contact lens.
- If the incident occurred in the workplace, notify the safety officer and/or emergency services.

Splashes of chemicals in the eye can cause serious injury if not treated quickly. Some chemicals damage the surface of the eye, resulting in scarring and even blindness.

Your priority is to wash out (irrigate) the eye so that the chemical is diluted and dispersed. When irrigating the eye, be careful that the contaminated rinsing water does not splash you or the casualty. Before beginning to treat the casualty, put on protective gloves if available.

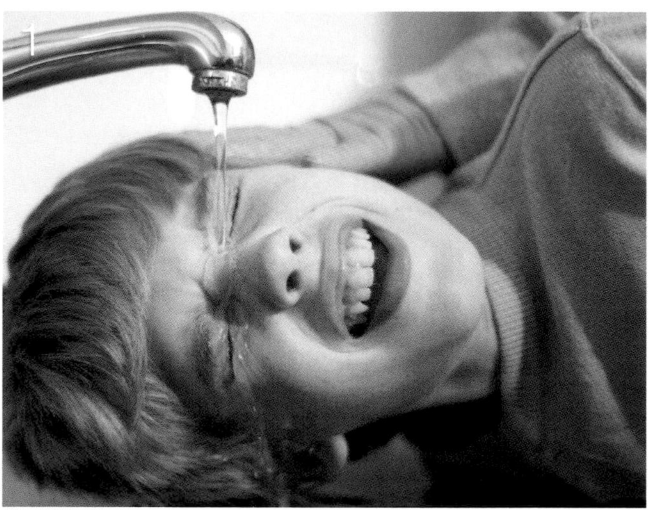

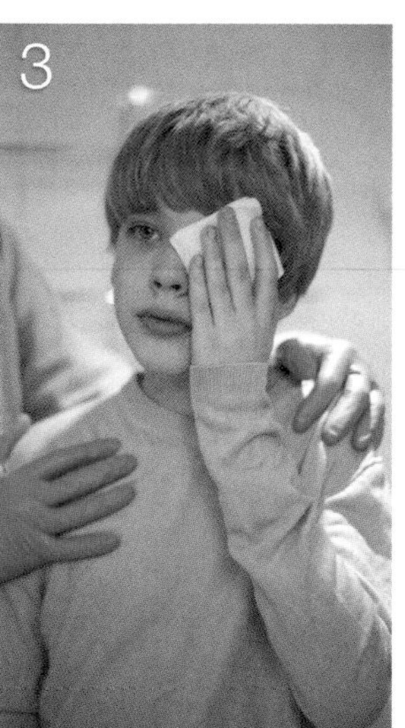

1 Put on protective gloves. Hold the casualty's affected eye under gently running cold water for at least ten minutes. Irrigate the eyelid thoroughly both inside and out; if the casualty's eye is shut in a spasm of pain, gently, but firmly, try to pull the eyelid open.

2 Make sure that contaminated water does not splash the uninjured eye. You may find it easier to pour the water over the eye using an eye irrigator or a glass.

3 Ask the casualty to hold a clean, non-fluffy pad over the injured eye. If it will be some time before the casualty receives medical attention, bandage the pad loosely in position.

4 Arrange to take or send the casualty to hospital. Identify the chemical if possible and pass on details to medical staff.

FLASH BURN TO THE EYE

RECOGNITION

- Intense pain in the affected eye(s).

There may also be:

- A "gritty" feeling in the eye(s);
- Sensitivity to light;
- Redness and watering of the eye(s).

YOUR AIMS

- To prevent further damage.
- To arrange transport to hospital.

CAUTION

- Do not remove the casualty's contact lenses.

This condition occurs when the surface (cornea) of the eye is damaged by exposure to ultraviolet light, such as prolonged glare from sunlight reflected off snow. Symptoms usually develop gradually, and recovery can take up to a week. Flash burns can also be caused by glare from a welder's torch.

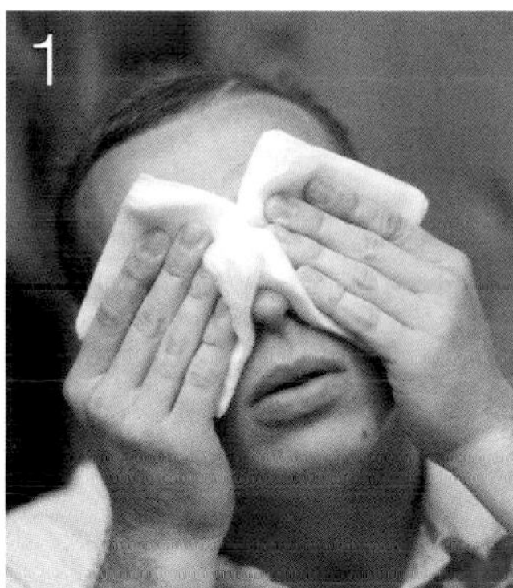

1 Reassure the casualty. Ask him to hold an eye pad against each injured eye. If it is likely to take some time to obtain medical attention, lightly bandage the pad(s) in place.

2 Arrange to take or send the casualty to hospital.

CS SPRAY INJURY

RECOGNITION

There may be:

- Watering of the eyes;
- Coughing and sneezing;
- A burning sensation in the skin, nose and throat;
- Chest tightness and difficulty with breathing;
- Reddening of the skin.

YOUR AIMS

- To get the casualty into fresh air.

CAUTION

- Do not wash any affected part since this will increase the effect of the spray.
- Do not rub any area affected by the spray.

This spray is employed by police forces for riot control and self-protection, and is sometimes used by unauthorised people as a weapon in assaults. CS spray irritates the eyes and upper airways and may cause vomiting. The effects usually wear off within minutes, although the eyes may remain sore for longer.

If CS spray is used on a person who suffers from asthma, it may induce an attack.

See also
Allergy **p.220**
Asthma **p.100**

1 Move the casualty to a well-ventilated area and reassure him that the symptoms will soon disappear – he may be very agitated. Try to prevent the casualty from rubbing his eyes.

2 If the casualty's eyes are painful, fan them to help speed up the vaporisation of any remaining CS chemical.

DEHYDRATION

RECOGNITION

There may be:

- Dry mouth and dry eyes;
- Dry and/or cracked lips;
- Headaches (light-headedness);
- Dizziness and confusion;
- Dark urine;
- Reduction in the amount of urine passed;
- Cramp, with a feeling of tightness in the most used muscles, such as the calves.
- In babies and young children, pale skin with sunken eyes. In young babies the soft spot on the head (the fontanelle) may be sunken.

YOUR AIMS

- To replace the lost body fluids and salts

See also
Cramp **p.159**
Heat exhaustion **p.192**

This condition occurs when the amount of fluids lost from the body is not adequately replaced. Dehydration can begin to develop when a person loses as little as one per cent of his bodyweight through fluid loss. A two to six per cent loss can occur during a typical period of exercise on a warm day; the average daily intake of fluids is 2.5 litres (4 pints). This fluid loss needs to be replaced. In addition to fluid, the body loses essential body salts through sweating.

Dehydration is mainly the result of: excessive sweating during sporting activities, especially in hot weather; prolonged exposure to sun, or hot, humid conditions; sweating through raised body temperature during a fever; and loss of fluid through severe diarrhoea and vomiting. Young children, older people or those involved in prolonged periods of activity are particularly at risk. Severe dehydration can cause muscle cramps through the loss of body salts. If untreated, dehydration can lead to heat exhaustion.

The aim of first aid is to replace the lost water and salts through rehydration. Water is usually sufficient but oral rehydration solutions can help to replace lost salt.

1 Reassure the casualty. Help him to sit down.

2 Give him plenty of fluids to drink. Water is usually sufficient but oral rehydration solutions can help with salt replacement.

3 If the casualty is suffering from cramp, stretch and massage the affected muscles (p.159). Advise the casualty to rest.

4 Monitor and record the casualty's condition. If he remains unwell, seek medical advice straightaway.

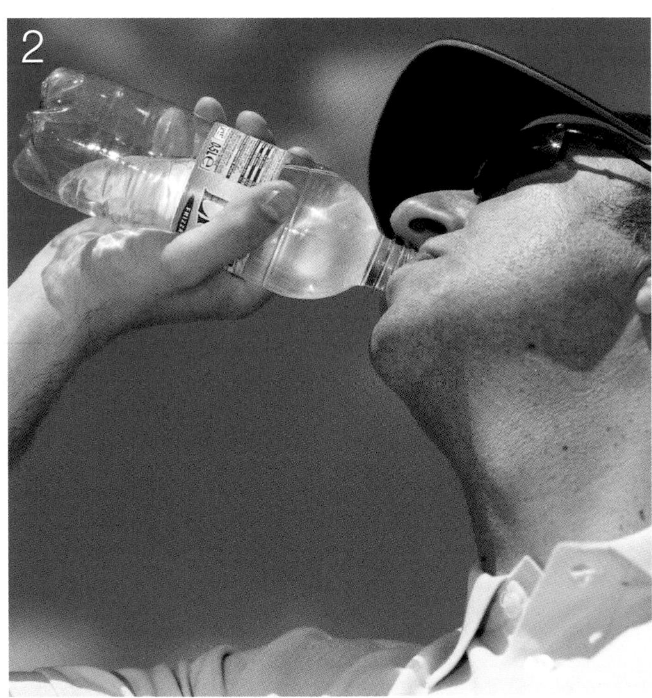
2

SUNBURN

RECOGNITION

- Reddened skin.
- Pain in the area of the burn.

Later there may be:

- Blistering of the affected skin.

YOUR AIMS

- To move the casualty out of the sun as soon as possible.
- To relieve discomfort and pain.

CAUTION

- If there is extensive blistering, or other skin damage, seek medical advice.

See also
Dehydration **opposite**
Heat exhaustion **p.192**
Heatstroke **p.193**
Minor burns and scalds **p.184**

Over-exposure to the sun or a sunlamp can result in sunburn. At high altitudes, sunburn can occur even on an overcast summer's day, or in the snow. Some medicines can trigger severe sensitivity to sunlight. Rarely, sunburn can be caused by exposure to radioactivity.

Sunburn can be prevented by staying in the shade, wearing protective clothing and by regularly applying high factor sunscreen.

Most sunburn is superficial; in severe cases, the skin is lobster-red and blistered. In addition, the casualty may suffer from heat exhaustion or heatstroke.

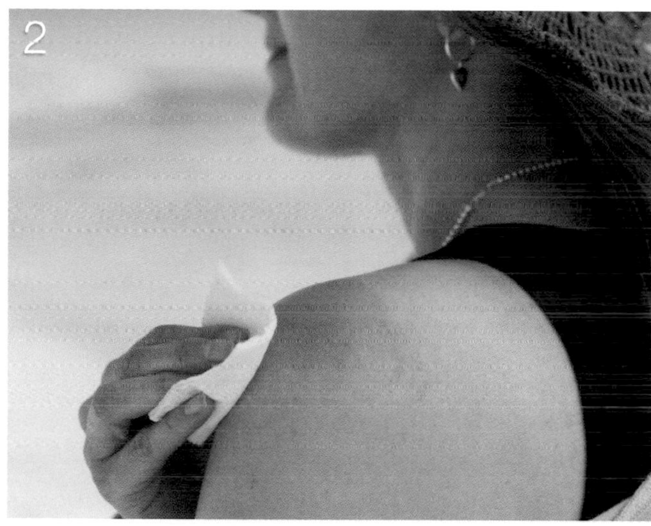

1 Cover the casualty's skin with light clothing or a towel. Help her to move out of the sun or, if at all possible, indoors.

2 Encourage the casualty to have frequent sips of cold water. Cool the affected skin by dabbing with cold water. If the area is extensive, the casualty may prefer to soak the affected skin in a cold bath for ten minutes.

3 If the burns are mild, calamine or an after-sun lotion may soothe them. Advise the casualty to stay inside or in the shade. If sunburn is severe, seek medical advice.

HEAT EXHAUSTION

RECOGNITION

As the condition develops, there may be:

- Headache, dizziness and confusion;
- Loss of appetite and nausea;
- Sweating, with pale, clammy skin;
- Cramps in the arms, legs or abdomen;
- Rapid, weakening pulse and breathing.

YOUR AIMS

- To cool the casualty down.
- To replace lost body fluids and salts.
- To obtain medical help if necessary.

See also
Dehydration **p.190**
Heatstroke **opposite**
The unconscious casualty **pp.54–85**

This disorder is caused by loss of salt and water from the body through excessive sweating. It usually develops gradually and often affects people who are not acclimatised to hot, humid conditions. People who are unwell, especially those with illnesses that cause vomiting and diarrhoea, are more susceptible than others to developing heat exhaustion.

A dangerous and common cause of heat exhaustion occurs when the body produces more heat than it can cope with. Some non-prescription drugs, such as ecstasy, can affect the body's temperature regulation system. This, combined with the exertion of dancing in a warm environment, can result in a person becoming overheated and dehydrated. These effects can lead to heatstroke and even death.

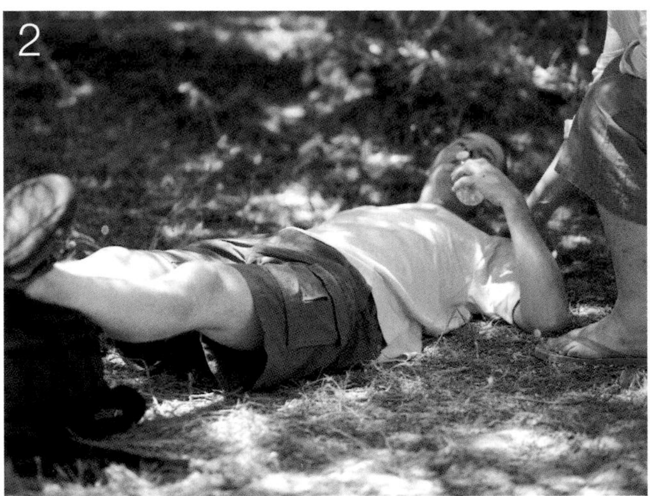

1 Help the casualty to a cool, shady place. Get him to lie down and raise and support his legs to improve blood flow to brain.

2 Give him plenty of water to drink. Oral rehydration salts or isotonic drinks will help with salt replacement.

3 Monitor and record vital signs – level of response, breathing and pulse (pp.52–53). Even if the casualty recovers quickly, advise him to seek medical help.

4 If the casualty's vital signs worsen, **call 999/112 for emergency help**. Monitor and record vital signs – level of response, breathing and pulse (pp.52–53) – while you are waiting for help to arrive.

HEATSTROKE

RECOGNITION

There may be:

- Headache, dizziness and discomfort;
- Restlessness and confusion;
- Hot, flushed and dry skin;
- Rapid deterioration in the level of response;
- Full, bounding pulse;
- Body temperature above 40°C (104°F).

YOUR AIMS

- To lower the casualty's body temperature as quickly as possible.
- To arrange urgent removal to hospital.

CAUTION

- If the casualty loses consciousness, open the airway and check breathing (The unconscious casualty pp.54–85).

See also
Drug poisoning **p.209**
The unconscious casualty **pp.54–85**

This condition is caused by a failure of the "thermostat" in the brain, which regulates body temperature. The body becomes dangerously overheated, usually due to a high fever or prolonged exposure to heat. Heatstroke can also result from the use of drugs such as ecstasy. In some cases, heatstroke follows heat exhaustion when sweating ceases, and the body then cannot be cooled by the evaporation of sweat.

Heatstroke can develop with little warning, resulting in unconsciousness within minutes of the casualty feeling unwell.

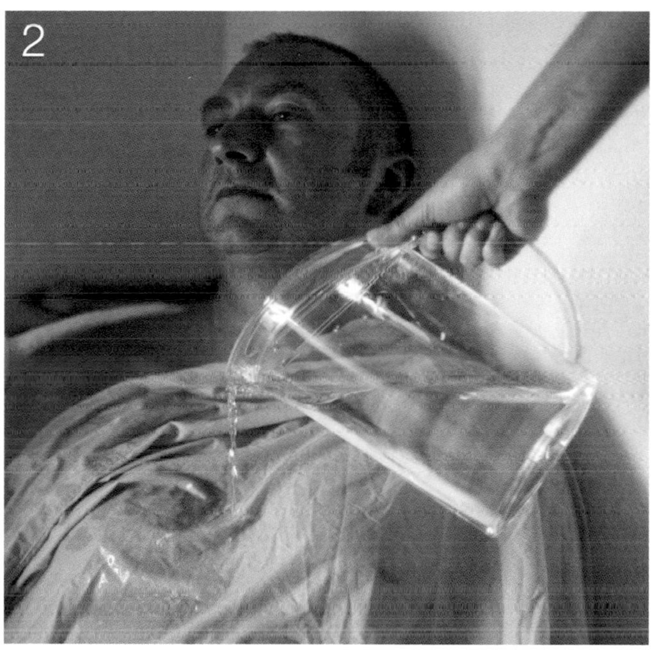

1 Quickly move the casualty to a cool place. Remove as much of his outer clothing as possible. **Call 999/112 for emergency help.**

2 Help the casualty to sit down, supported with cushions. Wrap him in a cold, wet sheet until his temperature falls to 38°C (100.4°F) under the tongue, or 37.5°C (99.5°F) under the armpit. Keep the sheet wet by continually pouring cold water over it. If there is no sheet available, fan the casualty, or sponge him with cold water.

3 Once the casualty's temperature appears to have returned to normal, replace the wet sheet with a dry one.

4 Monitor and record vital signs – level of response, breathing, pulse and temperature (pp.52–53) – while waiting for help. If the casualty's temperature rises again, repeat the cooling process.

HYPOTHERMIA

RECOGNITION

As hypothermia develops, there may be:

- Shivering, and cold, pale, dry skin;
- Apathy, disorientation or irrational behaviour;
- Lethargy or impaired consciousness;
- Slow and shallow breathing;
- Slow and weakening pulse. In extreme cases, the heart may stop.

YOUR AIMS

- To prevent the casualty losing more body heat.
- To re-warm the casualty slowly.
- To obtain emergency help if necessary.

CAUTION

- Do not give the casualty alcohol because it dilates superficial blood vessels and allows heat to escape, making hypothermia worse.
- Do not place any heat sources, such as hot-water bottles or fires, next to the casualty because these may mobilise blood too rapidly and divert it suddenly from the heart and brain to the skin. They could also burn the casualty.
- Do not warm an elderly casualty in a bath.
- If the casualty loses consciousness, open the airway and check breathing (The unconscious casualty pp.54–85). Persist with CPR until emergency help arrives to assess the casualty's condition.
- It is important that you stay warm yourself.

This condition develops when the body temperature falls below 35°C (95°F). The effects vary depending on the speed of onset and the level to which the body temperature falls. The blood supply to the superficial blood vessels in the skin, for example, shuts down to maintain the function of the vital organs such as the heart and brain. Moderate hypothermia can usually be reversed. Severe hypothermia – when the core body temperature falls below 30°C (86°F) – is often, although not always, fatal. No matter how low body temperature becomes, it is worth persisting with life-saving procedures until emergency help arrives.

WHAT CAUSES HYPOTHERMIA

Hypothermia can be caused by prolonged exposure to cold. Moving air has a much greater cooling effect than still air, so a high "wind-chill factor" in cold weather can substantially increase the risk of a person developing hypothermia. Immersion in cold water can cause death from hypothermia, not drowning. When surrounded by cold water, the body can cool up to 30 times faster than in dry air, and body temperature falls rapidly.

Hypothermia may also develop indoors in poorly heated houses. Elderly people, infants, homeless people and those who are thin and frail are particularly vulnerable. Lack of activity, chronic illness and fatigue all increase the risk; alcohol and drugs can exacerbate the condition.

See also
Drowning p.98
The unconscious casualty pp.54–85
Water rescue p.36

TREATMENT WHEN OUTDOORS

1 Take the casualty to a sheltered place as quickly as possible. Shield the casualty from the wind.

2 Remove and replace any wet clothing if possible; do not give him your clothes. Make sure his head is covered.

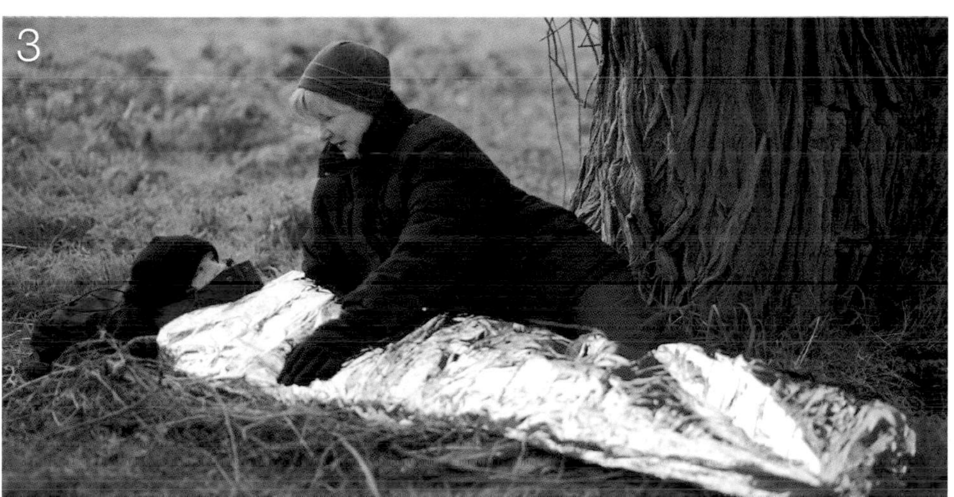

3 Protect the casualty from the ground. Lay him on a thick layer of dry insulating material, such as pine branches, heather or bracken. Put him in a dry sleeping bag and/or cover him with blankets or newspapers. Wrap him in a plastic or foil survival bag, if available. You can shelter and warm him with your body.

4 **Call 999/112 or send for emergency help.** Ideally, two people should go for help and stay together if you are in a remote area. It is important that you do not leave the casualty by himself; someone must remain with him at all times.

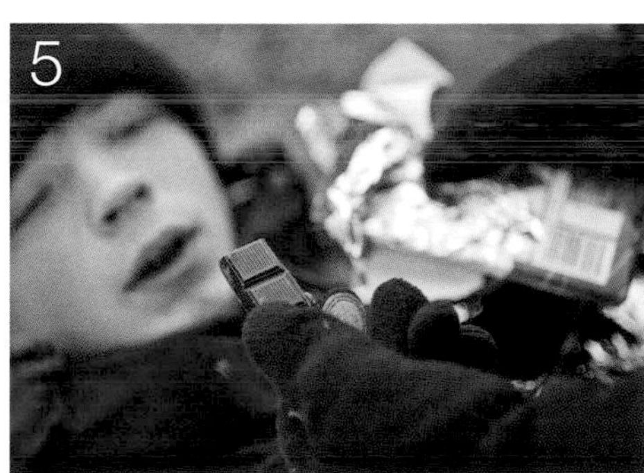

5 To help re-warm a casualty who is conscious, give him warm drinks and high-energy foods such as chocolate, if available.

6 The casualty must be re-warmed gradually. Monitor and record the casualty's vital signs – level of response, breathing, pulse and temperature (pp.52–52) – while waiting for help to arrive. When help arrives, the casualty should be taken to hospital by stretcher.

HYPOTHERMIA (continued)

TREATMENT WHEN INDOORS

1 The casualty must be re-warmed slowly. Cover an elderly person with layers of blankets and warm the room to about 25°C (77°F). If the casualty is warmed too rapidly, blood may be diverted suddenly from the heart and brain to the body surfaces. Handle the casualty gently because, in severe cases, rushed treatment or movement may cause an abnormal heart rhythm.

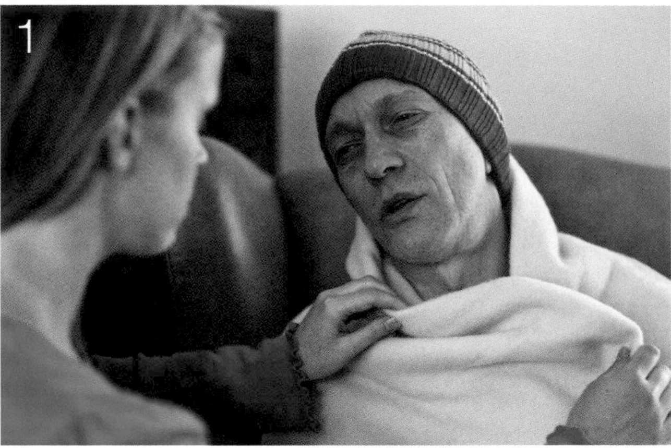
1

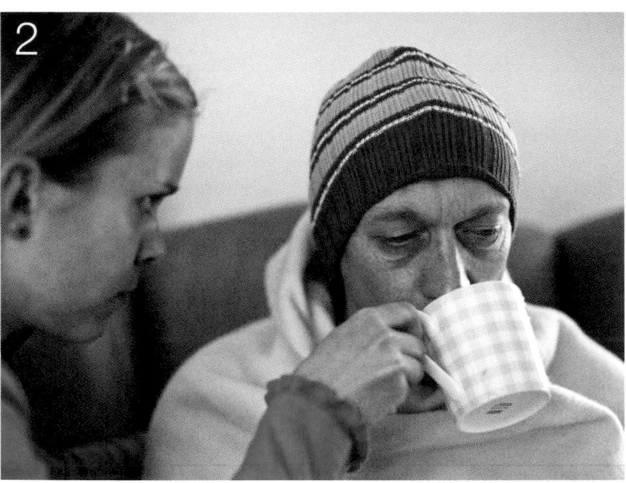
2

2 Give him a warm drink such as soup and/or high-energy foods such as chocolate to help re-warm him.

3 **Call 999/112 for emergency help.** Be aware that in the elderly, hypothermia may also be disguising the symptoms of a stroke (pp.174–75), a heart attack (p.110) or an underactive thyroid gland (hypothyroidism).

4 Monitor and record the casualty's vital signs – level of response, breathing, pulse and temperature (pp.52–53) – while waiting for help to arrive.

SPECIAL CASE HYPOTHERMIA IN INFANTS

A baby's mechanisms for regulating body temperature are under-developed, so she may develop hypothermia in a cold room. The baby's skin may look healthy but feel cold, and she may be limp, unusually quiet and refusing to feed. Re-warm a cold baby gradually, by wrapping her in blankets and warming the room. You should always seek medical advice if you suspect a baby has hypothermia.

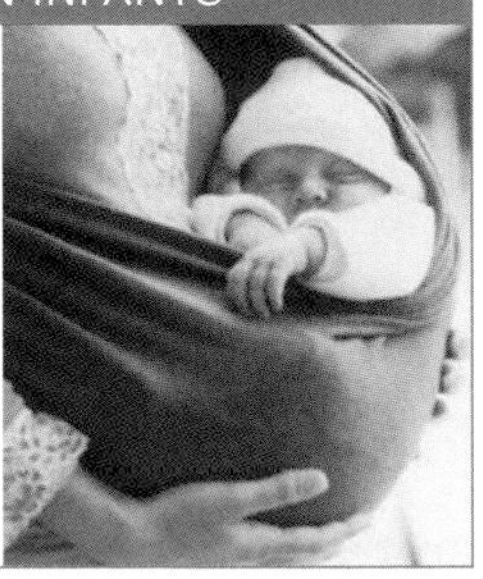

FROSTBITE

RECOGNITION

There may be:

- At first, "pins-and-needles";
- Paleness (pallor) followed by numbness;
- Hardening and stiffening of the skin;
- A colour change to the skin of the affected area: first white, then mottled and blue. On recovery, the skin may be red, hot, painful and blistered. Where gangrene occurs, the tissue may become black due to loss of blood supply.

YOUR AIMS

- To warm the affected area slowly to prevent further tissue damage.
- To arrange transport to hospital.

CAUTION

- Do not put the affected part near direct heat.
- Do not attempt to thaw the affected part if there is danger of it refreezing.
- Do not allow the casualty to smoke.

With this condition, the tissues of the extremities – usually the fingers and toes – freeze due to low temperatures. In severe cases, this freezing can lead to permanent loss of sensation and, eventually, tissue death and gangrene as the blood vessels and soft tissues become permanently damaged.

Frostbite usually occurs in freezing or cold and windy conditions. People who cannot move around to increase their circulation are particularly susceptible.

In many cases, frostbite is accompanied by hypothermia (pp.194–96), and this should be treated accordingly.

See also
Hypothermia **pp.194–96**

1 Advise the casualty to put his hands in his armpits. Move the casualty into warmth before you thaw the affected part further.

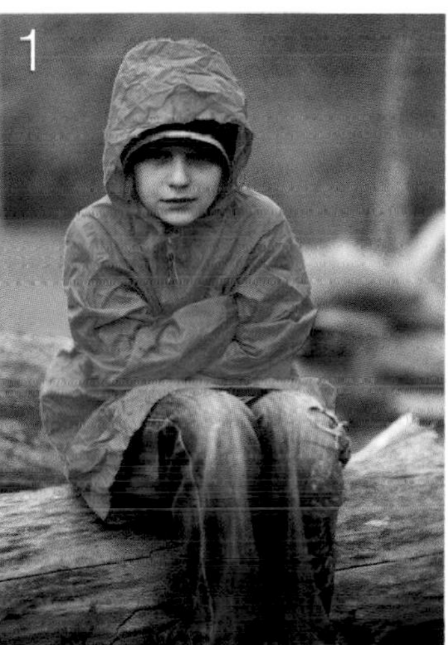

2 Once inside, gently remove gloves, rings and any other constrictions, such as boots. Warm the affected part with your hands, in your lap or continue to warm them in the casualty's armpits. Avoid rubbing the affected area because this can damage skin and other tissues.

3 Place the affected parts in warm water at around 40°C (104°F). Dry carefully, and apply a light dressing of dry gauze bandage.

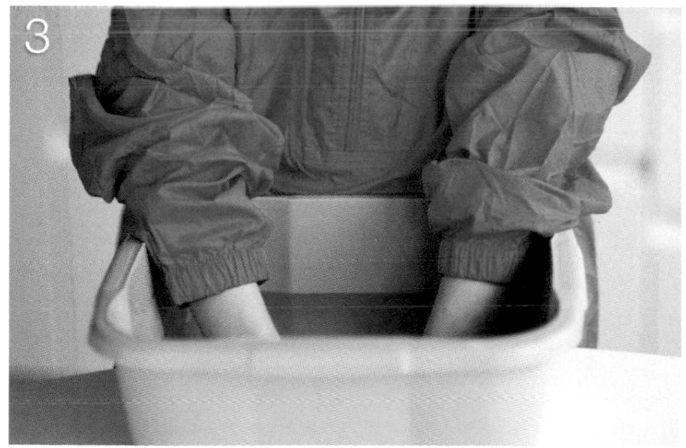

4 Raise the affected limb to reduce swelling. An adult may take the recommended dose of paracetamol or her own painkillers. A child may have the recommended dose of paracetamol syrup (not aspirin). Take or send the casualty to hospital.

10

Objects that find their way into the body, either through a wound in the skin or via an orifice, are known as "foreign objects". These range from grit in the eye to small objects that young children may push into their noses and ears. These can be distressing but do not usually cause serious problems for the casualty.

Poisoning may result from exposure to or ingestion of toxic substances, chemicals and contaminated food. The effects of poisons vary but medical advice will be needed in most cases.

Insect stings and marine stings can often be treated with first aid. However, multiple stings can produce a reaction that requires urgent medical help. Animal and human bites always require medical attention due to the risk of infection.

AIMS AND OBJECTIVES

- To ensure the safety of yourself and the casualty.
- To assess the casualty's condition quickly and calmly.
- To assess the potential danger of a foreign object.
- To identify the poisonous substance.
- To comfort and reassure the casualty.
- To look for and treat any injuries associated with the condition.
- To obtain medical help if necessary. Call 999/112 for emergency help if you suspect a serious illness or injury.
- To be aware of your own needs.

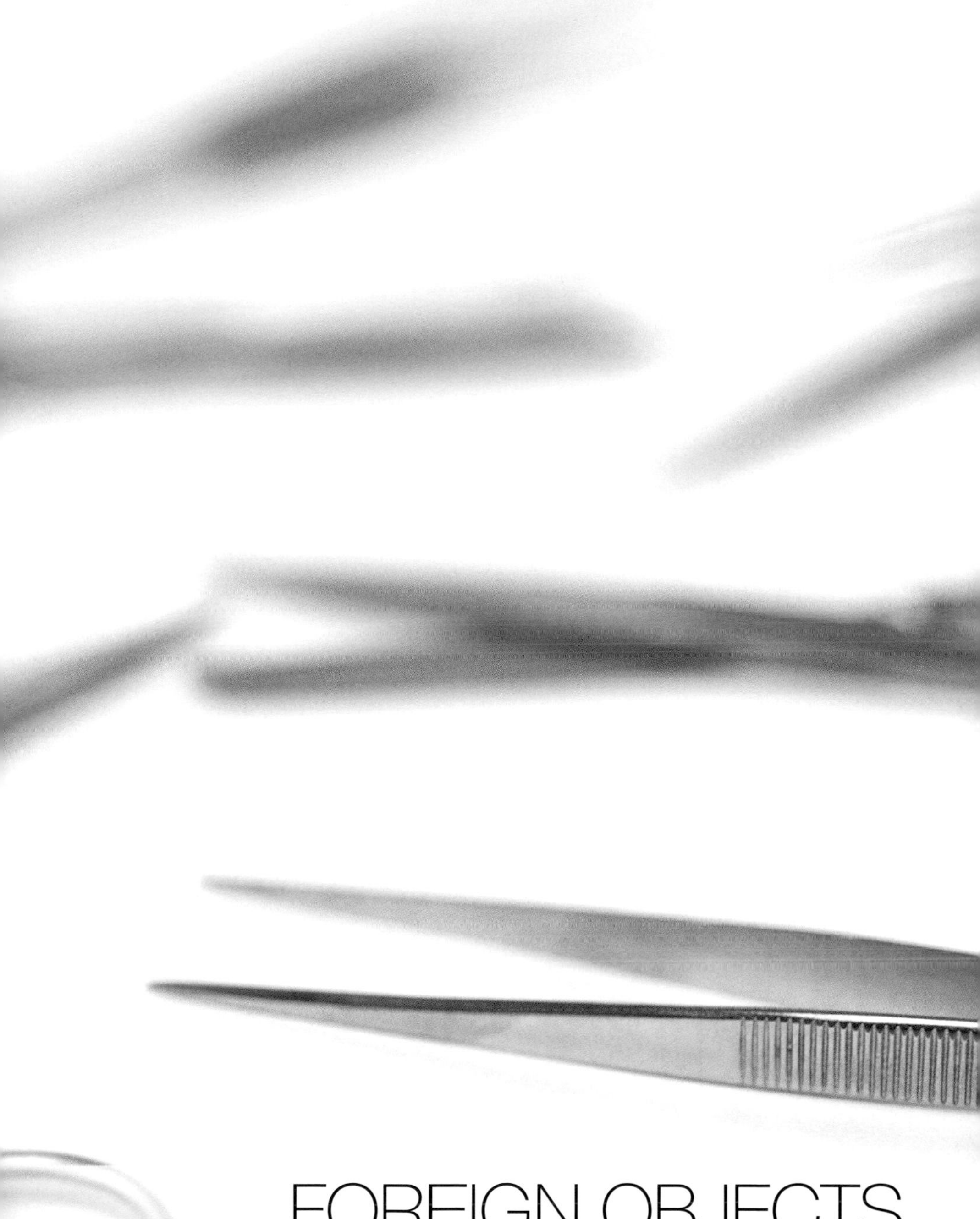

FOREIGN OBJECTS, POISONING, BITES & STINGS

THE SENSORY ORGANS

THE SKIN

The body is covered and protected by the skin. This is one of the body's largest organs and is made up of two layers: the outer layer, called the epidermis, and an inner layer, the dermis. The skin forms a barrier against harmful substances and germs. It is also an important sense organ, containing nerves that ensure the body is sensitive to heat, cold, pain and touch.

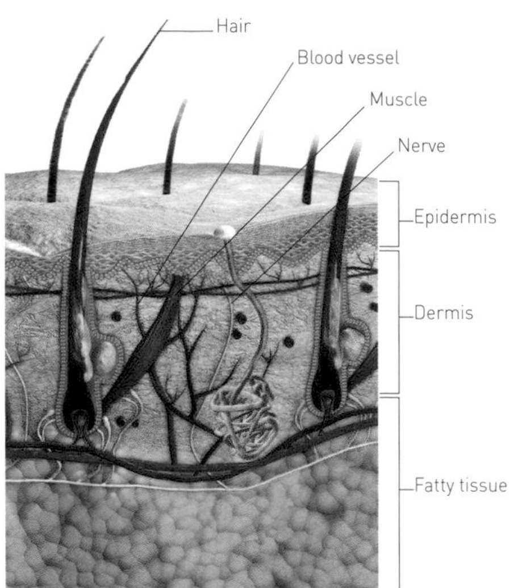

Structure of the skin
The skin consists of the thin epidermis and the thicker dermis, which sit on a layer of fatty tissue (subcutaneous fat). Blood vessels, nerves, muscles, sebaceous (oil) glands, sweat glands and hair roots (follicles) lie in the dermis.

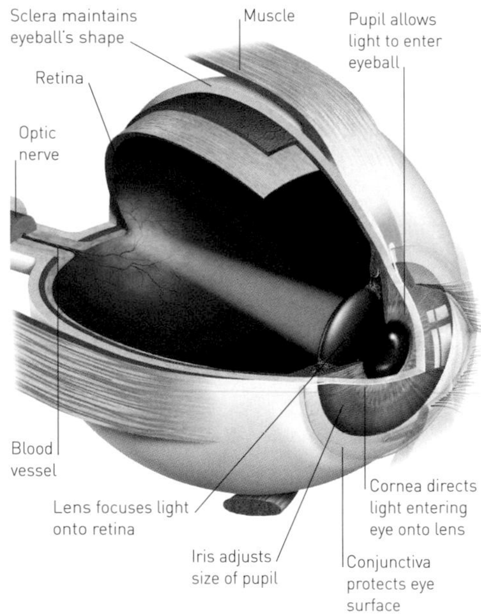

Structure of the eye
The eyes are fluid-filled, spherical structures about 2.5cm (1in) in diameter. They have focusing parts (cornea and lens), and light- and colour-sensitive cells in the retina.

THE EYES

These complex organs enable us to see the world around us. Each eye consists of a coloured part (iris) with a small opening (pupil) that allows rays of light to enter the eye. The size of the pupil changes according to the amount of light that is entering the eye.

Light rays are focused by the transparent lens onto a "screen" (retina) at the back of the eye. Special cells in the retina convert this information into electrical impulses that then travel, via the optic nerve that leads from the eye, to the part of the brain where the impulses are analysed.

Each eye is protected by a bony socket in the skull (p.133). The eyelids and delicate membranes called conjunctiva protect the front of the eyes.

Tears form a protective film across the front of the conjunctiva, lubricating the surface and flushing away dust and dirt.

THE EARS

As well as being the organs of hearing, the ears also play an important role in balance. The visible part of each ear, the auricle, funnels sounds into the ear canal to vibrate the eardrum. Fine hairs in the ear canal filter out dust, and glands secrete ear wax to trap any other small particles. The vibrations of the eardrum pass across the middle ear to the hearing apparatus (cochlea) in the inner ear. This structure converts the vibrations into nerve impulses and transmits them to the brain via the auditory nerve. The vestibular apparatus within the inner ear is involved in balance.

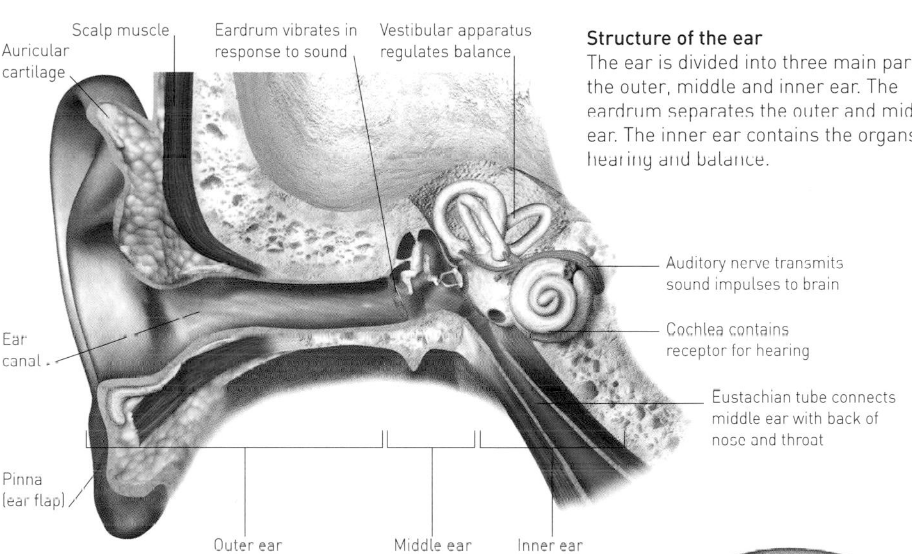

Structure of the ear
The ear is divided into three main parts: the outer, middle and inner ear. The eardrum separates the outer and middle ear. The inner ear contains the organs of hearing and balance.

THE MOUTH AND NOSE

These cavities form the entrances to the digestive and respiratory tracts respectively. The nasal cavities connect with the throat. They are lined with blood vessels and membranes that secrete mucus to trap debris as it enters the nose. Food enters the digestive tract via the mouth, which leads into the gullet (oesophagus). The epiglottis, a flap at the back of the throat, prevents food from entering the windpipe (trachea).

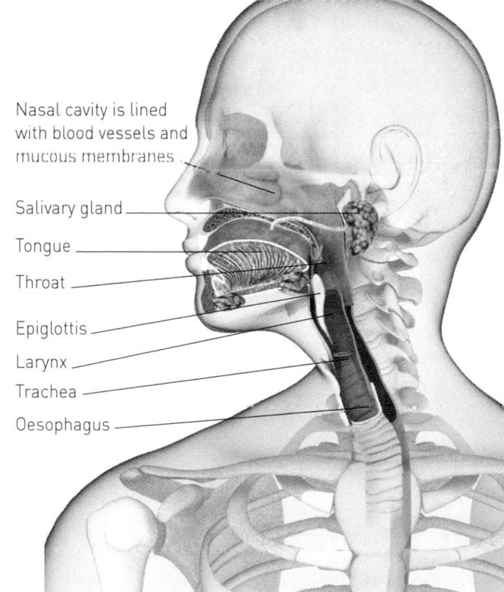

Structure of the mouth and nose
The nostrils lead into the two nasal cavities, which are lined with mucous membranes and blood vessels. The nasal cavities connect directly with the top of the throat, which is at the back of the mouth.

SPLINTER

YOUR AIMS

- To remove the splinter.
- To minimise the risk of infection.

CAUTION

- Ask the casualty about tetanus immunisation. Seek medical advice if he has a dirty wound; he has never been immunised; he is uncertain about number and timing of injections; he has not had at least five injections previously.

See also
Foreign object in a cut **p.122**
Infected wound **p.121**

Small splinters of wood, metal or glass may enter the skin. They carry a risk of infection because they are rarely clean. Often a splinter can be successfully withdrawn from the skin using tweezers. However, if the splinter is deeply embedded, lies over a joint, or is difficult to remove, you should leave it in place and advise the casualty to seek medical help.

1 Gently clean the area around the splinter with soap and warm water.

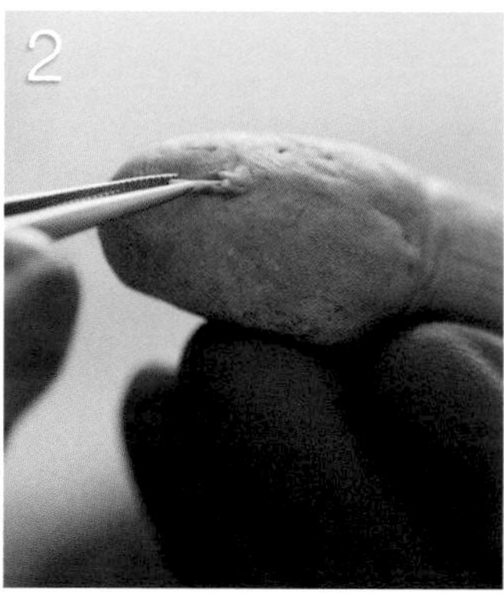

2 Hold the tweezers close to the end for a better grip. Grasp the splinter with tweezers as close to the skin as possible.

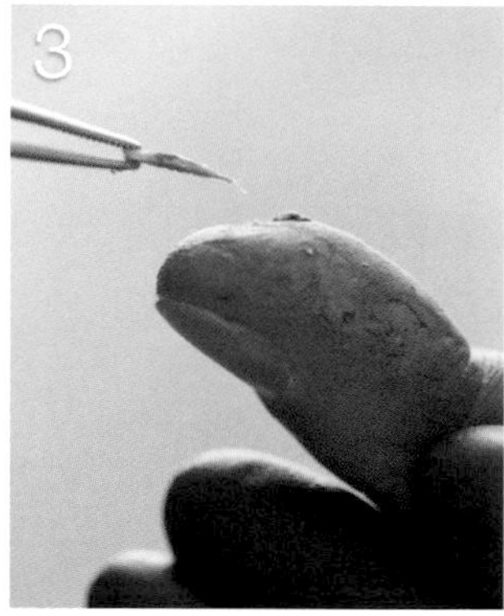

3 Draw the splinter out in a straight line at the same angle that it went into the skin; make sure it does not break.

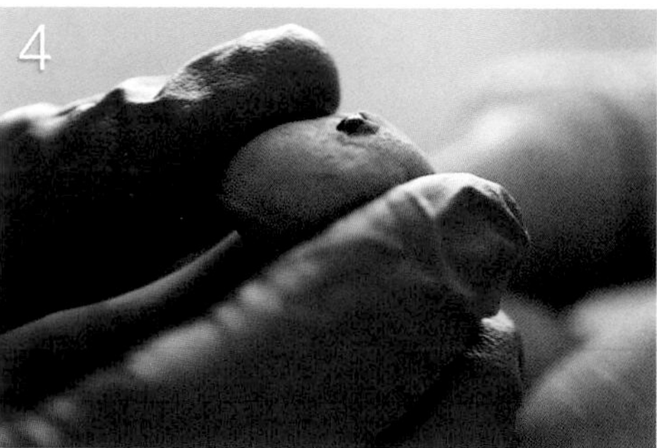

4 Carefully squeeze the wound to encourage a little bleeding. This will help to flush out any remaining dirt.

5 Clean and dry the wound and cover with a dressing.

SPECIAL CASE EMBEDDED SPLINTER

If a splinter is embedded or difficult to dislodge, do not probe the area with a sharp object, such as a needle, or you may introduce infection. Pad around the splinter until you can bandage over it without pressing on it, and seek medical help.

EMBEDDED FISH-HOOK

YOUR AIMS

- To obtain medical help.
- To minimise the risk of infection.
- If help is delayed, remove the fish-hook without causing the casualty any further injury and pain.

CAUTION

- Do not try to pull out a fish-hook unless you can cut off the barb. If you cannot, seek medical help.
- Ask the casualty about tetanus immunisation. Seek medical advice if: he has a dirty wound; he has never been immunised; he is uncertain about number and timing of injections; he has not had at least five injections previously.

A fish-hook that is embedded in the skin is difficult to remove because of the barb at the end of the hook. If possible, you should ensure that the hook is removed by a healthcare professional. Only attempt to remove a hook yourself if medical help is not readily available. Embedded fish-hooks carry a risk of infection, including tetanus.

1 **Support the injured area. If possible, cut off the fishing line as close to the hook as possible.**

2 **If medical help is readily available, build up pads of gauze around the hook until you can bandage over the top without pushing it in further. Bandage over the padding and the hook and arrange to take or send the casualty to hospital.**

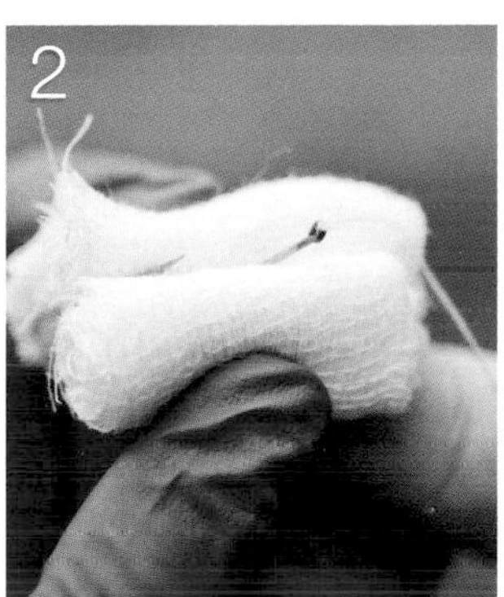

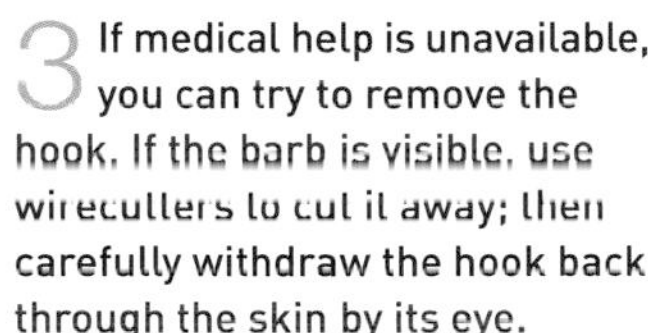

3 **If medical help is unavailable, you can try to remove the hook. If the barb is visible, use wirecutters to cut it away; then carefully withdraw the hook back through the skin by its eye.**

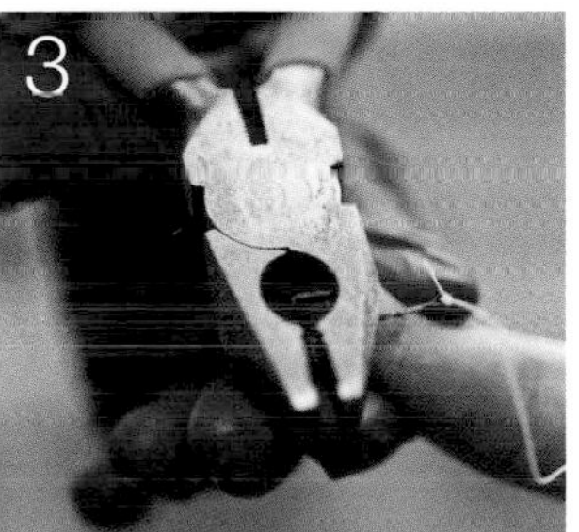

4 **Clean and dry the wound and cover with a dressing.**

SPECIAL CASE IF BARB IS NOT VISIBLE

If the barb is in the skin, gently ease the hook forwards until the barb emerges. Cut off the barb as in step 3, above, then withdraw the hook by its eye. If you cannot release the barb, pad around the hook, bandage in place and seek medical help as soon as possible.

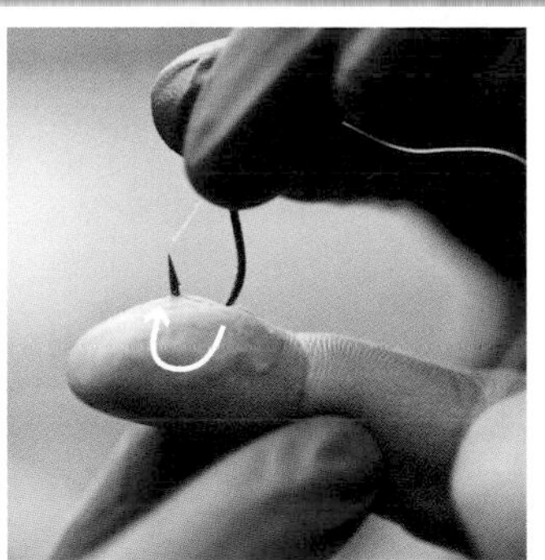

FOREIGN OBJECT IN THE EYE

RECOGNITION

There may be:

- Blurred vision;
- Pain or discomfort;
- Redness and watering of the eye;
- Eyelids screwed up in spasm.

YOUR AIMS

- To prevent injury to the eye.

CAUTION

- Do not touch anything that is sticking to, or embedded in, the eyeball. Cover the eye (p.124) and arrange to take or send casualty to hospital.

See also
Eye wound **p.124**

Foreign objects such as grit, a loose eyelash or a contact lens that are floating on the surface of the eye can easily be rinsed out. However, you must not attempt to remove anything that sticks to the eye or penetrates the eyeball because this may damage the eye. Instead, make sure that the casualty receives urgent medical attention.

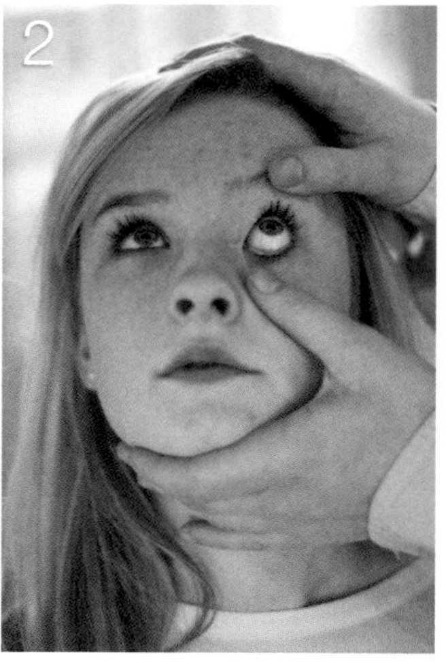

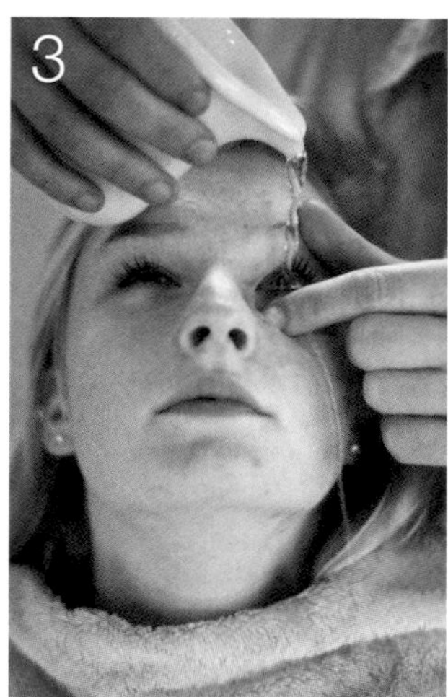

1 **Advise the casualty not to rub her eye. Ask her to sit down facing a light.**

2 **Stand beside, or just behind, the casualty. Gently separate her eyelids with your thumbs or finger and thumb. Ask her to look right, left, up and down. Examine every part of her eye as she does this.**

3 **If you can see a foreign object on the white of the eye, wash it out by pouring clean water from a glass or jug, or by using a sterile eyewash if you have one. Put a towel around the casualty's shoulders. Hold her eye open and pour the water from the inner corner so that it drains on to the towel.**

4 **If this is unsuccessful, try lifting the object off with a moist swab or the damp corner of a clean handkerchief or tissue. If you still cannot remove the object, seek medical help.**

SPECIAL CASE IF OBJECT IS UNDER UPPER EYELID

Ask the casualty to grasp the lashes on her upper eyelid and pull the upper lid over the lower lid; the lower lashes may brush the particle clear. If this is unsuccessful, ask her to try blinking under water since this may also make the object float off. Do not attempt to do this if the object is large or abrasive.

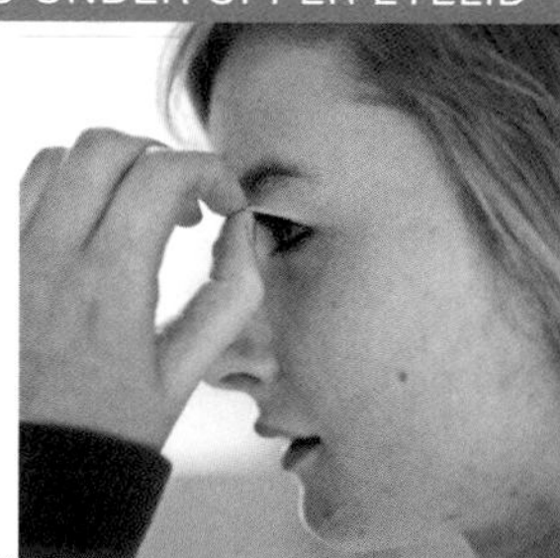

FOREIGN OBJECT IN THE EAR

YOUR AIMS

- To prevent injury to the ear.
- To remove a trapped insect.
- To arrange transport to hospital if a foreign object is lodged in the ear.

CAUTION

- Do not attempt to remove any object that is lodged in the ear. You may cause serious injury and push the foreign object in further.

If a foreign object becomes lodged in the ear, it may cause temporary deafness by blocking the ear canal. In some cases, a foreign object may damage the eardrum. Young children frequently push objects into their ears. The tips of cotton wool buds are often left in the ear. Insects can fly or crawl into the ear and may cause distress.

1 **Arrange to take or send the casualty to hospital as soon as possible. Do not try to remove a lodged foreign object yourself.**

2 **Reassure the casualty during the journey or until medical help arrives.**

SPECIAL CASE INSECT INSIDE THE EAR

Reassure the casualty and ask him to sit down. Support his head, with the affected ear uppermost. Gently flood the ear with tepid water; the insect should float out. If this flooding does not remove the insect, seek medical help.

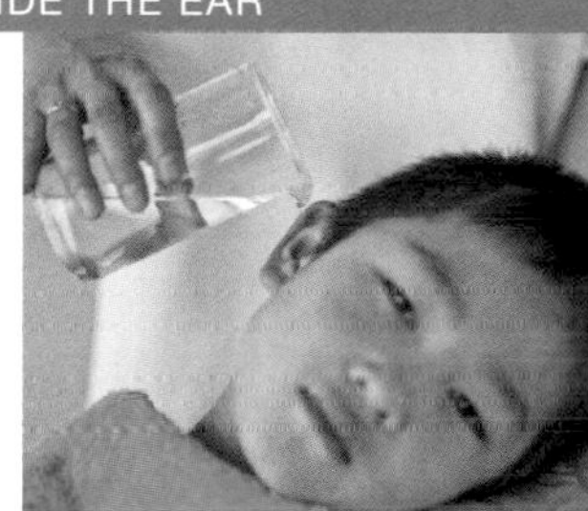

FOREIGN OBJECT IN THE NOSE

RECOGNITION

There may be:

- Difficult or noisy breathing through the nose;
- Swelling of the nose;
- Smelly or blood-stained discharge, indicating that an object may have been lodged for a while.

YOUR AIMS

- To arrange transport to hospital.

CAUTION

- Do not attempt to remove the foreign object, even if you can see it.

Young children may push small objects up their noses. Objects can block the nose and cause infection. If the object is sharp it can damage the tissues, and "button" batteries can cause burns and bleeding. Do not try to remove a foreign object; you may cause injury or push it further into the airway.

1 **Try to keep the casualty quiet and calm. Tell him to breathe through his mouth at a normal rate. Advise him not to poke inside his nose to try to remove the object himself.**

2 **Arrange to take or send the casualty to hospital, so that it can be safely removed by medical staff.**

HOW POISONS AFFECT THE BODY

A poison (toxin) is a substance that, if taken into or absorbed into the body in sufficient quantity, can cause either temporary or permanent damage.

Poisons can be swallowed, absorbed through the skin, inhaled, splashed into the eyes or injected. Once in the body, they may enter the bloodstream and be carried swiftly to all organs and tissues. Signs and symptoms of poisoning vary with the poison. They may develop quickly or over a number of days. Vomiting is common, especially when the poison has been ingested. Inhaled poisons often cause breathing difficulties.

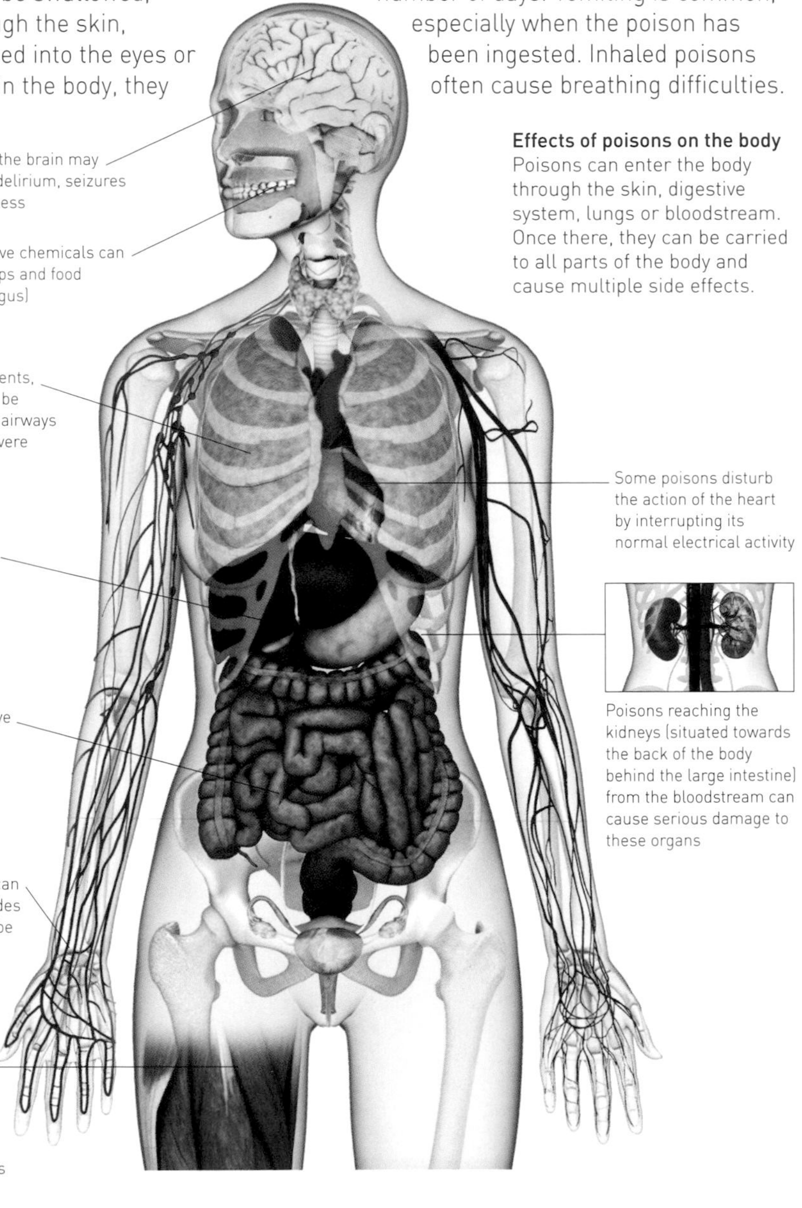

Effects of poisons on the body
Poisons can enter the body through the skin, digestive system, lungs or bloodstream. Once there, they can be carried to all parts of the body and cause multiple side effects.

TYPES OF POISON

Some poisons are man-made – for example, chemicals and drugs – and these are found in the home as well as in industry. Almost every household contains substances that are potentially poisonous, such as bleach and paint stripper, as well as prescribed or over-the-counter medicines, which may be dangerous if taken in excessive amounts.

Other poisons occur in nature: for example, plants produce poisons that may irritate the skin or cause more serious symptoms if ingested, and various insects and creatures produce venom in their bites and stings. Contamination of food by bacteria may result in food poisoning – one of the most common forms of poisoning.

RECOGNISING AND TREATING THE EFFECTS OF POISONING

ROUTE OF ENTRY INTO THE BODY	POISON	POSSIBLE EFFECTS	ACTION
Swallowed (ingested)	▪ Drugs and alcohol ▪ Cleaning products ▪ DIY and gardening products ▪ Plant poisons ▪ Bacterial food poisons ▪ Viral food poisons	▪ Nausea and vomiting ▪ Abdominal pain ▪ Seizures ▪ Irregular, or fast or slow, heartbeat ▪ Impaired consciousness	▪ Monitor casualty ▪ Call emergency help ▪ Commence CPR if necessary (pp.54–85) ▪ Use a face mask to protect yourself if you need to give rescue breaths
Absorbed through the skin	▪ Cleaning products ▪ DIY and gardening products ▪ Industrial poisons ▪ Plant poisons	▪ Pain ▪ Swelling ▪ Rash ▪ Redness ▪ Itching	▪ Remove contaminated clothing ▪ Wash with cold water for 20 minutes ▪ Seek medical help ▪ Commence CPR if necessary (pp.54–85)
Inhaled	▪ Fumes from cleaning and DIY products ▪ Industrial poisons ▪ Fumes from fires	▪ Difficulty breathing ▪ Hypoxia ▪ Grey-blue skin (cyanosis)	▪ Help casualty into fresh air ▪ Call emergency help ▪ Commence CPR if necessary (pp.54–85)
Splashed in the eye	▪ Cleaning products ▪ DIY and gardening products ▪ Industrial poisons ▪ Plant poisons	▪ Pain and watering of the eye ▪ Blurred vision	▪ Irrigate the eye for ten minutes (p.188) ▪ Call emergency help ▪ Commence CPR if necessary (pp.54–85)
Injected through the skin	▪ Venom from stings and bites ▪ Drugs	▪ Pain, redness and swelling at injection site ▪ Blurred vision ▪ Nausea and vomiting ▪ Difficulty breathing ▪ Seizures ▪ Impaired consciousness ▪ Anaphylactic shock	For sting/venom: ▪ Remove sting, if possible ▪ Call emergency help ▪ Commence CPR if necessary (pp.54–85) For injected drugs: ▪ Call emergency help ▪ Commence CPR if necessary (pp.54–85)

SWALLOWED POISONS

RECOGNITION

- History of ingestion/ exposure.

Depending on what has been swallowed, there may be:

- Vomiting, sometimes bloodstained, later diarrhoea;
- Cramping abdominal pains;
- Pain or a burning sensation;
- Empty containers in the vicinity;
- Impaired consciousness;
- Seizures.

YOUR AIMS

- To maintain an open airway, breathing and circulation.
- To remove any contaminated clothing.
- To identify the poison.
- To arrange urgent removal to hospital.

CAUTION

- Never attempt to induce vomiting.
- If a casualty is contaminated with chemicals, wear protective gloves, goggles and/or a mask.
- If the casualty loses consciousness, open the airway and check breathing (The unconscious casualty pp.54–85).
- If there are any chemicals on the casualty's mouth, protect yourself by using a face shield or pocket mask (adult p.69, child p.77) to give rescue breaths.

See also
Alcohol poisoning **p.210**
Chemical burn **p.187**
Drug poisoning **p.209**
Inhalation of fumes **pp.96–97**
The unconscious casualty **pp.54–85**

Chemicals that are swallowed may harm the digestive tract, or cause more widespread damage if they enter the bloodstream and are transported to other parts of the body. Hazardous chemicals include household substances such as bleach and paint stripper, which are poisonous or corrosive if swallowed. Drugs, both prescribed or those bought over the counter, can also be harmful if an overdose is taken. Some plants and their berries can also be poisonous.

1 **If the casualty is conscious, ask her what she has swallowed, and if possible how much and when. Look for clues – for example, poisonous plants, berries or empty containers. Try to reassure her.**

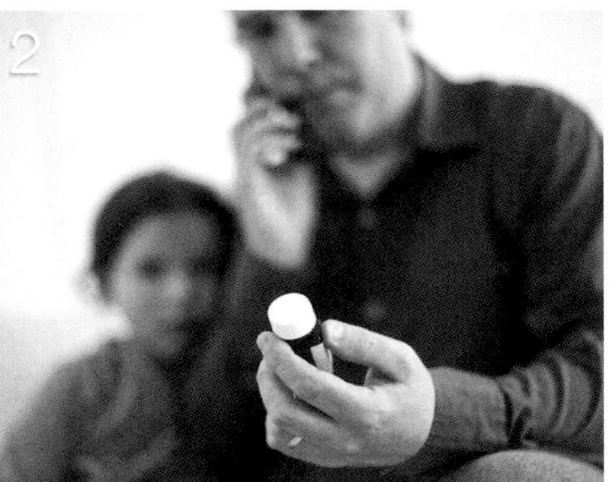
2

2 **Call 999/112 for emergency help.** Give ambulance control as much information as possible about the poison. This information will assist the medical team to treat the casualty.

3 Monitor and record the casualty's vital signs (pp.52–53) while waiting for help to arrive. Keep samples of any vomited material. Give these samples, containers and any others clues to the ambulance crew.

SPECIAL CASE IF LIPS ARE BURNT

If the casualty's lips are burnt by corrosive substances, give him frequent sips of cold milk or water while waiting for help to arrive.

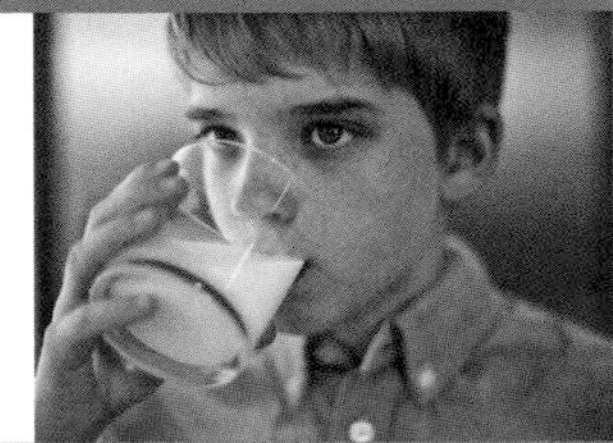

DRUG POISONING

YOUR AIMS

- To maintain breathing and circulation.
- To arrange removal to hospital.

CAUTION

- Do not induce vomiting.
- If the casualty loses consciousness, open the airway and check breathing, (The unconscious casualty pp.54–85).

See also
The unconscious casualty **pp.54–85**

Poisoning can result from an overdose of prescribed drugs, or drugs that are bought over the counter. It can also be caused by drug abuse or drug interaction. The effects vary depending on the type of drug and how it is taken (below). When you call the emergency services, give as much information as possible. While waiting for help to arrive, look for containers that might help you to identify the drug.

1 **If the casualty is conscious, help him into a comfortable position and ask him what he has taken. Reassure him while you talk to him.**

2 **Call 999/112 for emergency help.** **Tell ambulance control you suspect drug poisoning. Monitor and record vital signs – level of response, breathing and pulse (pp.52–53) – while waiting for help to arrive.**

3 **Keep samples of any vomited material. Look for evidence that might help to identify the drug, such as empty containers. Give these samples and containers to the ambulance personnel.**

RECOGNISING THE EFFECTS OF DRUG POISONING

CATEGORY	DRUG	EFFECTS OF POISONING
Painkillers	■ Aspirin (swallowed)	■ Upper abdominal pain, nausea and vomiting ■ Ringing in the ears ■ "Sighing" when breathing ■ Confusion and delirium ■ Dizziness
	■ Paracetamol (swallowed)	■ Little effect at first, but abdominal pain, nausea and vomiting may develop ■ Irreversible liver damage may occur within three days (alcohol and malnourishment increase the risk)
Nervous system depressants and tranquillisers	■ Barbiturates and benzodiazepines (swallowed)	■ Lethargy and sleepiness, leading to unconsciousness ■ Shallow breathing ■ Weak, irregular or abnormally slow or fast pulse
Stimulants and hallucinogens	■ Amphetamines (including ecstasy) and LSD (swallowed) ■ Cocaine (inhaled or injected)	■ Excitable, hyperactive behaviour, agitation ■ Sweating ■ Tremor of the hands ■ Hallucinations, in which the casualty may claim to "hear voices" or "see things" ■ Dilated pupils
Narcotics	■ Morphine, heroin (commonly injected)	■ Small pupils ■ Sluggishness and confusion, possibly leading to unconsciousness ■ Slow, shallow breathing, which may stop altogether ■ Needle marks, which may be infected
Solvents	■ Glue, lighter fuel (inhaled)	■ Nausea and vomiting ■ Headaches ■ Hallucinations ■ Possibly, unconsciousness ■ Rarely, cardiac arrest
Anaesthetic	■ Ketamine	■ Drowsiness ■ Shallow breathing ■ Hallucinations

ALCOHOL POISONING

RECOGNITION

There may be:

- A strong smell of alcohol;
- Empty bottles or cans;
- Impaired consciousness: the casualty may respond if roused, but will quickly relapse;
- Flushed and moist face;
- Deep, noisy breathing;
- Full, bounding pulse;
- Unconsciousness.

In the later stages of unconsciousness:

- Shallow breathing;
- Weak, rapid pulse;
- Dilated pupils that react poorly to light.

YOUR AIMS

- To maintain an open airway.
- To assess for other conditions.
- To seek medical help if necessary.

CAUTION

- Do not induce vomiting.
- If the casualty loses consciousness, open the airway and check his breathing (The unconscious casualty pp.54–85).

See also
Head injury **p.165**
Hypoglycaemia **p.219**
Hypothermia **pp.194–96**
The unconscious casualty **pp.54–85**

Alcohol (chemical name, ethanol) is a drug that depresses the activity of the central nervous system – in particular, the brain. Prolonged or excessive intake can severely impair all physical and mental functions, and the person may sink into deep unconsciousness.

There are other risks to a casualty from alcohol poisoning, for example: an unconscious casualty may inhale and choke on vomit; alcohol widens (dilates) the blood vessels so the body loses heat, and hypothermia may develop.

A casualty who smells of alcohol may be misdiagnosed and not receive appropriate treatment for an underlying cause of unconsciousness, such as a head injury, stroke, heart attack or hypoglycaemia.

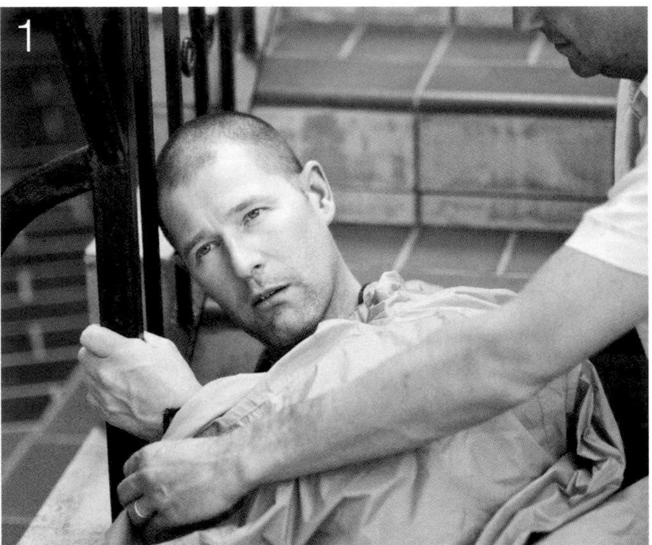

1 Cover the casualty with a coat or blanket to protect him from the cold.

2 Assess the casualty for any injuries, especially head injuries, or other medical conditions.

3 Monitor and record vital signs – level of response, pulse and breathing (pp.52–53) – until the casualty recovers or is placed in the care of a responsible person. If you are in any doubt about the casualty's condition, **call 999/112 for emergency help.**

ANIMAL AND HUMAN BITES

YOUR AIMS

- To control bleeding.
- To minimise the risk of infection.
- To obtain medical help if necessary.

CAUTION

- If you suspect rabies, arrange to take or send the casualty to hospital immediately.
- Ask the casualty about tetanus immunisation. Seek medical advice if he has a dirty wound; he has never been immunised; he is uncertain about the number and timing of injections, he has not had at least five injections previously.

See also
Cuts and grazes p.120
Infected wound p.121
Severe external bleeding pp.114–15
Shock pp.116–17

SPECIAL CASE
FOR A DEEP WOUND

If the wound is deep, control bleeding by applying direct pressure over a sterile pad and raise the injured part. Cover the wound and pad with a sterile dressing or large, clean non-fluffy pad and bandage firmly in place. Treat the casualty for shock and **call 999/112 for emergency help.**

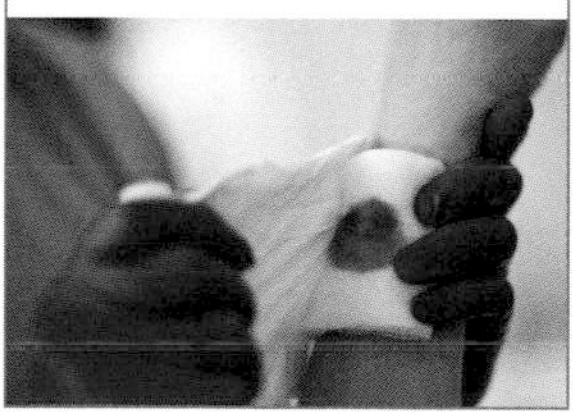

Bites from sharp, pointed teeth cause deep puncture wounds that can damage tissues and introduce germs. Bites also crush the tissue. Any bite that breaks the skin needs prompt first aid because of the increased risk of infection.

A serious infection risk is rabies, a potentially fatal viral infection of the nervous system. The virus is carried in the saliva of infected animals. If bitten in an area where there is a risk of rabies, seek medical advice since the casualty must be given anti-rabies injections. Try to identify the animal.

Tetanus is also a potential risk following any animal bite. There is probably only a small risk of hepatitis viruses being transmitted through a human bite – and an even smaller risk of transmission of the HIV/AIDS virus. However, medical advice should be sought straight away.

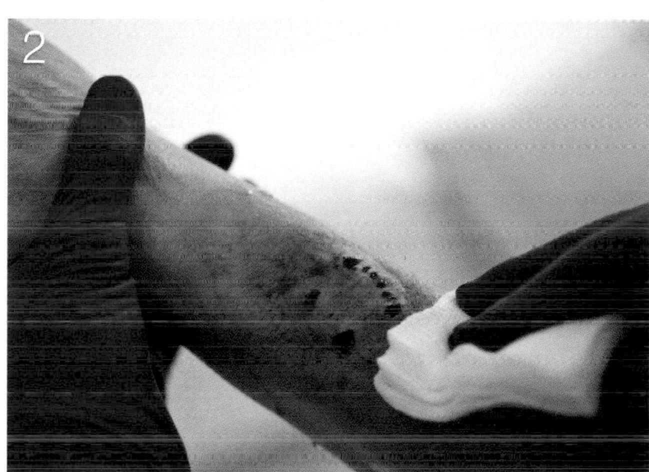

1 **Wash the bite wound thoroughly with soap and warm water in order to minimise the risk of infection.**

2 **Raise and support the wound and pat dry with clean gauze swabs. Then cover with a sterile wound dressing.**

3 **Arrange to take or send the casualty to hospital if the wound is large or deep.**

INSECT STING

RECOGNITION

- Pain at the site of the sting.
- Redness and swelling around the site of the sting.

YOUR AIMS

- To relieve swelling and pain.
- To arrange removal to hospital if necessary.

CAUTION

- **Call 999/112 for emergency help** if the casualty shows signs of anaphylactic shock (p.221), such as breathing difficulties and/or swelling of the face and neck. Monitor and record vital signs – level of response, breathing and pulse (pp.52–53) – while waiting for help to arrive.

See also
Anaphylactic shock **p.221**
The unconscious casualty **pp.54–85**

SPECIAL CASE
STINGS IN THE MOUTH AND THROAT

If a casualty has been stung in the mouth, there is a risk that swelling of tissues in the mouth and/or throat may occur, causing the airway to become blocked. To help prevent this, give the casualty an ice cube to suck or a glass of cold water to sip. **Call 999/112 for emergency help** if swelling starts to develop.

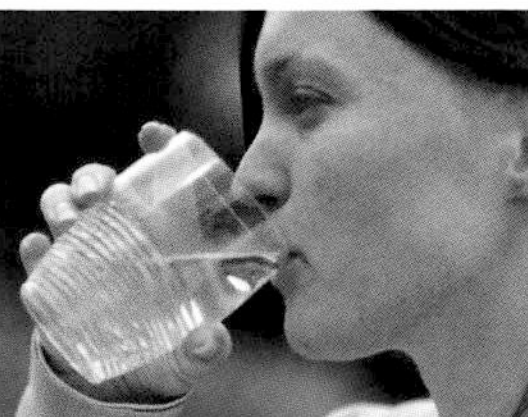

Usually, a sting from a bee, wasp or hornet is painful rather than dangerous. An initial sharp pain is followed by mild swelling, redness and soreness.

However, multiple insect stings can produce a serious reaction. A sting in the mouth or throat is potentially dangerous because swelling can obstruct the airway. With any bite or sting, it is important to watch for signs of an allergic reaction, which can lead to anaphylactic shock (p.221). Such reactions account for about ten deaths a year in the UK.

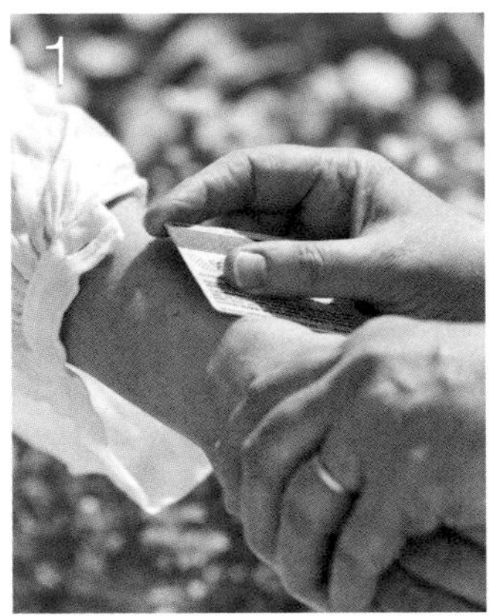

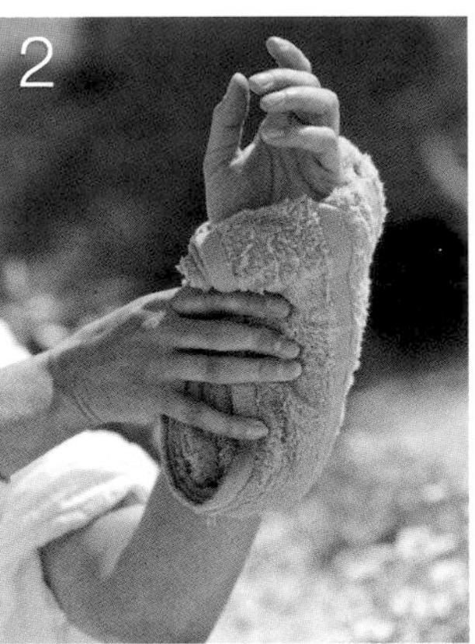

1 Reassure the casualty. If the sting is visible, brush or scrape it off sideways with the edge of a credit card or your fingernail. Do not use tweezers because you could squeeze the sting and inject more poison into the casualty.

2 Raise the affected part if possible, and apply a cold compress such as an ice pack (p.241) to minimise swelling. Advise the casualty to keep the compress in place for at least ten minutes. Tell her to seek medical advice if the pain and swelling persist.

3 Monitor vital signs – level of response, breathing and pulse (pp.52–53). Watch for signs of an allergic reaction, such as wheezing.

OTHER BITES AND STINGS

RECOGNITION

Depends on the species, but generally:

- Pain, redness and swelling at site of sting;
- Nausea and vomiting;
- Headache.

YOUR AIMS

- To relieve pain and swelling.
- To arrange removal to hospital if necessary.

CAUTION

- **Call 999/112 for emergency help** if a scorpion or a red back or funnel web spider has stung the casualty, or if the casualty is showing signs of anaphylactic shock (p.221).

Scorpion stings as well as bites from some spiders and mosquitoes can cause serious illness, and may even be fatal if not treated promptly.

Bites or stings in the mouth or throat are dangerous because swelling can obstruct the airway. Be alert to an allergic reaction, which may lead the casualty to suffer an anaphylactic shock (p.221).

See also
Anaphylactic shock **p.221**
The unconscious casualty **pp.54–85**

1 **Reassure the casualty and help him to sit or lie down.**

2 **Raise the affected part if possible. Place a cold compress such as an ice pack (p.241) on the affected area for at least ten minutes to minimise the risk of swelling.**

3 **Monitor vital signs – level of response, breathing and pulse (pp.52–53). Watch for signs of an allergic reaction, such as wheezing.**

TICK BITE

YOUR AIMS

- To remove the tick.

CAUTION

- Do not try to remove the tick with butter or petroleum jelly or burn or freeze it, since it may regurgitate infective fluids into the casualty.

Ticks are tiny, spider-like creatures found in grass or woodlands. They attach themselves to passing animals (including humans) and bite into the skin to suck blood. When sucking blood, a tick swells to about the size of a pea, and it can then be seen easily. Ticks can carry disease and cause infection, so they should be removed as soon as possible.

1 **Using tweezers, grasp the tick's head as close to the casualty's skin as you can. Pull the head upwards using steady even pressure. Do not use twisting or jerking movements as this may leave mouth parts embedded, or cause the tick to regurgitate infective fluids into the skin.**

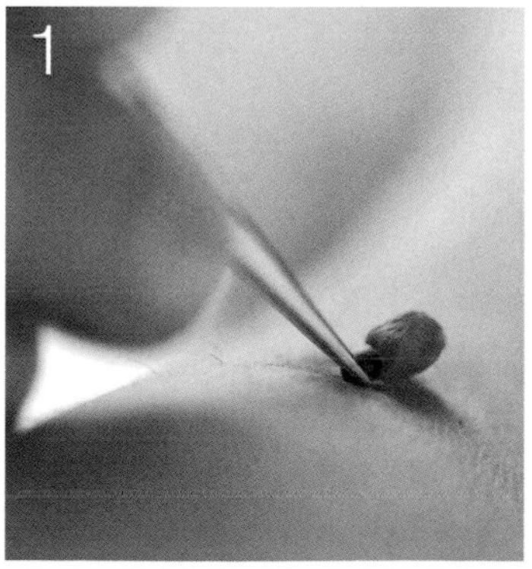

2 **Save the tick for identification; place it in a sealed plastic bag. The casualty should seek medical advice; tell him to take the tick since it may be required for analysis.**

SNAKE BITE

RECOGNITION

There may be:

- A pair of puncture marks – the bite may be painless;
- Severe pain, redness and swelling at the bite;
- Nausea and vomiting;
- Disturbed vision;
- Increased salivation and sweating;
- Laboured breathing; it may stop altogether.

YOUR AIMS

- To prevent venom spreading.
- To arrange urgent removal to hospital.

CAUTION

- Do not apply a tourniquet, slash the wound with a knife or try to suck out the venom.
- If the casualty loses consciousness, open the airway and check breathing (The unconscious casualty pp.54–85).

See also
Anaphylactic shock **p.221**
The unconscious casualty **pp.54–85**

Snake bites are uncommon in the UK. The only poisonous snake native to mainland Britain is the adder, and its bite is rarely fatal. However, poisonous snakes are sometimes kept as pets. People are also exposed to venomous snakes through travel.

While a snake bite is not usually serious, it is safer to assume that a snake is venomous. A venomous bite is often painless. Depending on the snake, venom may cause local tissue destruction, it may spread, blocking nerve impulses, causing heart and breathing to stop or it can cause blood clotting (coagulation) and then internal bleeding.

Note the time of the bite, as well as the snake's appearance to help doctors identify the correct antivenom. Take precautions to prevent others being bitten. Notify the authorities who will deal with the snake.

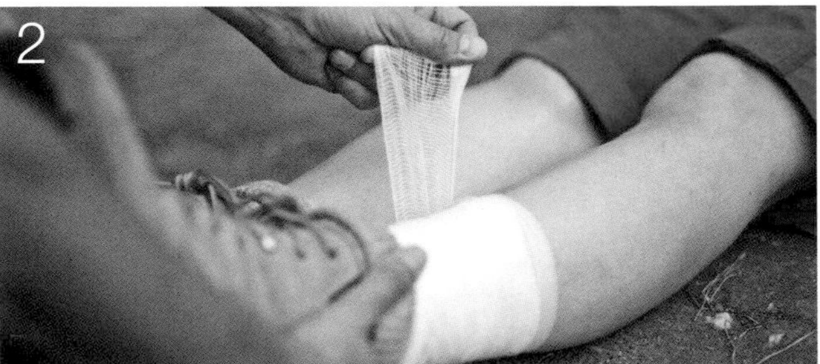

1 **Help the casualty to lie down, with head and shoulders raised. Reassure the casualty, tell her to keep calm and advise her not to move her limbs. Call 999/112 for emergency help.**

2 **If there is no pain, apply a pressure bandage at the site of the bite. Do not remove clothing from around the site since this can speed up the absorption of the venom.**

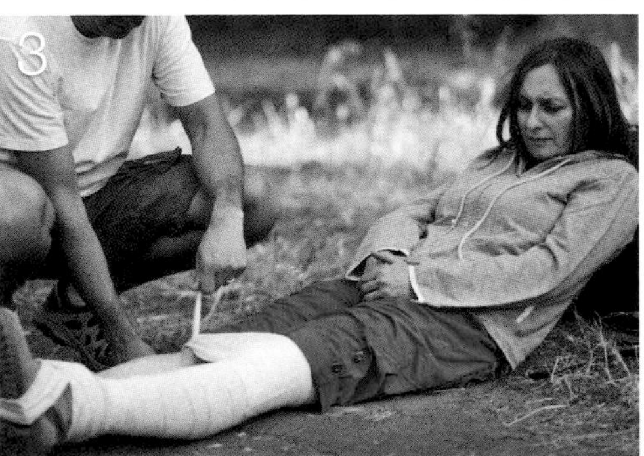

3 **Apply another pressure bandage to extend from the bite as far up the limb as possible. Tie it as for a sprained ankle, and check circulation after bandaging (p.243). If possible, mark the site of the bite. Immobilise the limb by securing it to the other leg with broad- and narrow-fold bandages (p.249).**

4 **Monitor and record vital signs (pp.52–53) while waiting for help to arrive. The casualty needs to remain still.**

STINGS FROM SEA CREATURES

RECOGNITION

Depends on the species, but generally:

- Pain, redness and swelling at site of sting;
- Nausea and vomiting;
- Headache.

YOUR AIMS

- To relieve pain and discomfort.
- To seek medical help if necessary.

CAUTION

- If the injury is extensive or there is a severe reaction, **call 999/112 for emergency help**. Monitor and record vital signs – level of response, breathing and pulse (pp.52–53) – while waiting for help to arrive.

See also
Anaphylactic shock **p.221**

Jellyfish, Portuguese men-of-war, sea anemones and corals can all cause stings. Their venom is contained in stinging cells that stick to the skin. Most marine species found in temperate regions of the world are not dangerous. However, some tropical marine creatures can cause severe poisoning. Occasionally, death results from paralysis of the chest muscles and, very rarely, from anaphylactic shock (p.221).

1 **Encourage the casualty to sit or lie down. Immerse the affected area in hot water (40–41°C/104–106°F) for ten minutes to relieve pain and swelling.**

2 **Alternatively, wash the area in copious quantities of cold water.**

3 **Monitor vital signs – level of response, breathing and pulse (pp.52–53). Watch for signs of an allergic reaction, such as wheezing.**

SPECIAL CASE
JELLYFISH STING

Pour copious amounts of vinegar or sea water over the area of the injury to incapacitate the stinging cells. Help the casualty to sit down and treat as for a snake bite (opposite). **Call 999/112 for emergency help.**

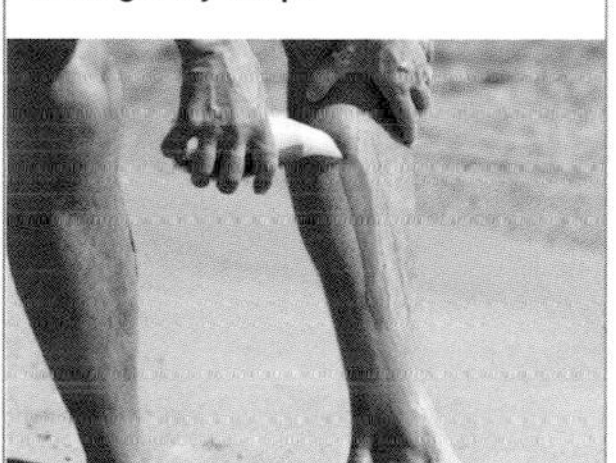

MARINE PUNCTURE WOUND

YOUR AIMS

- To relieve pain and discomfort.

CAUTION

- Do not bandage the wound.
- Do not scald the casualty.

Many marine creatures have spines that provide a mechanism against attack from predators but that can also cause painful wounds if trodden on. Sea urchins and weever fish have sharp spines that can become embedded in the sole of the foot. Wounds may become infected if the spines are not removed. Hot water breaks down fish venom.

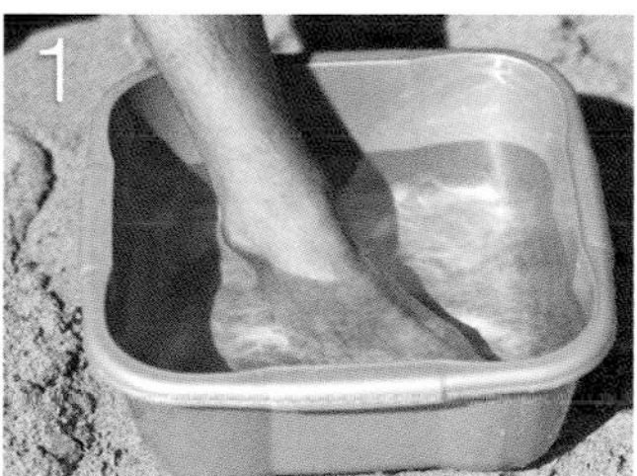

1 **Help the casualty to sit down. Immerse the injured part in water as hot as he can tolerate for about 30 minutes.**

2 **Take or send the casualty to hospital so that the spines can be safely removed.**

11

Many everyday conditions, such as fever and headache, need prompt treatment and respond well to first aid. However, a minor complaint can be the start of serious illness, so you should always be alert to this and seek medical advice if you are in doubt about the casualty's condition.

Other conditions such as diabetes-related hypoglycaemia (lower than normal blood sugar levels), severe allergic reaction (anaphylaxis) and meningitis are potentially life-threatening and require urgent medical attention.

Childbirth is a natural process and often takes many hours. So when a woman goes into labour unexpectedly, while it is important to call for emergency help, there is usually plenty of time to seek help and get her to hospital. In the rare event of a baby arriving quickly, do not try to deliver the baby – the birth will happen naturally without intervention.

Miscarriage, however, is a potentially serious problem due to the risk of severe bleeding. A woman who is miscarrying needs urgent medical help.

AIMS AND OBJECTIVES

- To assess the casualty's condition quietly and calmly.
- To comfort and reassure the casualty.
- To call 999/112 for emergency help if you suspect a serious illness.

MEDICAL CONDITIONS

DIABETES MELLITUS

This is a long-term (chronic) condition in which the body fails to produce sufficient insulin. Insulin is a chemical produced by the pancreas (a gland that lies behind the stomach), which regulates the blood sugar (glucose) level in the body. This condition can result in higher than normal blood sugar (hyperglycaemia) or lower than normal blood sugar (hypoglycaemia). If a person with diabetes is unwell, giving him sugar will rapidly correct hypoglycaemia and is unlikely to do harm in cases of hyperglycaemia.

TYPES OF DIABETES

There are two types: Type 1, or insulin-dependent diabetes, and Type 2, or non-insulin-dependent diabetes.

In Type 1 diabetes, the body produces little or no insulin. People with Type 1 diabetes need regular insulin injections throughout their lives. It is sometimes referred to as juvenile diabetes or early onset diabetes because it usually develops in childhood or teenage years. Insulin can be administered using a syringe or an injection pen (insulin pen). In some cases, it is given via a "pump", a small device about the size of a pack of cards that is strapped to the body. The insulin is administered via a piece of tubing that leads from the pump to a needle that sits just under the skin.

In Type 2 diabetes, the body does not make enough insulin or cannot use it properly. This type is usually linked with obesity, and is also known as maturity-onset diabetes, as it is more common in people over the age of 40. The risk of developing this type is increased if it runs in your family. Type 2 diabetes can normally be controlled with diet, weight loss and regular exercise. However, oral medication and, in some cases, insulin injections may be needed.

HYPERGLYCAEMIA

RECOGNITION

- Warm, dry skin.
- Rapid pulse and breathing.
- Fruity sweet breath and excessive thirst.
- Drowsiness, leading to unconsciousness if untreated.

YOUR AIMS

- To arrange urgent removal to hospital.

CAUTION

- If the casualty loses consciousness, open the airway and check breathing (The unconscious casualty pp.54–85).

High blood sugar (hyperglycaemia) develops slowly over a period of days.Those who suffer from hyperglycaemia may wear warning bracelets, cards or medallions alerting a first aider to the condition. If it is not treated, hyperglycaemia will result in unconsciousness (diabetic coma) and so requires urgent treatment in hospital.

See also
The unconscious casualty **pp.54–85**

1 **Call 999/112 for emergency help;** tell ambulance control that you suspect hyperglycaemia.

2 **Monitor and record vital signs – level of response, breathing and pulse (pp.52–53) – while waiting for help to arrive.**

HYPOGLYCAEMIA

RECOGNITION

There may be:

- A history of diabetes – the casualty may recognise the onset of a hypo attack himself;
- Weakness, faintness or hunger;
- Confusion and irrational behaviour;
- Sweating with cold, clammy skin;
- Rapid pulse;
- Palpitations and muscle tremors;
- Deteriorating level of response.
- Diabetic identity bracelet or necklace, glucose gel, medication such as tablets or an insulin syringe.

YOUR AIMS

- To raise the sugar content of the blood as quickly as possible
- To obtain appropriate medical help.

CAUTION

- If consciousness is impaired, do not give the casualty anything to eat or drink.
- If the casualty loses consciousness, open the airway and check breathing (The unconscious casualty pp.54–85).

See also
Impaired consciousness **p.164**
The unconscious casualty **pp.54–85**

This condition occurs when the blood sugar level falls below normal. It is characterised by a rapidly deteriorating level of response. Hypoglycaemia develops if the insulin–sugar balance is incorrect; for example, when a person with diabetes misses a meal or takes too much exercise. It is more common in a person with newly diagnosed diabetes while he is becoming used to balancing sugar levels. More rarely, hypoglycaemia may develop following an epileptic seizure (pp.168–69) or after an episode of binge drinking. It can also occur with heat exhaustion or hypothermia.

People with diabetes may carry their own blood-testing kits to check their blood sugar levels, as well as their insulin medication, so are well prepared for emergencies; for example, many carry sugar lumps or a tube of glucose gel.

If the hypoglycaemic attack is at an advanced stage, consciousness may be impaired and you must seek emergency help.

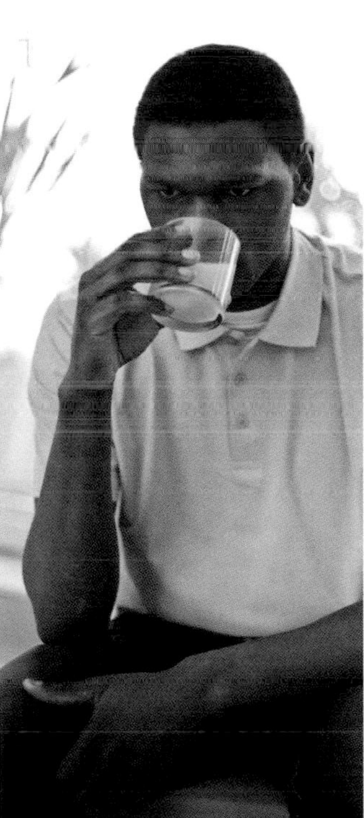

1 **Help the casualty to sit down. Give him a sugary drink, sugar lumps or sweet food. If he has his own glucose gel, help him to take it.**

2 **If the casualty responds quickly, give him more food or drink and let him rest until he feels better. Help him find his glucose testing kit so that he can check his glucose level. Monitor him until he is completely recovered.**

3 **If his condition does not improve, look for other possible causes. Call 999/112 for emergency help and monitor and record vital signs – level of response, breathing and pulse (pp.52–53) – while waiting for help to arrive.**

ALLERGY

RECOGNITION

Features of mild allergy vary depending on the trigger and the person. There may be:

- Red, itchy rash or raised areas of skin (weals);
- Red, itchy eyes;
- Wheezing and/or difficulty breathing;
- Swelling of hands, feet and/or face;
- Abdominal pain, vomiting and diarrhoea.

YOUR AIMS

- To assess the severity of the allergic reaction.
- To seek medical advice if necessary.

CAUTION

- **Call 999/112 for emergency help** if the casualty does not improve, she has difficulty in breathing or is becoming distressed. Monitor and record vital signs (pp.52–53) while waiting for help.

An allergy is an abnormal reaction of the body's defence system (immune response) to a normally harmless "trigger" substance (or allergen). An allergy can present itself as a mild itching, swelling, wheezing or digestive condition, or can progress to full-blown anaphylaxis, or anaphylactic shock (opposite), which can occur within seconds or minutes of exposure to an offending allergen.

Common triggers include pollen, dust, nuts, shellfish, eggs, wasp and bee stings, latex and certain medications. Skin changes can be subtle, absent or variable in up to 20 per cent of allergic reactions.

See also
Anaphylactic shock **opposite**
Asthma **p.100**

1 **Assess the casualty's signs and symptoms. Ask if she has any known allergy.**

2 **Remove the trigger if possible, or move the casualty from the trigger.**

3 **Treat any symptoms. Allow the casualty to take her own medication for a known allergy.**

4 **If you are at all concerned about the casualty's condition, seek medical advice.**

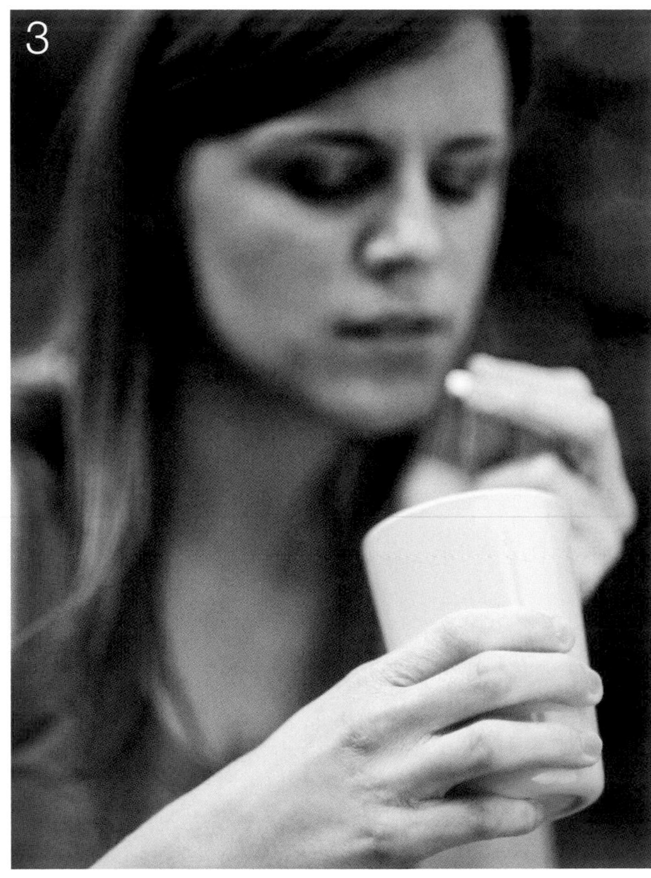

ANAPHYLACTIC SHOCK

RECOGNITION

Features of allergy (opposite) may be present:

- Red, itchy rash or raised areas of skin (weals);
- Red itchy, watery eyes;
- Swelling of hands, feet and/ or face;
- Abdominal pain, vomiting and diarrhoea.

There may also be:

- Difficulty breathing, ranging from a tight chest to severe difficulty, causing the casualty to wheeze and gasp for air;
- Pale or flushed skin;
- Visible swelling of tongue and throat with puffiness around the eyes;
- Feeling of terror;
- Confusion and agitation;
- Signs of shock, leading to collapse and loss of consciousness.

YOUR AIMS

- To ease breathing.
- Treat shock.
- To arrange urgent removal to hospital.

CAUTION

- If a pregnant casualty needs to lie down, lean her towards her left side to prevent her baby restricting blood flow back to the heart.
- If the casualty loses consciousness, open the airway and check breathing (The unconscious casualty pp.54–85).

See also
Hypoxia **p.90**
Shock **pp.116–17**
The unconscious casualty **pp.54–85**

This is a severe allergic reaction affecting the whole body. It may develop within seconds or minutes of contact with a trigger and is potentially fatal. In an anaphylactic reaction, chemicals are released into the blood that widen (dilate) blood vessels. This causes blood pressure to fall and air passages to narrow (constrict), resulting in breathing difficulties. In addition, the tongue and throat can swell, obstructing the airway. The amount of oxygen reaching the vital organs can be severely reduced, causing hypoxia (p.90). Common triggers include: nuts, shellfish, eggs, wasp and bee stings, latex and certain medications.

A casualty with anaphylactic shock needs emergency treatment with an injection of adrenaline (epinephrine).

1 **Call 999/112 for emergency help. Tell ambulance control that you suspect anaphylaxis.**

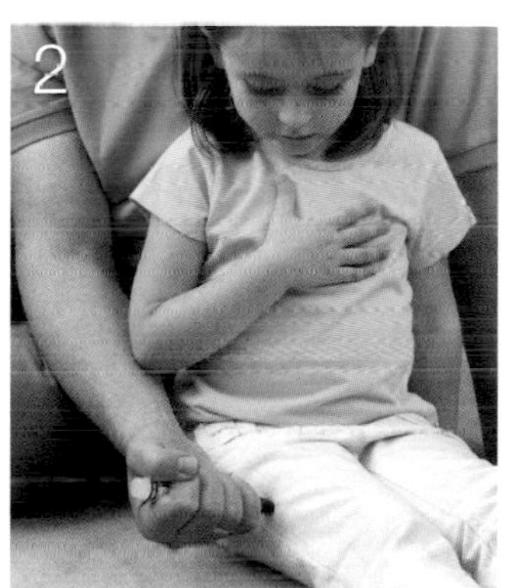

2 **Check whether the casualty is carrying any medication – a syringe or an auto-injector of adrenaline (epinephrine) – and help her to use it. If she is unable to administer it, and you have been trained to use an auto-injector, you may give it to her. Pull off the safety cap and, holding the injector with your fist, place the tip firmly against the casualty's thigh to release the medication (it can be delivered through clothing).**

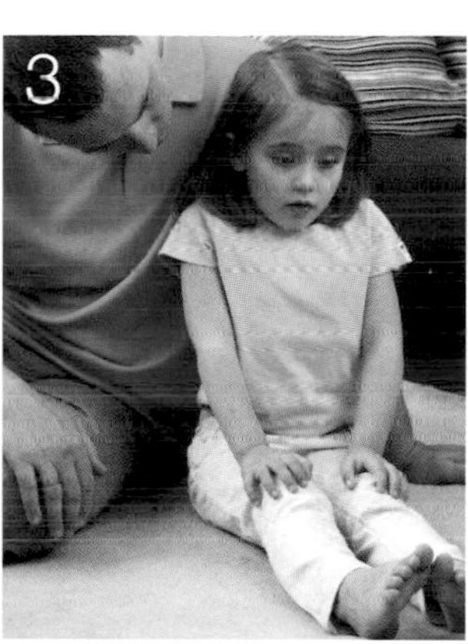

3 **Help the casualty to sit up in the position that best relieves any breathing difficulty. If she becomes pale with a weak pulse, help her to lie down with legs raised and treat for shock (pp.116–17).**

4 **Monitor and record vital signs – level of response, breathing and pulse (pp.52–53) – while waiting for help to arrive. Repeated doses of adrenaline (epinephrine) can be given at five-minute intervals if there is no improvement or the symptoms return.**

FEVER

RECOGNITION

- Raised body temperature above 37°C (98.6°F).
- Pallor; casualty may feel cold with goose pimples, shivering and chattering teeth.

Later:

- Hot, flushed skin and sweating;
- Headache;
- Generalised aches and pains.

YOUR AIMS

- To bring down the fever.
- To obtain medical aid if necessary.

CAUTION

- If you are concerned about the casualty's condition, seek medical advice.
- Do not over- or underdress a child with fever; do not sponge a child to cool her.
- Do not give aspirin to any person under 16 years of age.

See also
Seizures in children **p.170**

A sustained body temperature above the normal level of 37°C (98.6°F) is known as fever. It is usually caused by a bacterial or viral infection, but may be associated with earache, sore throat, measles, chickenpox, meningitis (opposite) or local infection, such as an abscess. The infection may have been acquired during overseas travel.

Moderate fever is not harmful to adults, but in young children a temperature above 37°C (98.6°F) can be dangerous and may trigger seizures. If you are in any doubt about a casualty's condition, seek medical advice.

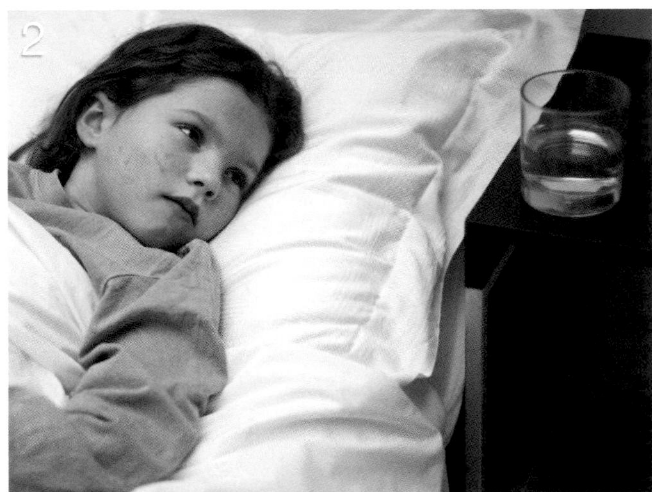

1 **Keep casualty cool and comfortable – preferably in bed with a light covering.**

2 **Give her plenty of cool drinks to replace body fluids lost through sweating.**

3 **If the child appears distressed or unwell, she may have the recommended dose of paracetamol syrup (not aspirin). An adult may take the recommended dose of paracetamol tablets or her own painkillers.**

4 **Monitor and record a casualty's vital signs – level of response, breathing, pulse and temperature (pp.52–53) – until she recovers.**

SPECIAL CASE IF A CHILD BECOMES VERY HOT

If there is a risk of seizure because of the raised temperature, cool the child further by removing his clothes and bed covering.

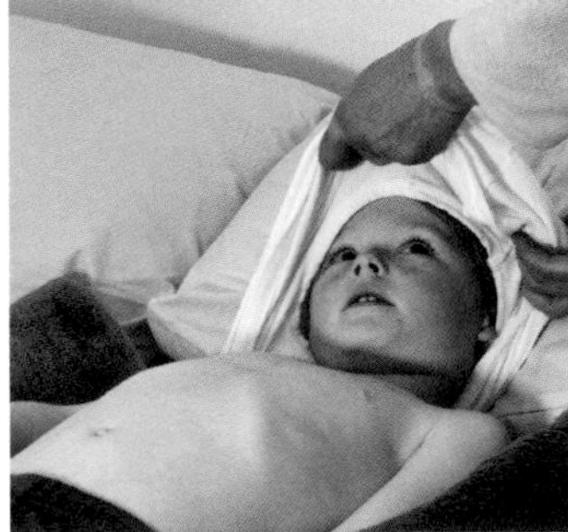

MENINGITIS

RECOGNITION

The symptoms and signs are usually not all present at the same time. They include:

- Flu-like illness with a high temperature;
- Cold hands and feet;
- Joint and limb pain;
- Mottled or very pale skin.

As the infection develops:

- Severe headache;
- Neck stiffness (the casualty will not be able to touch her chest with her chin);
- Vomiting;
- Eyes become very sensitive to any light – daylight, electric light or even the television;
- Drowsiness;
- In infants, there may also be high-pitched moaning or a whimpering cry, floppiness and a tense or bulging fontanelle (soft part of the skull).

Later:

- A distinctive rash of red or purple spots that do not fade when pressed.

YOUR AIMS

- To obtain urgent medical help.

CAUTION

- If a casualty's condition is deteriorating, and you suspect meningitis, **call 999/112 for emergency help** even if she has already seen a doctor.

This is a condition in which the linings that surround the brain and the spinal cord become inflamed. It can be caused by bacteria or a virus and can affect any age group.

Meningitis is potentially a very serious illness and the casualty may deteriorate very quickly. If you suspect meningitis, you must seek urgent medical assistance as prompt treatment in hospital is vital. For this reason it is important that you are able to recognise the symptoms of meningitis, which may include a high temperature, headache and a distinctive rash. With early diagnosis and treatment most people make a full recovery.

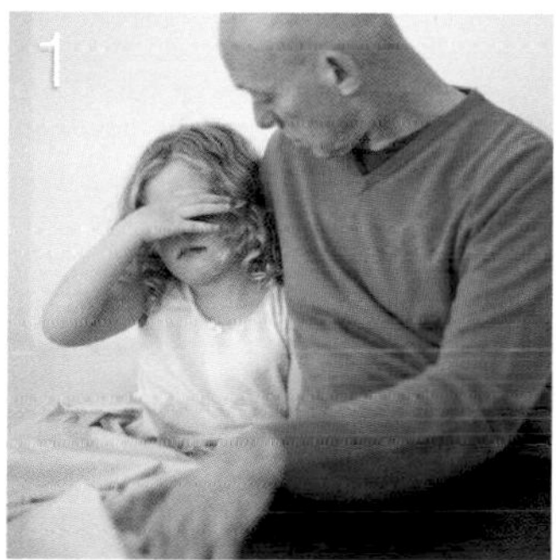

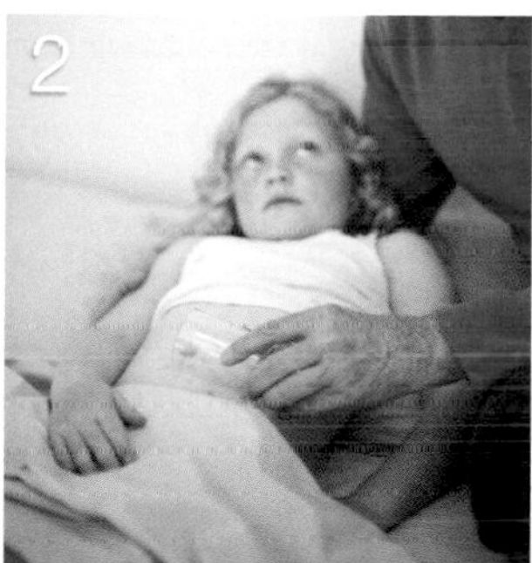

1 **Seek urgent medical advice if you notice any of the signs of meningitis; for example, shielding eyes from the light. Do not wait for all the symptoms and signs to appear because they may not all develop. Treat the fever (opposite).**

2 **Check the casualty for signs of a rash. On dark skin, check on lighter parts of the body; for example, the inner eyelids or fingertips. If you see any signs, call 999/112 for emergency help.**

3 **While waiting for help to arrive, reassure the casualty and keep her cool. Monitor and record vital signs – level of response, breathing and pulse (pp.52–53).**

IMPORTANT MENINGITIS RASH

Accompanying the later stage of meningitis is a distinctive red or purple rash that does not fade if you press it. If you press the side of a glass firmly against most rashes they will fade; if a rash does not fade, **call 999/112 for emergency help** immediately.

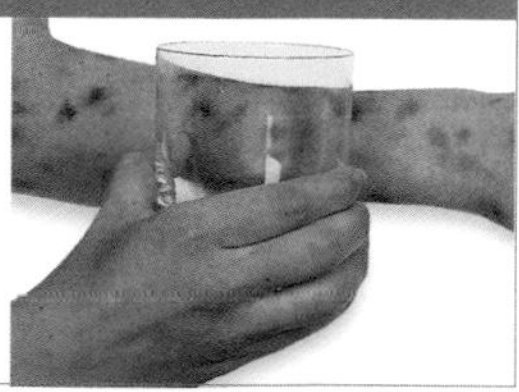

HEADACHE

YOUR AIMS

- To relieve the pain.
- To obtain medical advice if necessary.

CAUTION

- Do not give aspirin to anyone under 16 years of age.

Seek urgent medical advice if the pain:

- Develops very suddenly;
- Is severe and incapacitating;
- Is accompanied by fever or vomiting;
- Is recurrent or persistent;
- Is accompanied by loss of strength or sensation, or by impaired consciousness;
- Is accompanied by a stiff neck and sensitivity to light;
- Follows a head injury.

A headache may accompany any illness, particularly a feverish ailment such as flu. It may develop for no reason, but can often be traced to tiredness, tension, stress or undue heat or cold. Mild "poisoning" caused by a stuffy or fume-filled atmosphere, or by excess alcohol or any other drug, can also induce a headache. However, a headache may also be the most prominent symptom of meningitis or a stroke.

See also
Head injury p.165
Meningitis p.223
Stroke pp.174–75

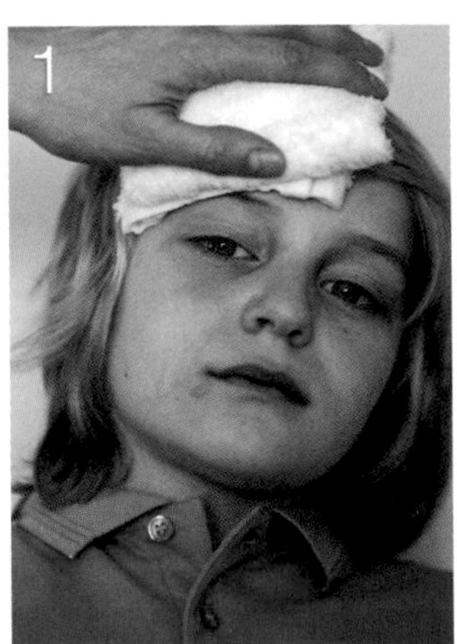

1 **Help the casualty to sit or lie down in a quiet place. Give him a cold compress to hold against his head (p.241).**

2 **An adult may take the recommended dose of paracetamol tablets or his own painkillers. A child may have the recommended dose of paracetamol syrup (not aspirin).**

MIGRAINE

RECOGNITION

- Before the attack there may be disturbance of vision in the form of flickering lights and/or a "blind patch".
- Intense throbbing headache, which is sometimes on just one side of the head.
- Abdominal pain, nausea and vomiting.
- Inability to tolerate bright light or loud noise.

YOUR AIMS

- To relieve the pain.
- To obtain medical aid if necessary.

Migraine attacks are severe, "sickening" headaches and can be triggered by a variety of causes, such as allergy, stress or tiredness. Other triggers include lack of sleep, missed meals, alcohol and some foods – for example, cheese or chocolate. Migraine sufferers usually know how to recognise and deal with attacks and may carry their own medication.

1 **Help the casualty to take any medication that he may have for migraine attacks.**

2 **Advise the casualty to lie down or sleep for a few hours in a quiet, dark room. Provide him with some towels and a container in case he vomits.**

3 **If this is the first attack, advise the casualty to seek medical advice.**

EARACHE AND TOOTHACHE

YOUR AIMS

- To relieve the pain.
- To obtain medical or dental advice if necessary.

CAUTION

- Do not give aspirin to anyone under 16 years of age.
- If there is a discharge from an ear, fever or hearing loss, obtain medical help.

Earache can result from inflammation of the outer, middle or inner ear, often caused by an infection associated with a cold, tonsillitis or flu. It can also be caused by a boil, an object stuck in the ear canal or transmitted pain from a tooth abscess. There may also be temporary hearing loss. Earache often occurs when flying as a result of the changes in air pressure during ascent and descent. Infection can cause pus to collect in the middle ear; the eardrum may rupture, allowing the pus to drain, which temporarily eases the pain.

Toothache can develop when pulp inside a tooth becomes inflamed due to dental decay. If untreated, the pulp becomes infected, leading to an abscess, which causes a throbbing pain. Infection may cause swelling around the tooth or jaw.

1 **An adult may take the recommended dose of paracetamol tablets or her own painkillers. A child may have the recommended dose of paracetamol syrup (not aspirin).**

2 **Give her a source of heat, such as a hot water bottle wrapped in a towel, to hold against the affected side of her face.**

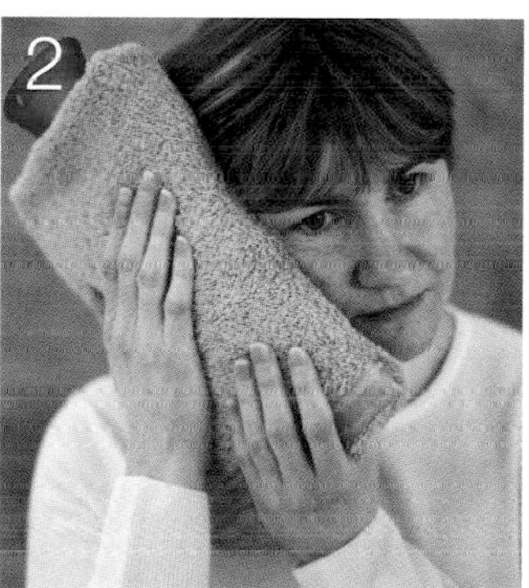

3 **In addition for toothache, you can soak a plug of cotton wool in oil of cloves to hold against the affected tooth.**

4 **Advise a casualty to seek medical advice if you are concerned, particularly if the casualty is a child. If a casualty has toothache, advise her to see her dentist.**

SORE THROAT

YOUR AIMS

- To relieve the pain.
- To obtain medical advice if necessary.

CAUTION

- Do not give aspirin to anyone under 16 years of age.
- If you suspect tonsillitis or glandular fever, tell the casualty to seek medical advice.

The most common sore throat is a "raw" feeling caused by inflammation, which is often the first sign of a cough or cold. Tonsillitis occurs when the tonsils at the back of the throat are infected. The tonsils become red and swollen and white spots of pus may be seen. Swallowing may be difficult and the glands at the angle of the jaw may be enlarged and sore.

1 **Give the casualty plenty of fluids to help ease the pain and stop the throat from becoming dry.**

2 **An adult may take the recommended dose of paracetamol tablets or his own painkillers. A child may have the recommended dose of paracetamol syrup (not aspirin).**

ABDOMINAL PAIN

YOUR AIMS

- To relieve pain and discomfort.
- To obtain medical help if necessary.

CAUTION

- If the pain is severe, or occurs with fever and vomiting, **call 999/112 for emergency help**. Treat the casualty for shock (pp.116–17). Do not give her medicine or allow her to eat or drink, because an anaesthetic may be needed.

See also
Angina **p.111**
Shock **pp.116–17**

SPECIAL CASE STITCH

This common condition is a form of cramp, usually associated with exercise, which occurs in the trunk or the sides of the chest. The most likely cause is a build-up in the muscles of chemical waste products, such as lactic acid, during physical exertion. Help the casualty to sit down and reassure him. The pain will usually ease quickly. If the pain does not disappear within a few minutes, or if you are concerned about the casualty's condition, seek medical advice.

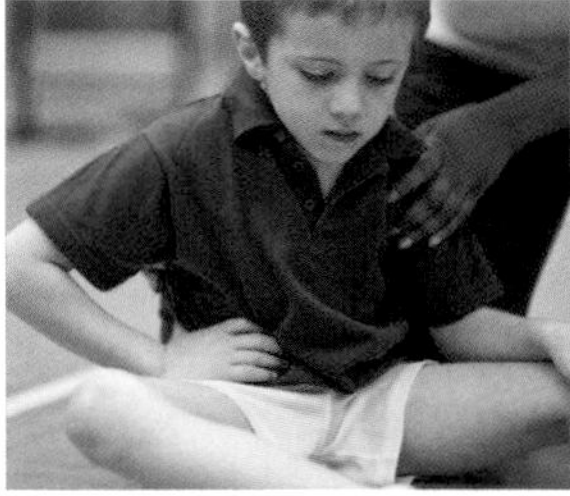

Pain in the abdomen often has a relatively minor cause, such as food poisoning. The pain of a stitch usually occurs during exercise and is sharp. Distension (widening) or obstruction of the intestine causes colic – pain that comes and goes in waves – which often makes the casualty double up in agony and may be accompanied by vomiting.

Occasionally abdominal pain is a sign of a serious disorder affecting the organs and other structures in the abdomen. If the appendix bursts, or the intestine is damaged, the contents of the intestine can leak into the abdominal cavity, causing inflammation of the cavity lining. This life-threatening condition, called peritonitis, causes intense pain, which is made worse by movement or pressure on the abdomen, and will lead to shock (pp.116–17).

An inflamed appendix (appendicitis) is especially common in children. Symptoms include pain (often starting in the centre of the abdomen and moving to the lower right-hand side), loss of appetite, nausea, vomiting, bad breath and fever. If the appendix bursts, peritonitis will develop. The treatment is urgent surgical removal of the appendix.

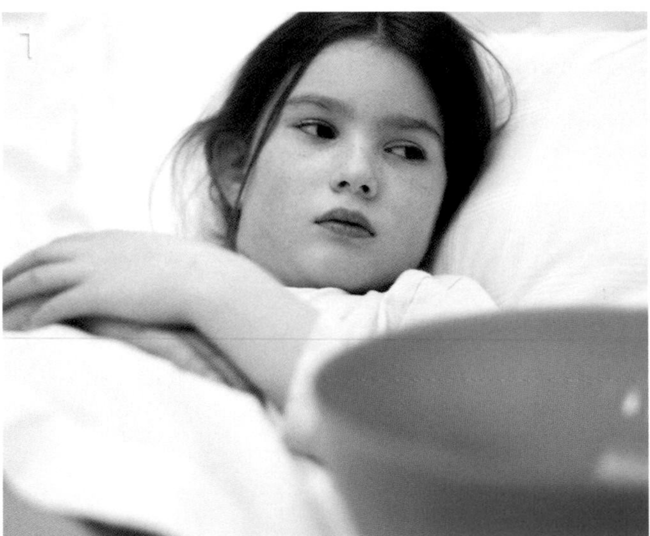

1 **Reassure the casualty and make her comfortable. Prop her up if she finds breathing difficult. Give her a container to use if she is vomiting.**

2 **Give the casualty a hot-water bottle wrapped in a towel to hold against her abdomen. If in doubt about her condition, seek medical advice.**

VOMITING AND DIARRHOEA

RECOGNITION

There may be:

- Nausea;
- Vomiting and later diarrhoea;
- Stomach pains;
- Fever.

YOUR AIMS

- To reassure the casualty.
- To restore lost fluids and salts.

CAUTION

- Do not give anti-diarrhoea medicines.
- If you are concerned about a casualty's condition, particularly if the vomiting or diarrhoea is persistent, or the casualty is a young child or an older person, seek medical advice.

See also
Drug poisoning **p.209**
Swallowed poisons **p.208**

1 Reassure the casualty if she is vomiting and give her a warm damp cloth to wipe her face.

2 Help her to sit down and when the vomiting stops give her water or unsweetened fruit juice to sip slowly and often.

3 When the casualty is hungry again, advise her to eat easily digested foods such as pasta, bread or potatoes for the first 24 hours.

These problems are usually due to irritation of the digestive system. Diarrhoea and vomiting can be caused by a number of different organisms, including viruses, bacteria and parasites. They usually result from eating contaminated food or drinking contaminated water, but infection can be passed directly from person to person. Cleanliness and good hygiene help prevent infectious diarrhoea.

Vomiting and diarrhoea may occur either separately or together. Both conditions can cause the body to lose vital fluids and salts, resulting in dehydration. When they occur together, the risk of dehydration is increased and can be serious, especially in infants, young children and elderly people.

The aim of treatment is to prevent dehydration by giving frequent sips of water or unsweetened fruit juice, even if the casualty is vomiting. Rehydration powder, which is added to water, provides the correct balance of water and salt to replace those lost through the vomiting and diarrhoea.

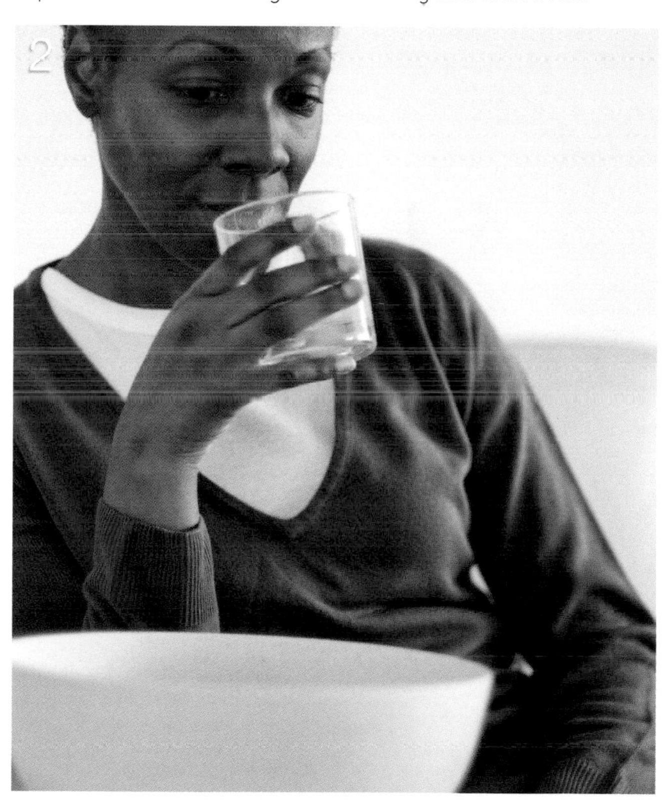
2

CHILDBIRTH

YOUR AIMS

- To obtain medical help or arrange for the woman to be taken to hospital.
- To ensure privacy, reassure the woman and make her comfortable.
- To prevent infection in the mother, baby and yourself.
- To care for the baby during and after delivery.

See also
Shock **pp.116–17**
Vaginal bleeding **p.128**

Childbirth is a natural and often lengthy process that normally occurs at about the 40th week of pregnancy. There is usually plenty of time to get a woman to hospital, or get help to her, before the baby arrives. Most pregnant women are aware of what happens during childbirth, but a woman who goes into labour unexpectedly or early may be very anxious. You will need to reassure her and make her comfortable. Miscarriage, however, is potentially serious because there is a risk of severe bleeding. A woman who is miscarrying needs urgent medical help (p.128).

There are three distinct stages to childbirth. In the first stage, the baby gets into position for the birth. The baby is born in the second stage, and in the third stage, the afterbirth (placenta and umbilical cord) is delivered.

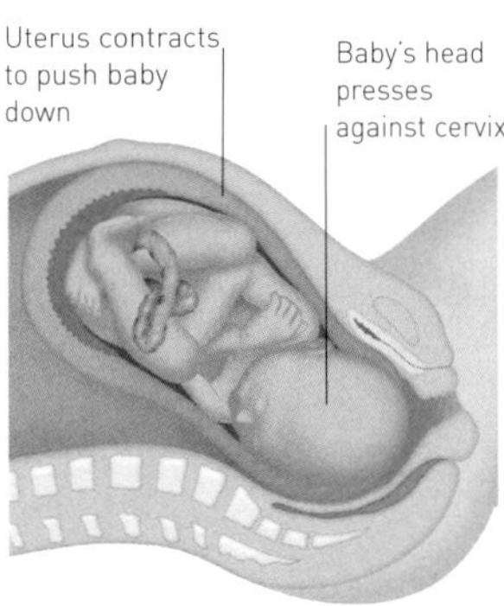

First stage
In this stage, a woman's body begins to experience contractions, which, together with the pressure of the baby's head, cause the cervix (neck of the uterus/womb) to open. The contractions become stronger and more frequent until the cervix is fully dilated (open) – about 10cm (4in) – and ready for the baby to be born. During this first stage, the mucus plug that protects the uterus from infection is expelled and the amniotic fluid surrounding the baby leaks out from the vagina. This stage can take several hours for a first baby but is normally shorter in any subsequent pregnancies.

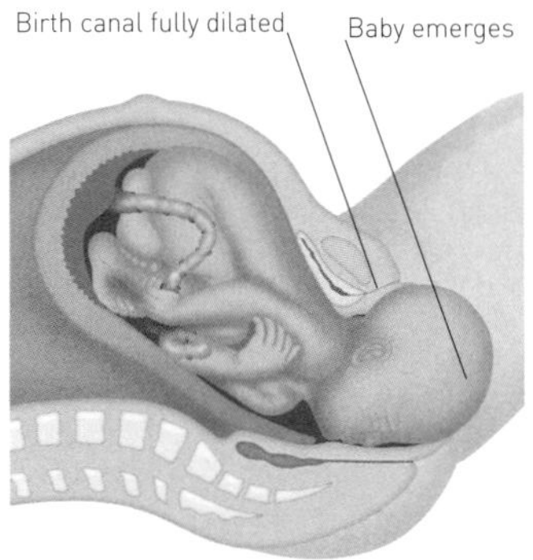

Second stage
Once the cervix is fully dilated, the baby's head will press down on the mother's pelvic floor, triggering a strong urge to push. The birth canal (vagina) stretches as the baby travels through it. The baby's head normally emerges first, and the body is delivered soon afterwards. This stage of labour normally lasts about an hour.

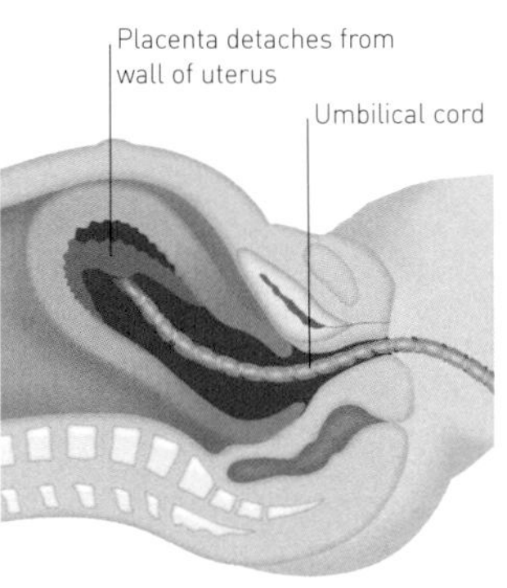

Third stage
About 10–30 minutes after the baby is born, the placenta (the organ that nourishes the unborn baby) and the umbilical cord will be expelled from the uterus. The uterus begins to contract again, pushing the placenta out, then it closes down the area where it was attached; this reduces the bleeding.

EMERGENCY CHILDBIRTH

CAUTION

- Do not give the mother anything to eat because there is a risk that she may vomit. If she is thirsty give her sips of water.
- Do not pull on the baby's head or shoulders during delivery.
- If the umbilical cord is wrapped around the baby's neck as he is born, check that it is loose, and then very carefully ease it over the head to protect the baby from strangulation.
- If a newborn baby does not cry, open the airway and check breathing (Unconscious infant pp.78–81). Do not smack the baby.
- Do not pull or cut the umbilical cord, even when the placenta has been delivered.

In the rare event of a baby arriving quickly, you should not try to "deliver" the baby; the birth will happen naturally without intervention. Your role is to comfort and listen to the wishes of the mother and care for her and her baby.

1 **Call 999/112 for emergency help.** Give ambulance control details of the stage the mother has reached, the length of each contraction and the intervals between them. Call the mother's midwife too if she requests it.

2 During the first stage, help her sit or kneel on the floor in a comfortable position. Support her with cushions or let her move around. Stay calm, and encourage her to breathe deeply during her contractions.

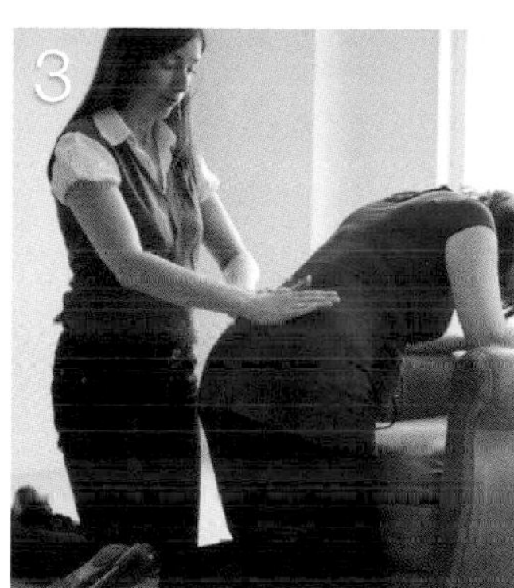

3 Massage her lower back gently using the heel of your hand. She may find having her face and hands wiped soothing, or you can spray her face with cool water and give her ice cubes to suck.

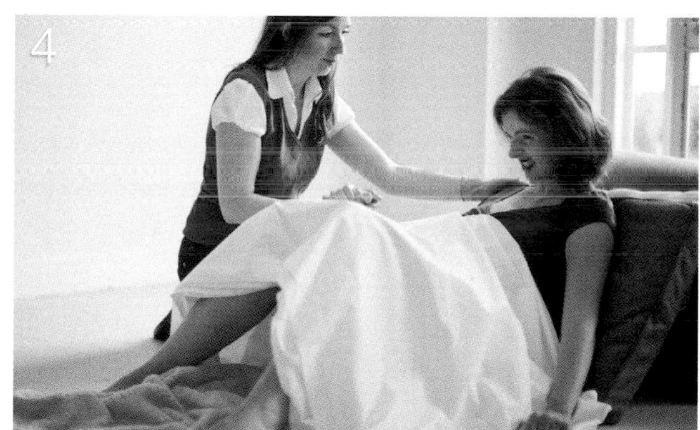

4 When the second stage starts, the mother will want to push. Make sure the surroundings are as clean as possible to reduce the risk of infection. The mother should remove any items of clothing that could interfere with the birth. Put clean sheets or towels under the woman; she may also want to be covered. Encourage her to stay as upright as possible.

5 As the baby is born, handle him carefully, as newborn babies are very slippery. Give him to the mother; lay him on her stomach or wrap him in a clean cloth, towel or blanket.

6 As the third stage begins, reassure the mother. Support her as she delivers the afterbirth; do not cut the cord. Keep the placenta and the umbilical cord intact as the midwife, doctor or ambulance crew need to check that it is complete. If bleeding or pain is severe, treat for shock (pp.116–17). Help the mother to lie down and raise her legs.

12

This chapter outlines the techniques and procedures that underpin first aid, including moving a casualty and applying dressings and bandages. Usually, a first aider is not expected to move an injured person, but in some circumstances – such as when a casualty is in immediate danger – it may be necessary. The key principles for moving casualties are described here. Information is also given on making an assessment of the risks involved in moving a casualty or assisting a casualty to safety.

A guide to the equipment and materials commonly found in a first aid kit is given, with information on how and when to use them. Applying dressings and bandages effectively is an essential part of first aid: wounds usually require a dressing, and almost all injuries benefit from the support that bandages can give.

AIMS AND OBJECTIVES

- To assess the casualty's condition.
- To comfort and reassure the casualty.
- To maintain a casualty's privacy and dignity.
- To use a first aid technique relevant to the injury.
- To use dressings and bandages as needed.
- To apply good handling techniques if moving a casualty.
- To obtain appropriate help: call 999/112 for emergency help if you suspect serious injury or illness.

TECHNIQUES AND EQUIPMENT

REMOVING CLOTHING

To make a thorough examination of a casualty, obtain an accurate diagnosis or give treatment, you may have to remove some of his clothing. This should be done with the minimum of disturbance to the casualty and with his agreement if possible. Remove as little clothing as possible and do not damage clothing unless it is necessary. If you need to cut a garment, try to cut along the seams, keeping the clothing clear of the casualty's injury. Maintain the casualty's privacy and prevent exposure to cold. Stop if removing clothing increases the casualty's discomfort or pain.

REMOVING CLOTHING IN LOWER BODY INJURIES

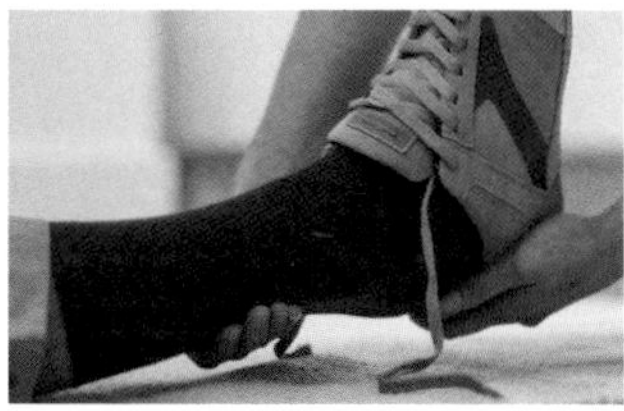

SHOES
Untie any laces, support the ankle and carefully pull the shoe off by the heel. To remove long boots, you may need to cut them down the back seam.

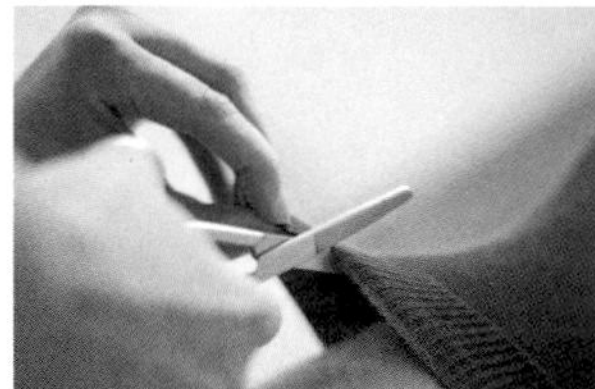

SOCKS
Remove socks by pulling them off gently. If this is not possible, lift each sock away from the leg and cut the fabric with a pair of scissors.

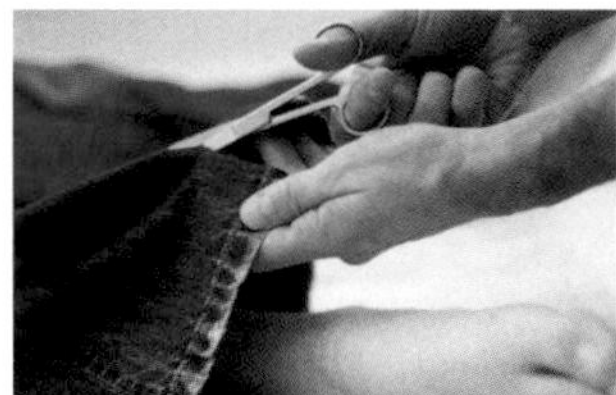

TROUSERS
Gently pull up the trouser leg to expose the calf and knee or pull down from the waist. If you need to cut clothing, lift it clear of the casualty's injury.

REMOVING CLOTHING IN UPPER BODY INJURIES

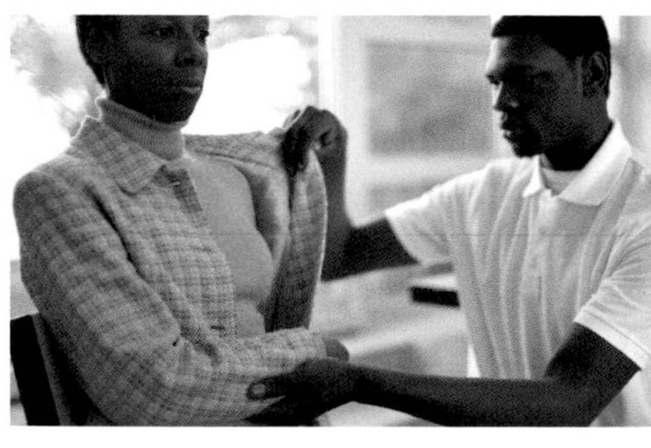

JACKETS
Support the injured arm. Undo any fastenings on the jacket and gently pull the garment off the casualty's shoulders. Remove the arm on the uninjured side from its sleeve. Pull the garment round to the injured side of the body and ease it off the injured arm.

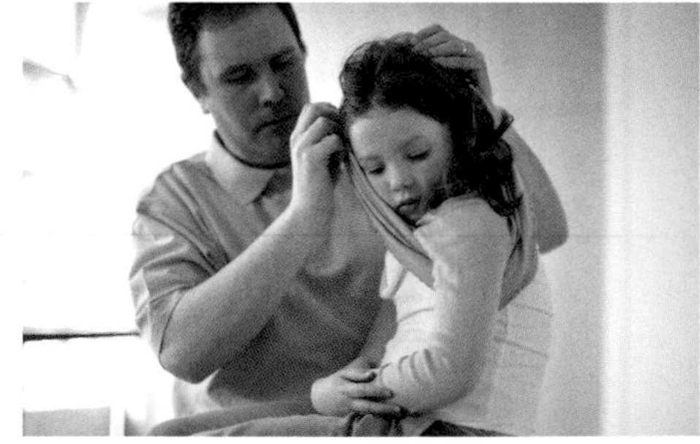

SWEATERS AND SWEATSHIRTS
With clothing that cannot be unfastened, begin by easing the arm on the uninjured side out of its sleeve. Next, roll up the garment and stretch it over the casualty's head. Finally, slip off the other sleeve of the garment, taking care not to disturb her arm on the injured side.

REMOVING HEADGEAR

CAUTION

Do not remove a helmet unless absolutely necessary.

See also
Spinal injury **pp.171–73**

Protective headgear, such as a riding hat or a motorcyclist's crash helmet, is best left on; it should be removed only if absolutely necessary, for example, if you cannot maintain an open airway. If the item does need to be removed, the casualty should do this herself if possible; otherwise, you and a helper should remove it. Take care to support the head and neck at all times and keep the head aligned with the spine.

REMOVING AN OPEN-FACE OR RIDING HELMET

1 Undo or cut through the chinstrap. Support the casualty's head and neck, keeping them aligned with the spine. Hold the lower jaw with one hand and support the neck with the other hand.

2 Ask a helper to grip the sides of the helmet and pull them apart to take pressure off the head, then lift the helmet upwards and backwards.

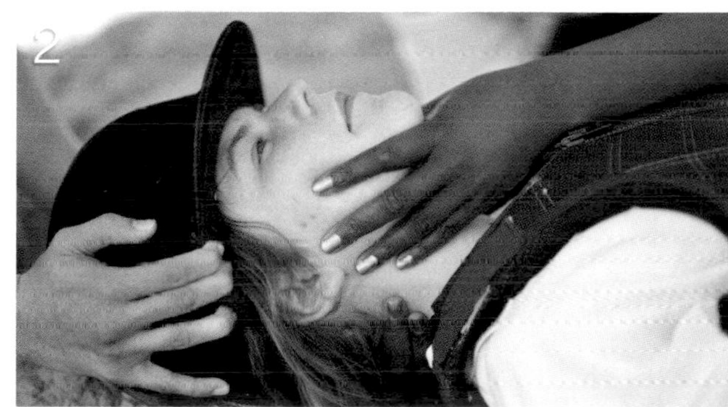

REMOVING A FULL-FACE HELMET

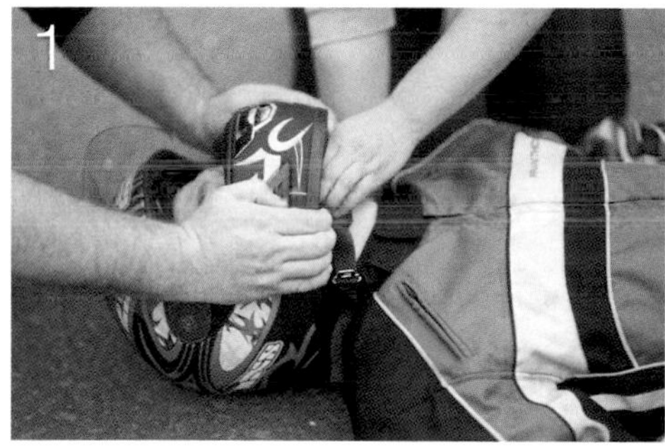

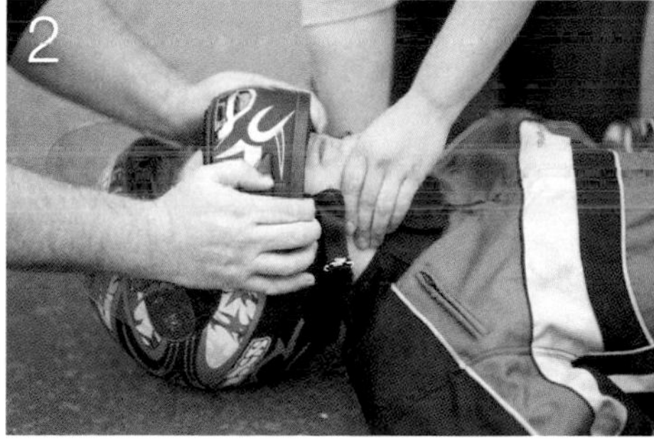

1 Undo or cut the straps. Working from the base of the helmet, ease your fingers underneath the rim. Support the back of the neck with one hand and hold the lower jaw firmly. Ask a helper to hold the helmet with both hands.

2 Continue to support the casualty's neck and lower jaw. Ask your helper, working from above, to tilt the helmet backwards (without moving the head) and gently lift the front of the helmet clear of the casualty's chin.

3 Maintain support on the head and neck. Ask your helper to tilt the helmet forwards slightly so that it will pass over the base of the skull, and then to lift it straight off the casualty's head.

CASUALTY HANDLING

CAUTION

- Do not approach a casualty if doing so puts your own life in danger.
- Do not move a casualty unless there is an emergency situation that demands you take immediate action.

When giving first aid you should leave a casualty in the position in which you find him until medical help arrives. Only move him if he is in imminent danger, and even then only if it is safe for you to approach and you have the training and equipment to carry out the move. A casualty should be moved quickly if he is in imminent danger from:

- **Drowning** (p.36);
- **Fire** or he is in an area that is filling with smoke (pp.32–33);
- **Explosion or gunfire**;
- **A collapsing building** or other structure.

ASSESSING THE RISK OF MOVING A CASUALTY

If it is necessary to move a casualty, consider the following before you start.

- **Is the task necessary?** Usually, the casualty can be assessed and treated in the position in which you find him.
- **What are his injuries or conditions**, and will a move make them worse?
- **Can the casualty move himself?** Ask the casualty if he feels able to move.
- **The weight and size** of the casualty.
- **Can anyone help?** If so, are you and any helpers trained and physically fit?
- **Will you need protective equipment** to enter the area, and do you have it?
- **Is there any equipment available** to assist with moving the casualty and are you trained to use it?
- **Is there enough space** around the casualty to move him safely?
- **What sort of ground** will you be crossing?

ASSISTING A CASUALTY SAFELY

If you need to move a casualty, take the following steps to ensure safety.

- **Select a method relevant** to the situation, the casualty's condition and the help and equipment that is available.
- **Use a team.** Appoint one person to coordinate the move and make sure that the team understands exactly what to do.
- **Plan your move** carefully and make sure that everyone is prepared.
- **Prepare any equipment** and make sure that the team and equipment are in position.
- **Use the correct technique** to avoid injuring the casualty, yourself or any helpers.
- **Ensure the safety** and comfort of the casualty, yourself and any helpers.
- **Always explain** to the casualty what is happening, and encourage him to cooperate as much as possible.
- **Position yourself** as close as possible to the casualty's body.
- **Adopt a stable base,** with your feet shoulder-width apart, so that you remain well balanced and maintain good posture at all times during the procedure.
- **Use the strongest muscles** in your legs and arms to power the move. Bend your knees.

FIRST AID MATERIALS

All workplaces, leisure centres, homes and cars should have first aid kits. The kits for workplaces or public places must conform to legal requirements and be clearly marked in a green box with a white cross and easily accessible. For home or the car, you can either buy a kit or put together first aid items yourself and keep them in a clean, waterproof container. Any first aid kit must be kept in a dry place, and checked and replenished regularly. The items on these pages form the basis of a first aid kit for the home. You may wish to add pain-relief tablets such as paracetamol.

STERILE DRESSINGS

WOUND DRESSINGS

The most useful dressings consist of a dressing pad attached to a roller bandage, and are sealed in a protective wrapping. They are easy to apply, so are ideal in an emergency. Various sizes are available. Individual sterile dressing pads are also available that can be secured with tape or bandages.

STERILE WOUND DRESSING

STERILE PAD

STERILE EYE PAD

FABRIC PLASTERS

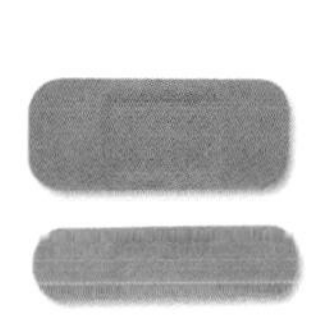

WATERPROOF PLASTERS

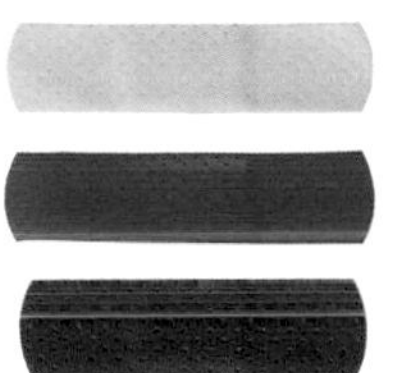

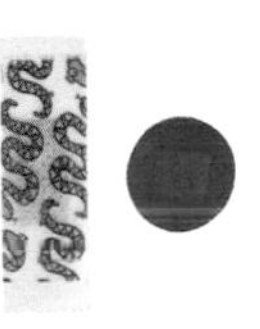

NOVELTY PLASTERS FOR CHILDREN

ADHESIVE DRESSINGS OR PLASTERS

These are applied to small cuts and grazes and are made of fabric or waterproof plastic. Use hypoallergenic plasters for anyone who is allergic to the adhesive in regular ones. People who work with food are required to use blue plasters. Special gel plasters can protect blisters.

CLEAR PLASTERS

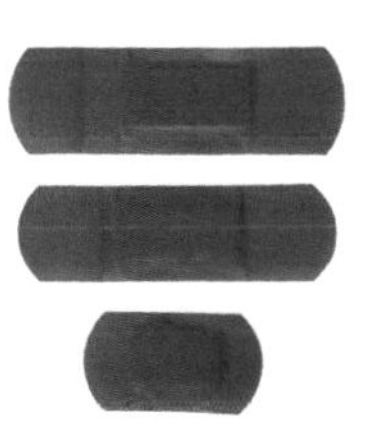

BLUE CATERING PLASTERS

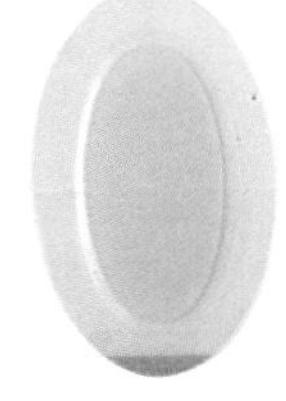

GEL BLISTER PLASTER

FIRST AID MATERIALS (continued)

BANDAGES

ROLLER BANDAGES

These items are used to give support to injured joints, secure dressings in place, maintain pressure on wounds and limit swelling.

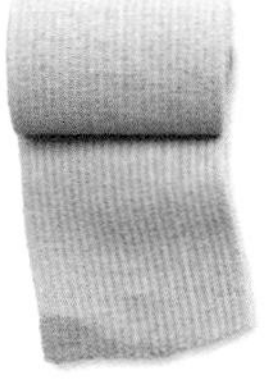

CONFORMING ROLLER BANDAGE

OPEN-WEAVE ROLLER BANDAGE

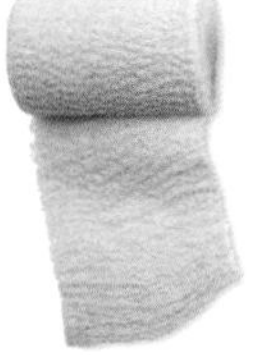

CRÊPE ROLLER BANDAGE

SELF-ADHESIVE BANDAGE

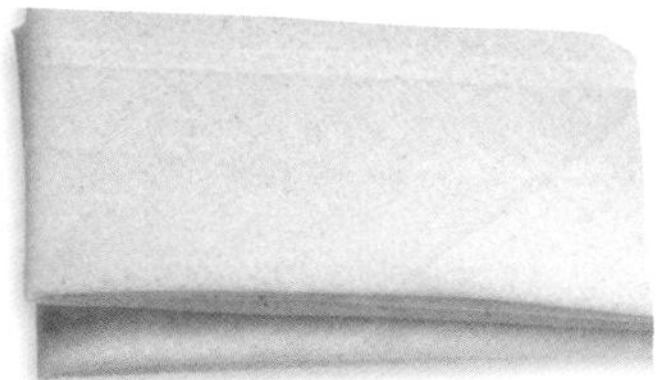

FOLDED TRIANGULAR BANDAGE

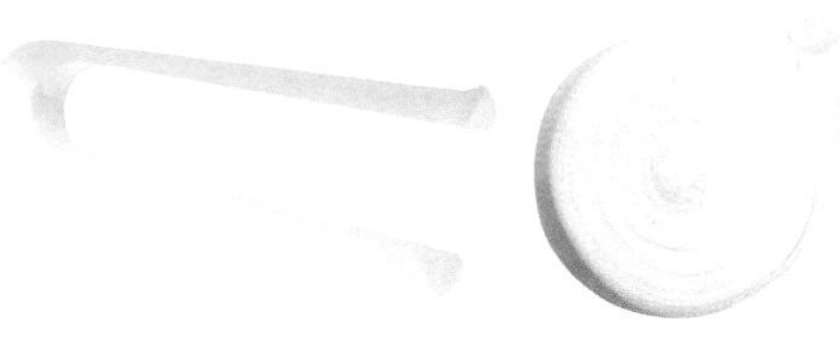

GAUZE TUBULAR BANDAGE AND APPLICATOR

TRIANGULAR BANDAGES

Made of cloth, these items can be used folded as bandages or slings. If they are sterile and individually wrapped, they may also be used as dressings for large wounds and burns.

GAUZE TUBULAR BANDAGES

Gauze tubular bandages are used with an applicator to secure dressings on fingers and toes. Elasticated tubular bandages are sometimes used to support injured joints such as the knee or elbow.

PROTECTIVE ITEMS

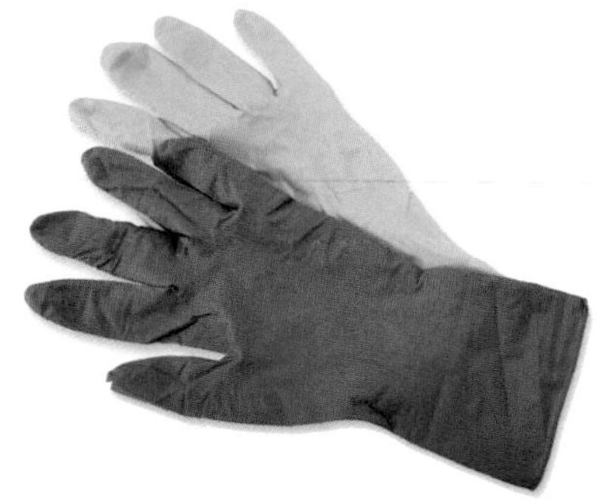

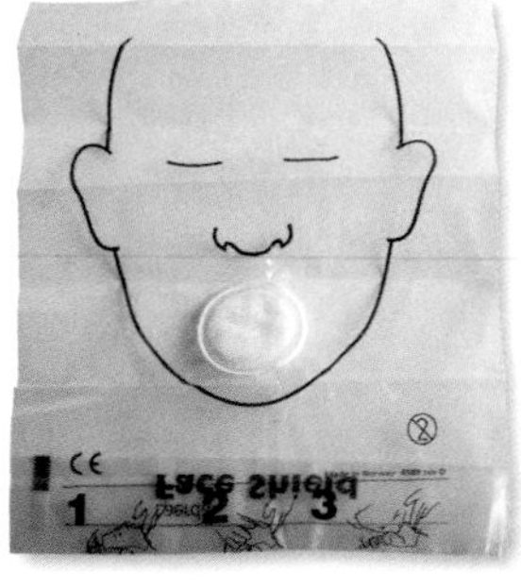

FACE SHIELD

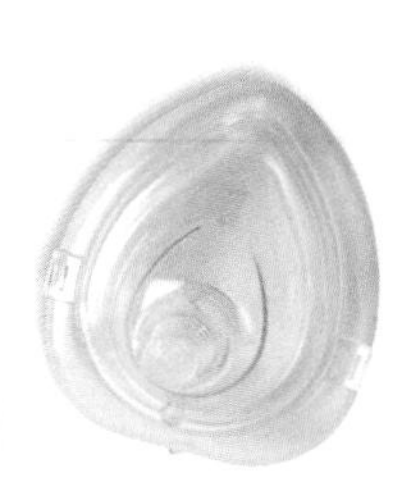

POCKET MASK

DISPOSABLE GLOVES

Wear gloves, if available, whenever you dress wounds or when you handle body fluids or other waste materials. Use latex-free gloves because some people are allergic to latex.

PROTECTION FROM INFECTION IN CPR

You can use a plastic face shield or a pocket mask to protect you and the casualty from cross infections when giving rescue breaths.

ADDITIONAL ITEMS

CLEANSING WIPES
Alcohol-free wipes can be used to clean skin around wounds.

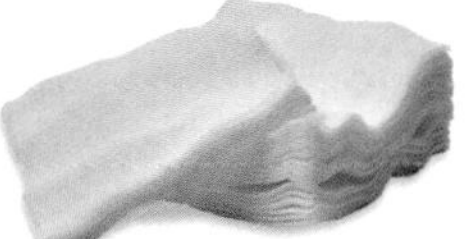

GAUZE PADS
Use these pads as dressings, as padding, or as swabs to clean around wounds.

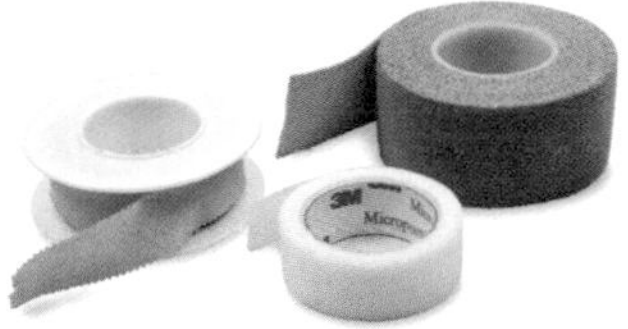

ADHESIVE TAPE
Use tape to secure dressings or the loose ends of bandages. If the casualty is allergic to the adhesive on the tape, use a hypoallergenic tape.

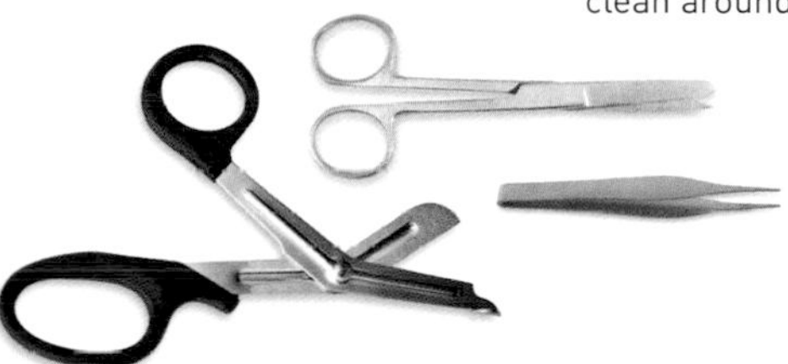

SCISSORS, SHEARS AND TWEEZERS
Choose items that are blunt-ended so that they will not cause injuries. Use shears to cut clothing.

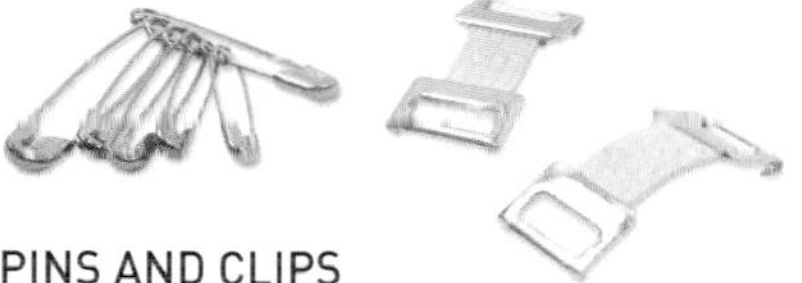

PINS AND CLIPS
Use these to secure the ends of bandages.

USEFUL ITEMS
Kitchen film or clean plastic bags can be used to dress burns and scalds. Non-stick dressings can be kept for larger wounds. Keep alcohol gel to clean your hands when no water is available.

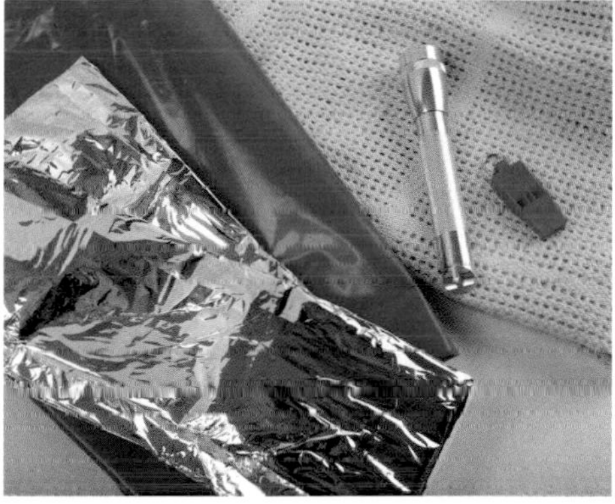

FOR USE OUTDOORS
A blanket can protect a casualty from cold. Survival bags are very compact and will keep a person warm and dry in an emergency. A torch helps visibility, and a whistle can be used to summon help.

BASIC MATERIALS FOR A GENERAL FIRST AID KIT

- Easily identifiable watertight box
- 20 adhesive dressings (plasters) in assorted sizes
- Six medium sterile dressings
- Two large sterile dressings
- One sterile eye pad
- Six triangular bandages
- Six safety pins
- Disposable gloves
- Two roller bandages
- Scissors
- Tweezers
- Alcohol-free wound cleansing wipes
- Adhesive tape
- Plastic face shield or pocket mask
- Notepad and pencil
- Alcohol gel

Other useful items:

- Blanket, survival bag, torch, whistle
- Warning triangle and high visibility jacket to keep in the car

DRESSINGS

You should always cover a wound with a dressing because this helps to prevent infection. With severe bleeding, dressings are used to help the blood-clotting process by exerting pressure on the wound.

Use a pre-packed sterile wound dressing with a bandage attached (opposite) whenever possible. If no such dressing is available, use a sterile pad. Alternatively, any clean, non-fluffy material can be used to improvise a dressing (p.240). Protect small cuts with an adhesive dressing (p.241).

See also
Cuts and grazes **p.120**
First aid materials **pp.235–37**
Severe external bleeding **p.114**

RULES FOR USING DRESSINGS

When handling or applying a dressing, there are a number of rules to follow. These enable you to apply dressings correctly; they also protect the casualty and yourself from cross infection.

- **Always wear disposable gloves,** if these are available, before handling any dressing.
- **Cover the wound** with a dressing that extends beyond the wound's edges.
- **Hold the edge of the dressing,** keeping your fingers well away from the area that will be in contact with the wound.
- **Place the dressing** directly on top of the wound; do not slide it on from the side.
- **Remove and replace** any dressing that slips out of position.
- **If you only have one sterile dressing,** use this to cover the wound, and put other clean materials on top of it.
- **If blood seeps through** the dressing, do not remove it; instead, place another dressing over the top. If blood seeps through the second dressing, remove both dressings completely and then apply a fresh dressing, making sure that you put pressure on the bleeding point.
- **After treating a wound,** dispose of gloves, used dressings and soiled items in a suitable plastic bag, such as a yellow biohazard bag (below). Keep disposable gloves on until you have finished handling any materials that may be contaminated, then put them in the bag.

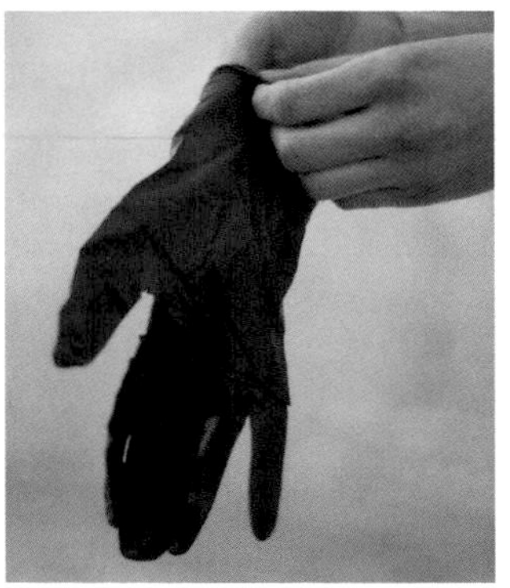

WEAR DISPOSABLE GLOVES

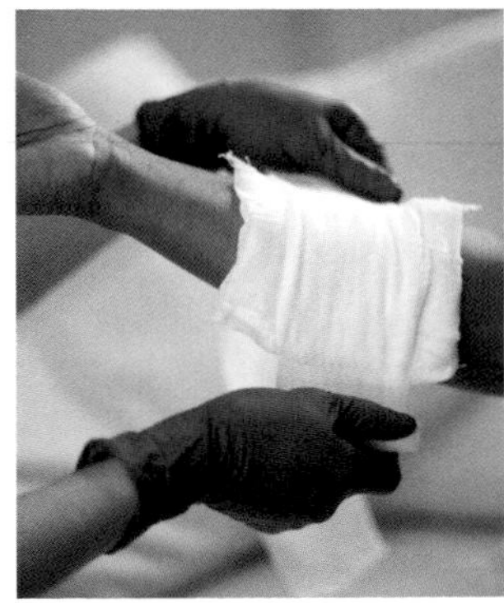

USE DRESSING LARGER THAN WOUND

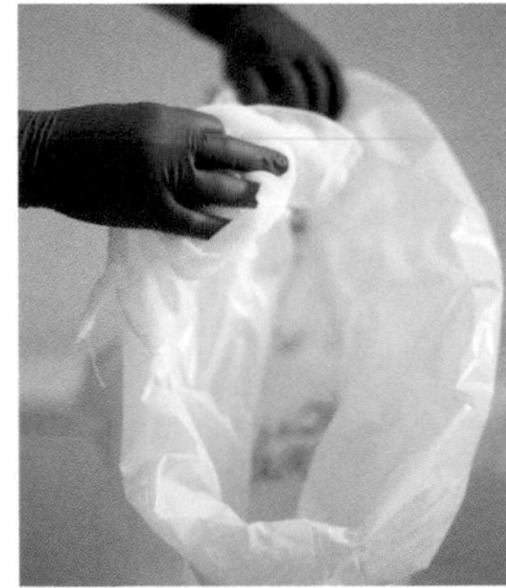

DISPOSE OF WASTE

HOW TO APPLY A STERILE WOUND DRESSING

CAUTION

- If the dressing slips out of place, remove it and apply a new dressing.
- Take care not to impair the circulation beyond the dressing (p.243).

This type of dressing consists of a dressing pad attached to a roller bandage. The pad is a piece of gauze backed by a layer of cotton wool or padding.

Sterile dressings are available individually wrapped in various sizes. They are sealed in protective wrappings to keep them sterile. Once the seal on this type of dressing has been broken, the dressing is no longer sterile.

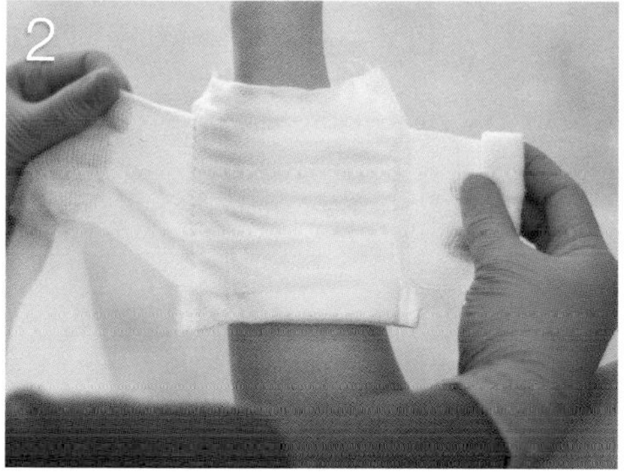
2

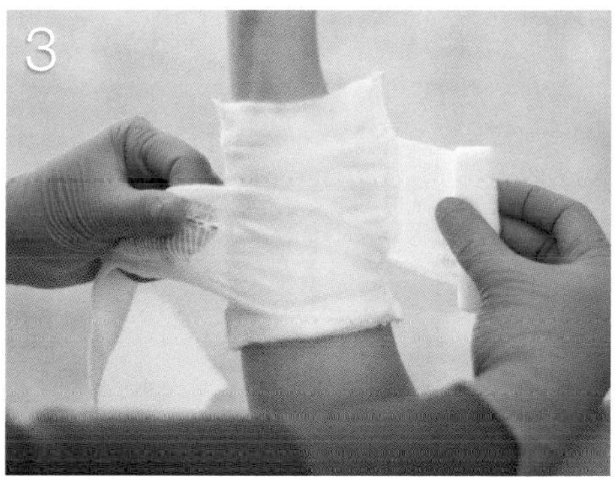
3

1 Break the seal and remove the wrapping. Unwind some of the bandage, taking care not to drop the roll or touch the dressing pad.

2 Unfold the dressing pad, and lay it directly on the wound. Hold the bandage on each side of the pad as you place it over the wound.

3 Wind the short end of the bandage once around the limb and the pad to secure the dressing.

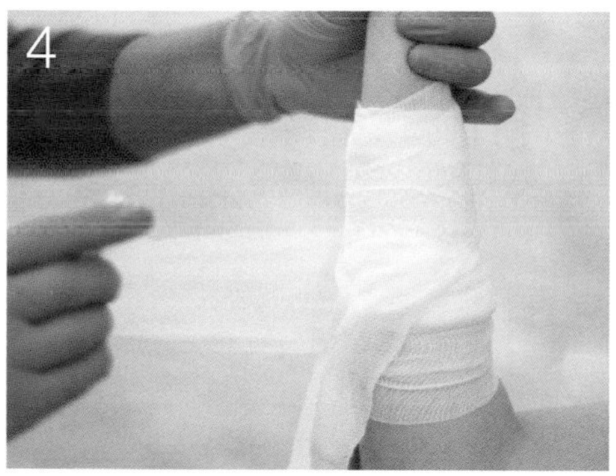
4

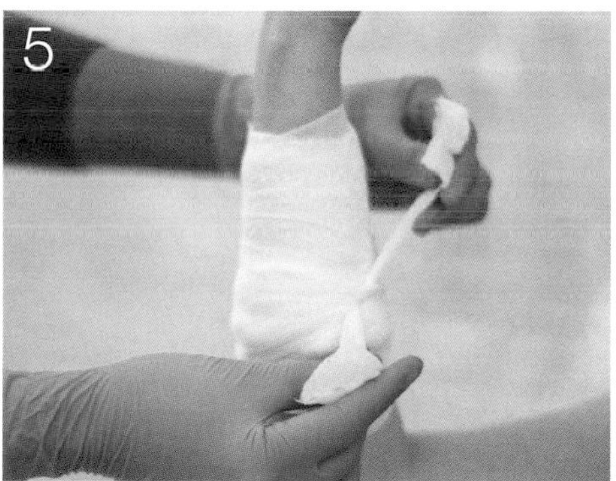
5

4 Wind the other end (head) of the bandage around the limb to cover the whole pad. Leave the short end of the bandage hanging free.

5 To secure the bandage, tie the ends in a reef knot (p.250). Tie the knot directly over the pad to maintain firm pressure on the wound.

6 Once you have secured the bandage, check the circulation in the limb beyond it (p.243). Loosen the bandage if it is too tight, then reapply. Recheck every ten minutes.

DRESSINGS (continued)

STERILE PAD AND GAUZE DRESSINGS

CAUTION

- Never apply adhesive tape all the way around a limb or digit since this can impair circulation.
- Check that the casualty is not allergic to the adhesive before using adhesive tape; if there is any allergy, use a pad and bandage.

If there is no sterile wound dressing with a bandage available, use a sterile pad or make a pad with pieces of gauze. Make sure the pad is large enough to extend well beyond the edges of the wound. Hold the dressing face down; never touch the part of the dressing that will be in contact with a wound. Secure the dressing with tape. If you need to maintain pressure to control bleeding, use a bandage.

See also
Roller bandages **pp.244–47**

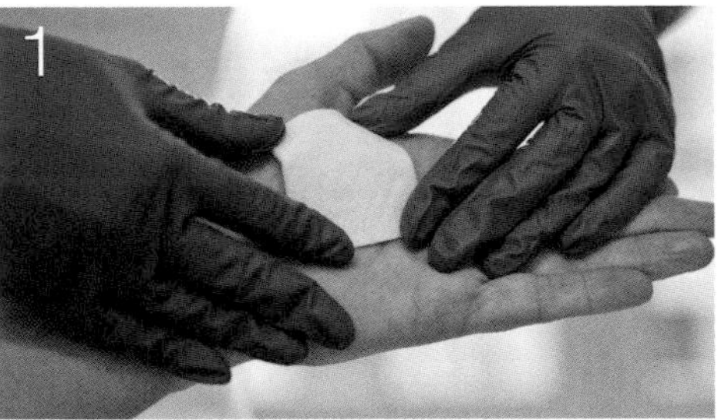

1 **Holding the dressing or pad by the edges, place it directly on to the wound.**

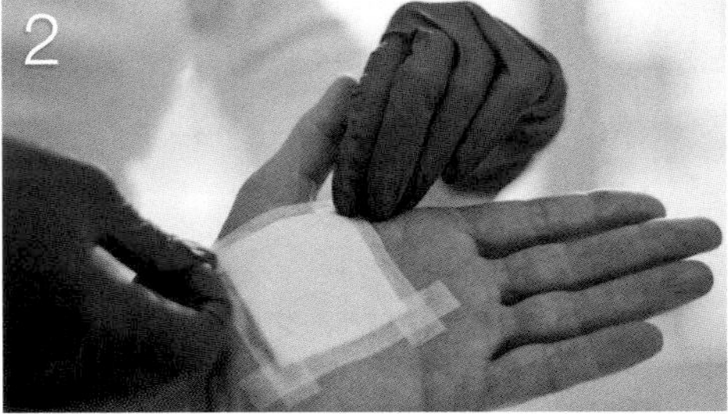

2 **Secure the pad with adhesive tape or a roller bandage.**

IMPROVISED DRESSINGS

If you have no suitable dressings, any clean non-fluffy material can be used in an emergency. If using a piece of folded cloth, hold it by its edges, unfold it, then refold it so that the clean inner side can be placed against the wound.

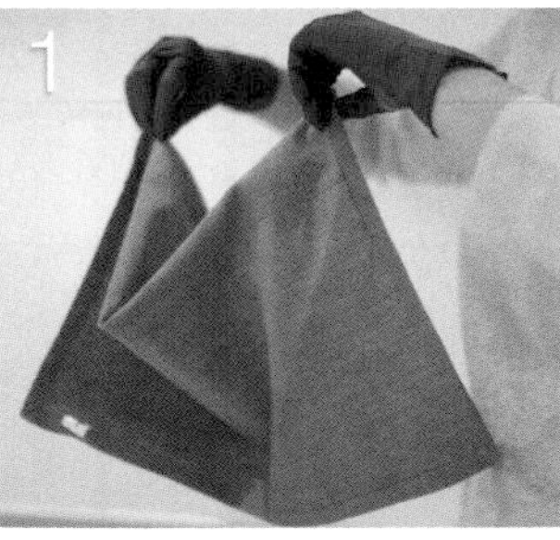

1 **Hold the material by the edges. Open it out and refold it so that the inner surface faces outwards.**

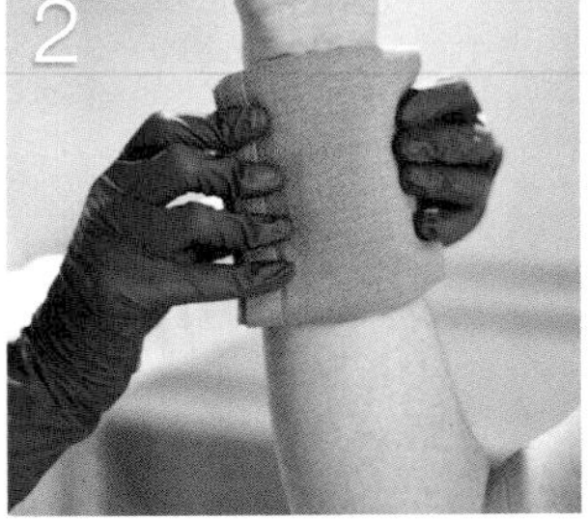

2 **Place the cloth pad directly on to the wound. If necessary, cover the pad with more material.**

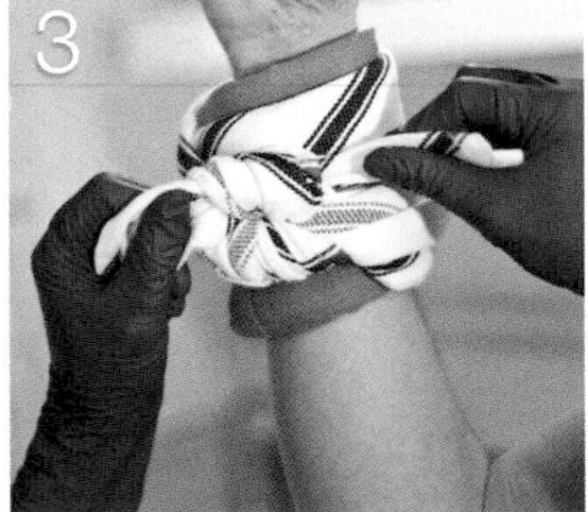

3 **Secure the pad with a bandage or a clean strip of cloth, such as a scarf. Tie the ends in a reef knot (p.250).**

ADHESIVE DRESSINGS

CAUTION

- Check that the casualty is not allergic to the adhesive dressings. If he is, use hypoallergenic tape or a pad and bandage.

Plasters are useful for dressing small cuts and grazes. They consist of a gauze or cellulose pad and an adhesive backing, and are often wrapped singly in sterile packs. There are several sizes available, as well as special shapes for use on fingertips, heels and elbows; some types are waterproof. Blister plasters have an oval cushioned pad. People who work with food must cover any wounds with visible, blue, waterproof plasters.

1 Clean and dry the skin around the wound. Unwrap the plaster and hold it by the protective strips over the backing, with the pad side facing downwards.

2 Peel back the strips to expose the pad, but do not remove them. Without touching the pad surface, place the pad on the wound.

3 Carefully pull away the protective strips, then press the edges of the plaster down.

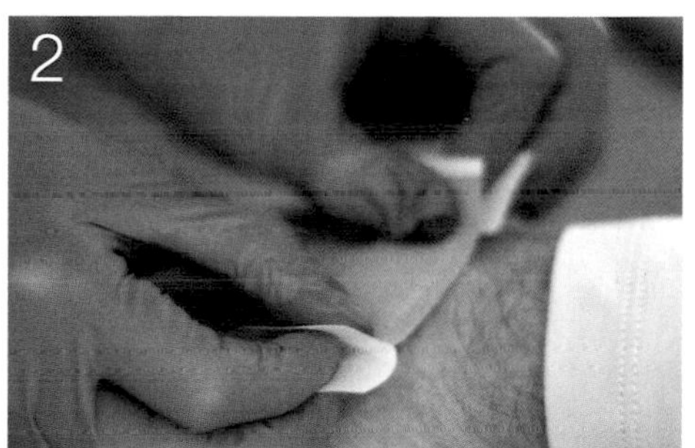

COLD COMPRESSES

CAUTION

To prevent cold injuries, always wrap an ice pack in a cloth. Do not leave it on for more than ten minutes at a time.

Cooling an injury such as a bruise or sprain can reduce swelling and pain. There are two types of compress: cold pads, which are made from material dampened with cold water, and ice packs. An ice pack can be made using ice cubes (or packs of frozen peas or other small vegetables) wrapped in a dry cloth.

COLD PAD

1 Soak a clean flannel or towel in cold water. Wring it out lightly and fold it into a pad. Hold it firmly against the injury (right).

2 Re-soak the pad in cold water every few minutes to keep it cold. Cool the injury for at least ten minutes.

ICE PACK

1 Partly fill a plastic bag with small ice cubes or crushed ice, or use a pack of frozen vegetables. Wrap the bag in a dry cloth.

2 Hold the pack firmly on the area. Cool for ten minutes, topping up the ice as needed.

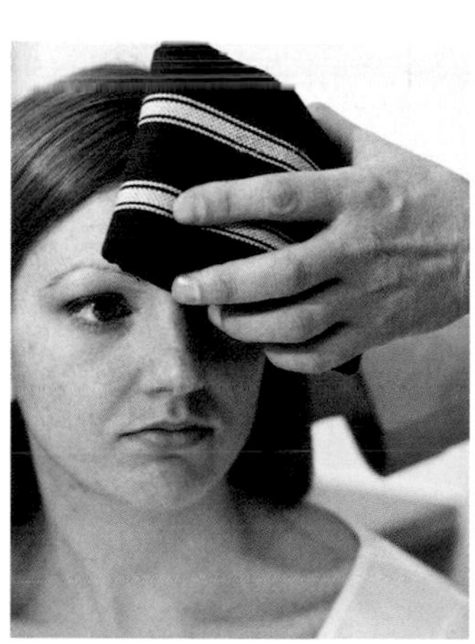

PRINCIPLES OF BANDAGING

There are a number of different first aid uses for bandages: they can be used to secure dressings, control bleeding, support and immobilise limbs and reduce swelling in an injured limb. There are three main types of bandage. Roller bandages secure dressings and support injured limbs. Tubular bandages hold dressings on fingers or toes, or support injured joints. Triangular bandages can be used as large dressings, as slings, to secure dressings or to immobilise limbs. If you have no bandage available, you can improvise from everyday items; for example, you can fold a square of fabric, such as a headscarf, diagonally to make a triangular bandage (p.249).

See also
Roller bandages pp.244–47
Triangular bandages p.249
Tubular gauze bandages p.248

RULES FOR APPLYING A BANDAGE

- **Reassure the casualty** before applying a bandage and explain clearly what you are going to do.
- **Help the casualty** to sit or lie down in a comfortable position.

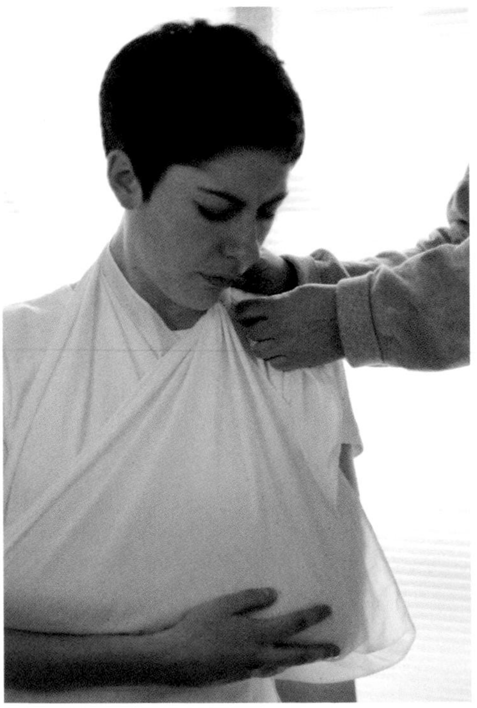

- **Support the injured part** of the body while you are working on it. Ask the casualty or a helper to do this.
- **Work from the front** of the casualty, and from the injured side where possible.
- **Pass the bandages** through the body's natural hollows at the ankles, knees, waist and neck, then slide them into position by easing them back and forth under the body.
- **Apply bandages firmly,** but not so tightly that they interfere with circulation to the area beyond the bandage (opposite).
- **Fingers or toes** should be left exposed, if possible, so that you can check the circulation afterwards.
- **Use reef knots** to tie bandages (p.250). Ensure that the knots do not cause discomfort, and do not tie the knot over a bony area. Tuck loose ends under a knot if possible, to provide additional padding.
- **Check the circulation** in the area beyond the bandage (opposite) every ten minutes once it is secure. If necessary, unroll the bandage until the blood supply returns, and reapply it more loosely.

IMMOBILISING A LIMB

When applying bandages to immobilise a limb you also need to use soft, bulky material, such as towels or clothing, as padding. Place the padding between the legs, or between an arm and the body, so that the bandaging does not displace broken bones or press bony areas against each other. Use folded triangular bandages and tie them at intervals along the limb, avoiding the injury site. Secure with reef knots (p.250) tied on the uninjured side. If both sides of the body are injured, tie knots in the middle or where there is least chance of causing further damage.

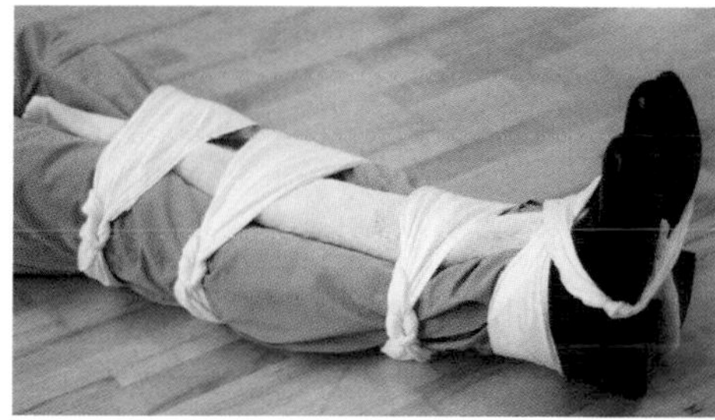

TIE KNOTS ON THE UNINJURED SIDE

CHECKING CIRCULATION AFTER BANDAGING

RECOGNITION

If circulation is impaired there may be:

- A swollen and congested limb;
- Blue skin with prominent veins;
- A feeling that the skin is painfully distended.

Later there may be:

- Pale, waxy skin;
- Skin cold to touch;
- Numbness and tingling followed by severe pain;
- Inability to move affected fingers or toes.

When bandaging a limb or using a sling, you must check the circulation in the hand or foot immediately after you have finished bandaging, and every ten minutes thereafter. These checks are essential because limbs swell after an injury, and a bandage can rapidly become too tight and interfere with blood circulation to the area beyond it. The symptoms of impaired circulation change as first the veins and then the arteries become constricted.

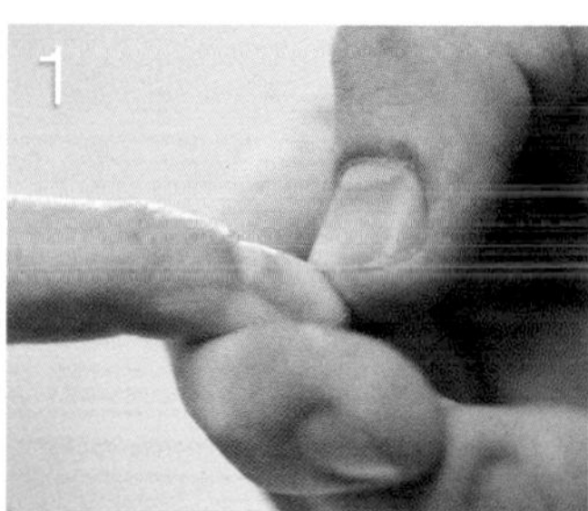

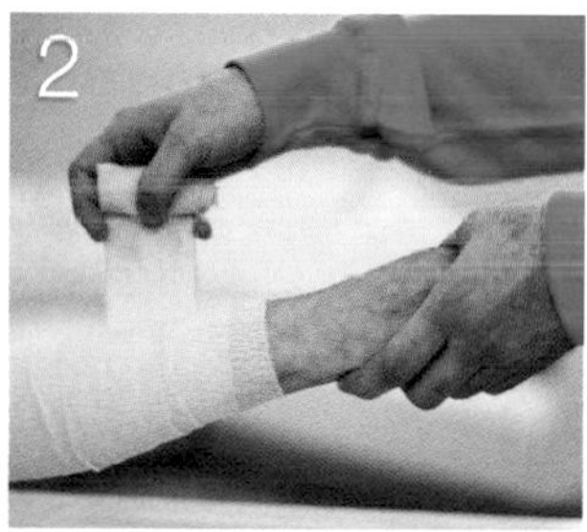

1 Briefly press one of the nails or the skin, until it turns pale, then release the pressure. If the colour does not return, or returns slowly, the bandage may be too tight.

2 Loosen a tight bandage by unrolling enough turns for warmth and colour to return to the skin. The casualty may feel a tingling sensation. If necessary loosen and reapply the bandage. Recheck every ten minutes.

ROLLER BANDAGES

These bandages are made of cotton, gauze, elasticated fabric or linen and are wrapped around the injured part of the body in spiral turns. There are three main types of roller bandage.

- **Open-weave bandages** are used to hold dressings in place. Because of their loose weave they allow good ventilation, but they cannot be used to exert direct pressure on the wound to control bleeding or to provide support to joints.
- **Self-adhesive support bandages** are used to support muscle (and joint) injuries and do not need pins or clips.
- **Crêpe bandages** are used to give firm, even support to injured joints.

SECURING ROLLER BANDAGES

There are several ways to fasten the end of a roller bandage. Safety pins or adhesive tape are usually included in first aid kits. Some bandage packs may contain bandage clips. If you do not have any of these, a simple tuck should keep the bandage end in place.

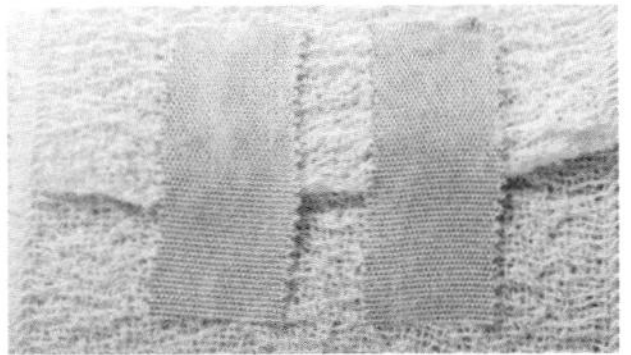

ADHESIVE TAPE
The ends of bandages can be folded under and then stuck down with small strips of adhesive tape.

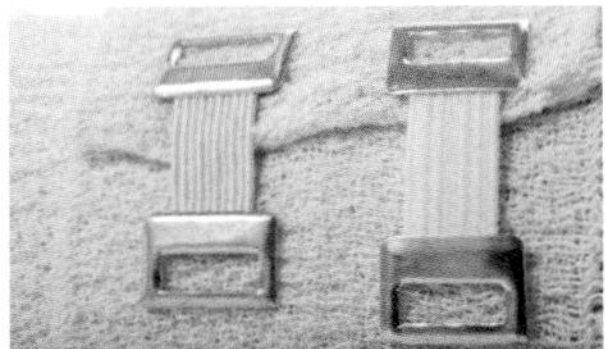

BANDAGE CLIP
Metal clips are sometimes supplied with crêpe roller bandages for securing the ends.

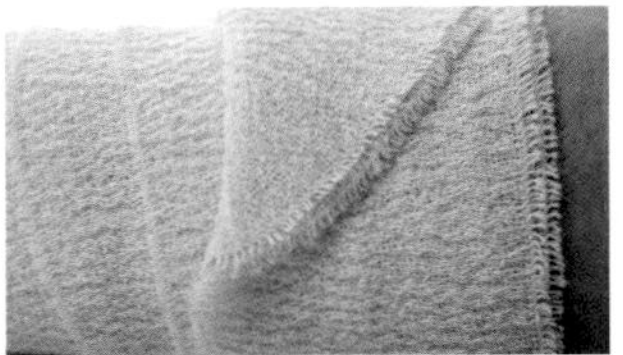

TUCKING IN THE END
If you have no fastening, secure the bandage by passing the end around the limb once and tucking it in.

SAFETY PIN
These pins can secure all types of roller bandage. Fold the end of the bandage under, then put your finger under the bandage to prevent injury as you insert the pin (right). Make sure that, once fastened, the pin lies flat (far right).

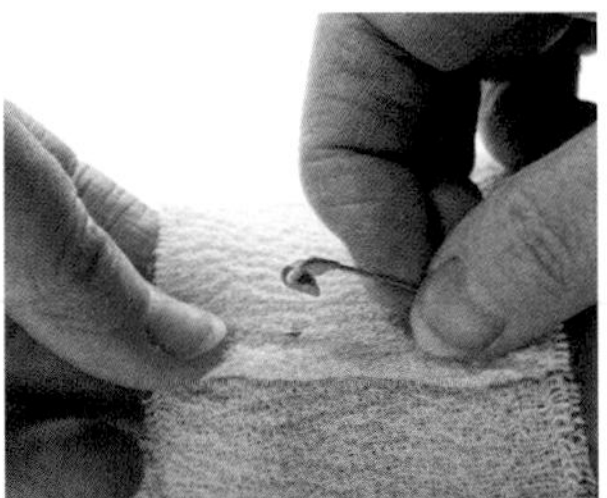

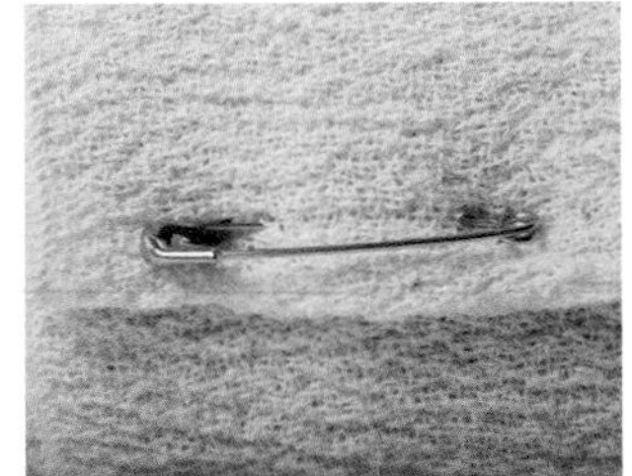

CHOOSING THE CORRECT SIZE OF BANDAGE

Before applying a roller bandage, check that it is tightly rolled and of a suitable width for the injured area. Small areas such as fingers require narrow bandages of approximately 2.5cm (1in) wide, while wider bandages of 10–15cm (4–6in) are more suitable for large areas such as legs. It is better for a roller bandage to be too wide than too narrow. Smaller sizes may be needed for a child.

ROLLER BANDAGES

APPLYING A ROLLER BANDAGE

CAUTION

Once you have applied the bandage, check the circulation in the limb beyond it (p.243). This is especially important if you are applying an elasticated or crêpe bandage since these mould to the shape of the limb and may become tighter if the limb swells.

Follow the general rules below when applying a roller bandage to an injury.

- **Keep the rolled** part of the bandage (the "head") uppermost as you work. (The unrolled short end is called the "tail".)
- **Position yourself** in front of the casualty, on the injured side.
- **Support the injured** part while you apply the bandage.

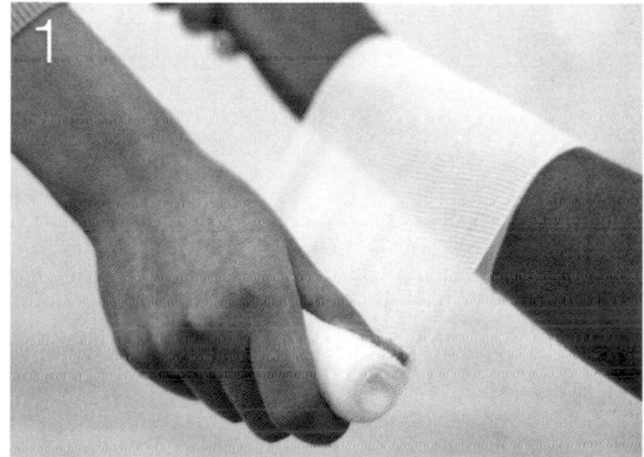

1 Place the tail of the bandage below the injury. Working from the inside of the limb outwards, make two straight turns with the bandage to anchor the tail in place.

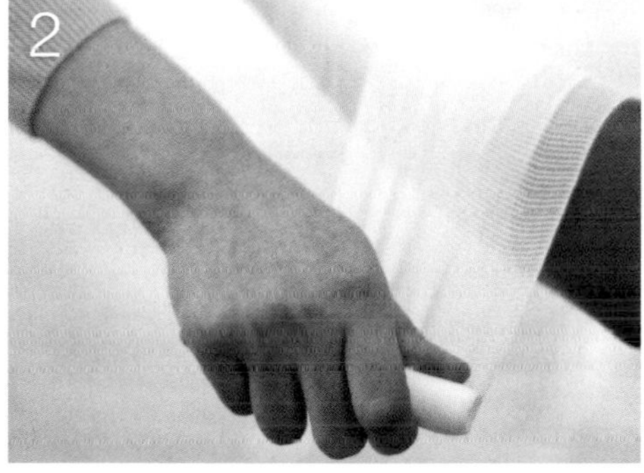

2 Wind the bandage in spiralling turns working from the inner to the outer side of the limb, and work up the limb. Cover one half to two-thirds of the previous layer of bandage with each new turn.

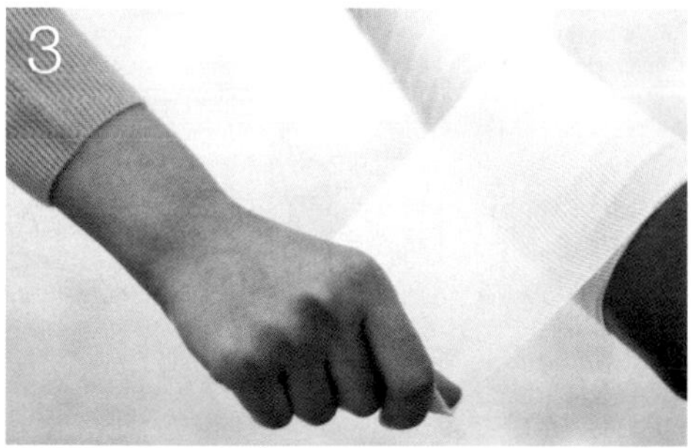

3 Finish with one straight turn. If the bandage is too short, apply another one in the same way so that the injured area is covered.

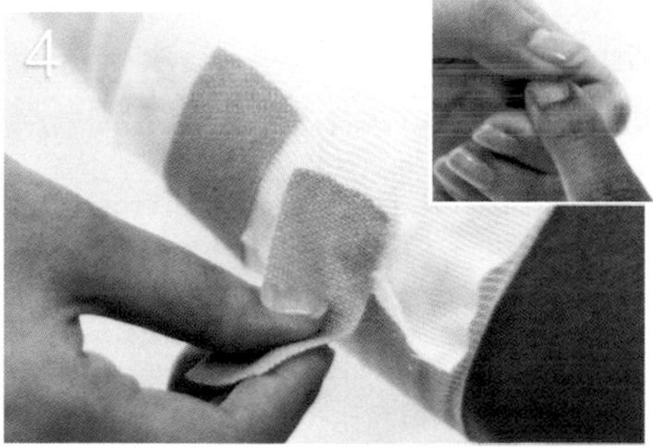

4 Secure the end of the bandage, then check the circulation beyond the bandage (p.243). If necessary, unroll the bandage until the blood supply returns, and reapply it more loosely. Recheck every ten minutes.

ROLLER BANDAGES (continued)

ELBOW AND KNEE BANDAGES

CAUTION

Do not apply the bandage so tightly that the circulation to the limb beyond is impaired.

Roller bandages can be used on elbows and knees to support soft tissue injuries such as strains or sprains. To ensure that there is effective support, flex the joint slightly, then apply the bandage in figure-of-eight turns rather than the standard spiralling turns (p.245). Work from the inside to the outside of the upper surface of the joint. Extend the bandaging far enough on either side of the joint to exert an even pressure.

1 Support the injured limb in a comfortable position for the casualty, with the joint partially flexed. Place the tail of the bandage on the inner side of the joint. Pass the bandage over and around to the outside of the joint. Make one-and-a-half turns, so that the tail end of the bandage is fixed and the joint is covered.

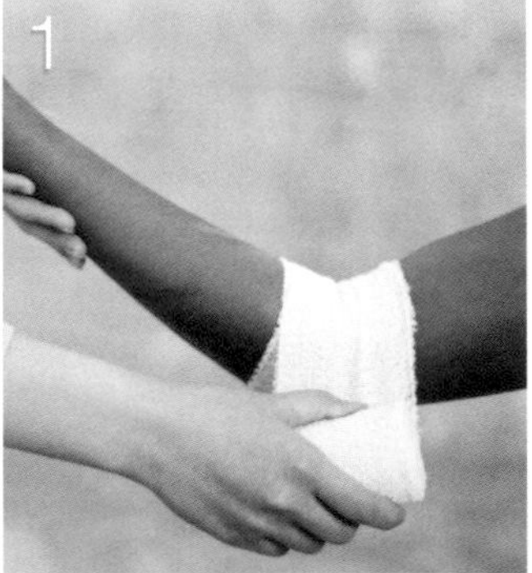

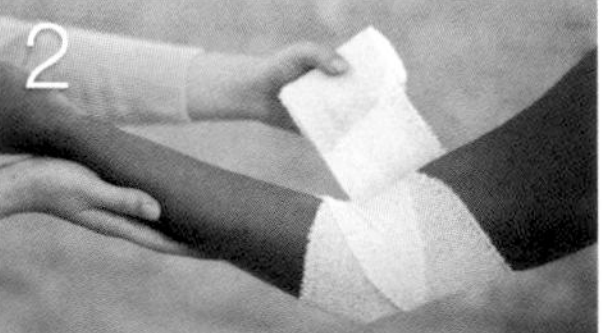

2 Pass the bandage to the inner side of the limb, just above the joint. Make a turn around the limb, covering the upper half of the bandage from the first turn.

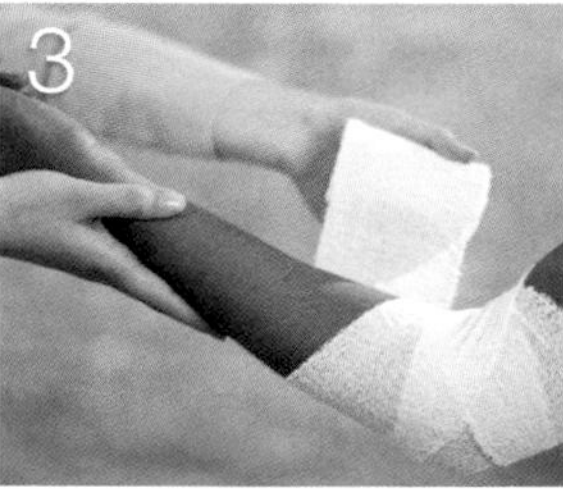

3 Pass the bandage from the inner side of the upper limb to just below the joint. Make one diagonal turn below the elbow joint to cover the lower half of the bandaging from the first straight turn.

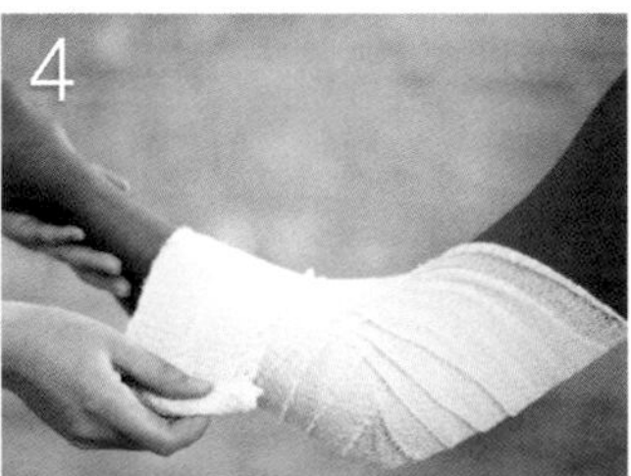

4 Continue to bandage diagonally above and below the joint in a figure-of-eight. Increase the bandaged area by covering about two-thirds of the previous turn with each new layer.

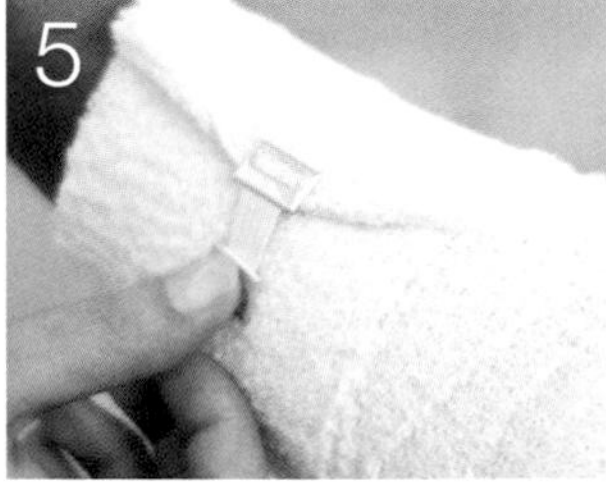

5 To finish bandaging the joint, make two straight turns around the limb, then secure the end of the bandage (p.244). Check the circulation beyond the bandage as soon as you have finished, then recheck every ten minutes (p.243). If necessary unroll the bandage and reapply more loosely.

HAND BANDAGES

A roller bandage may be applied to hold dressings in place on a hand, or to support a wrist in soft tissue injuries. A support bandage should extend well beyond the injury site to provide pressure over the whole of the injured area.

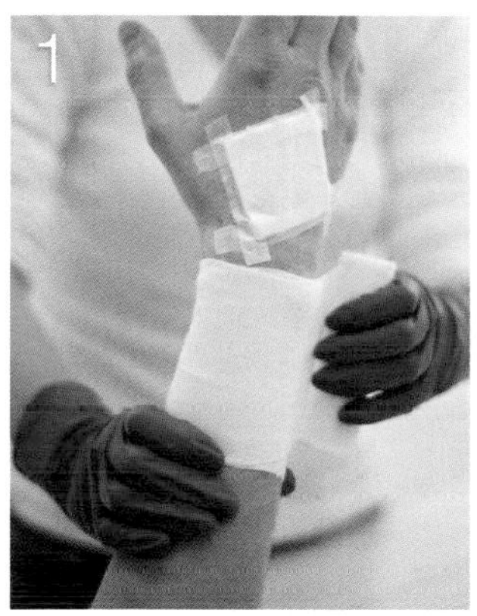

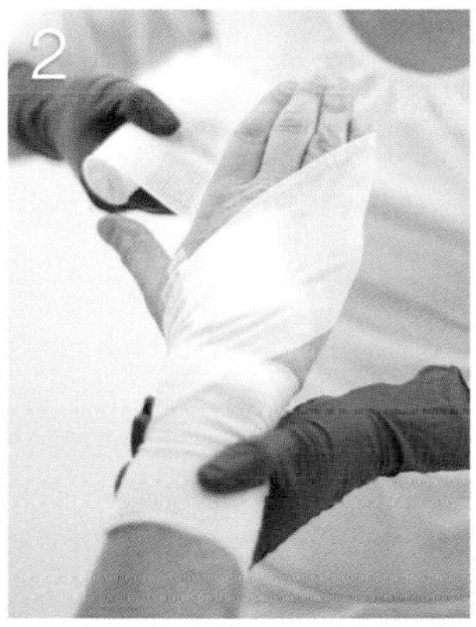

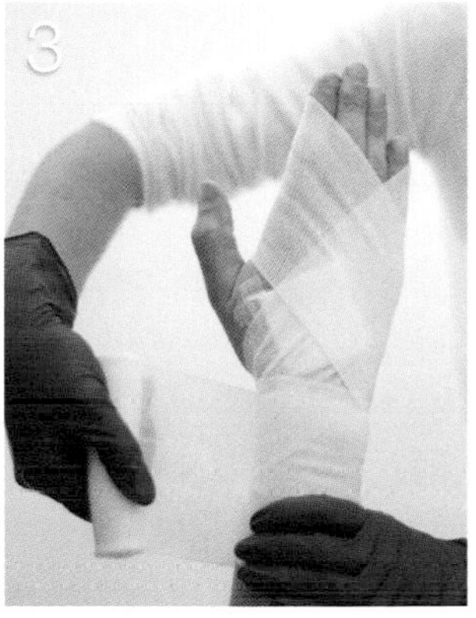

1 Place the tail of the bandage on the inner side of the wrist, by the base of the thumb. Make two straight turns around the wrist.

2 Working from the inner side of the wrist, pass the bandage diagonally across the back of the hand to the nail of the little finger, and across the front of the casualty's fingers.

3 Pass the bandage diagonally across the back of the hand to the outer side of the wrist. Take the bandage under the wrist. Then repeat the diagonal over the back of the hand.

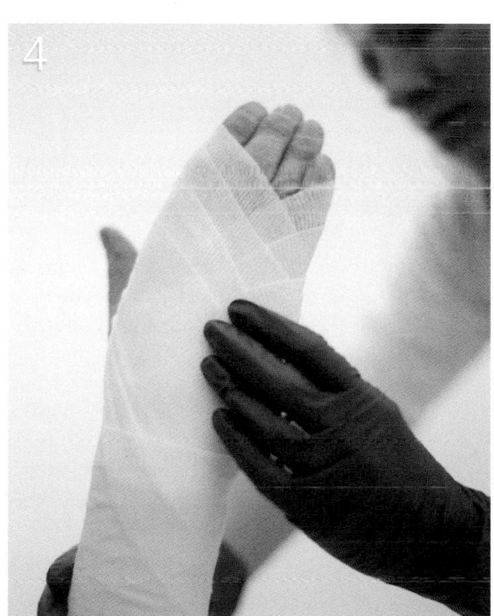

4 Repeat the sequence of figure-of-eight turns. Extend the bandaging by covering about two-thirds of the bandage from the previous turn with each new layer. When the hand is completely covered, finish with two straight turns around the wrist.

5 Secure the end (p.244). As soon as you have finished, check the circulation beyond the bandage (p.243), then recheck every ten minutes. If necessary, unroll the bandage until the blood supply returns and reapply it more loosely.

TUBULAR GAUZE BANDAGES

CAUTION

Do not encircle the finger completely with tape because this may impair circulation.

These bandages are rolls of seamless, tubular fabric. The tubular gauze bandage is used with a special applicator which is supplied with the bandage. It is suitable for holding dressings in place on a finger or toe, but not to control bleeding.

APPLYING A TUBULAR GAUZE

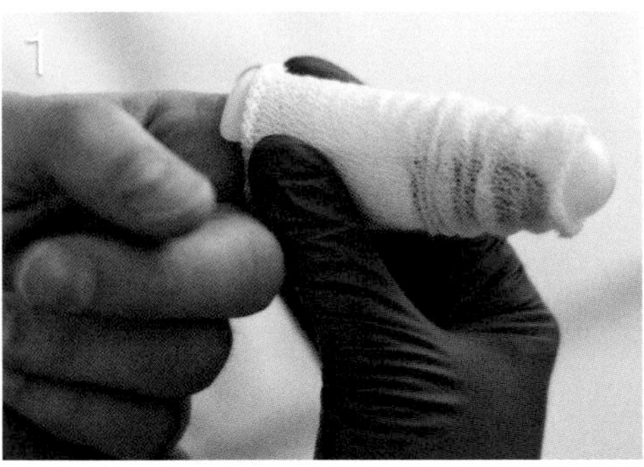

1 Cut a piece of tubular gauze about two-and-a-half times the length of the injured finger. Push the whole length of the tubular gauze on to the applicator, then gently slide the applicator over the casualty's finger.

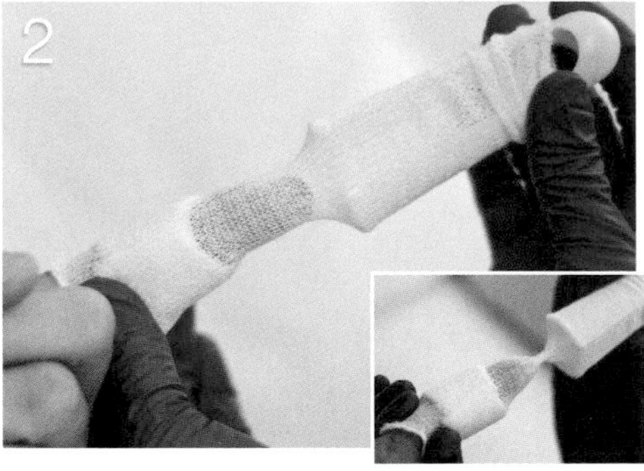

2 Holding the end of the gauze on the finger, pull the applicator slightly beyond the fingertip to leave a gauze layer on the finger. Twist the applicator twice to seal the bandage over the end of the finger.

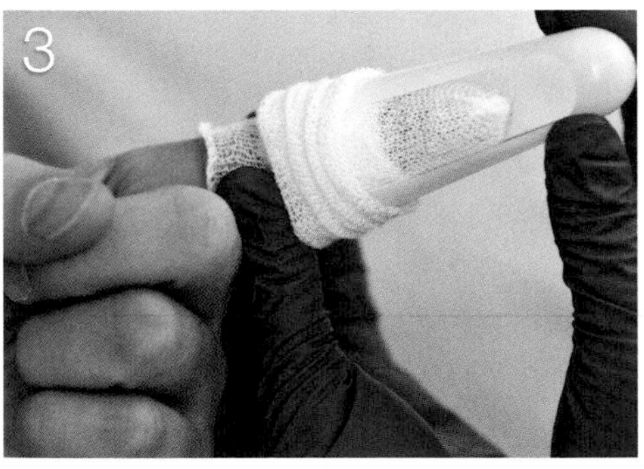

3 While still holding the gauze at the base of the finger, gently push the applicator back over the finger to apply a second layer of gauze. Once the gauze has been applied, remove the applicator from the finger.

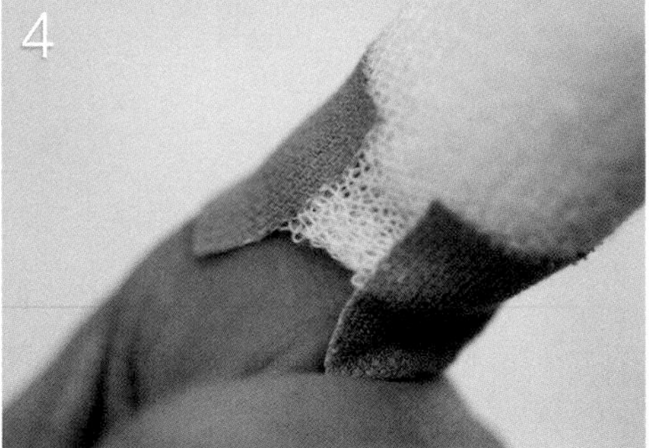

4 Secure the gauze at the base of the finger with adhesive tape. Check the circulation to the finger immediately (p.243) and then again every ten minutes. Ask the casualty if the finger feels cold or tingly. If it does, remove the gauze and reapply it more loosely.

TRIANGULAR BANDAGES

This type of bandage may be supplied in a sterile pack as part of a first aid kit. You can also make one by cutting or folding a square metre of sturdy fabric (such as linen or calico) diagonally in half. The bandage can be used in the following three ways.

- **Folded as a broad-fold bandage** or narrow-fold bandage (below) to immobilise and support a limb or to secure a splint or bulky dressing.
- **Opened to form a sling,** or to hold a hand, foot or scalp dressing in place.
- **From a sterile pack,** folded into a pad and used as a sterile dressing.

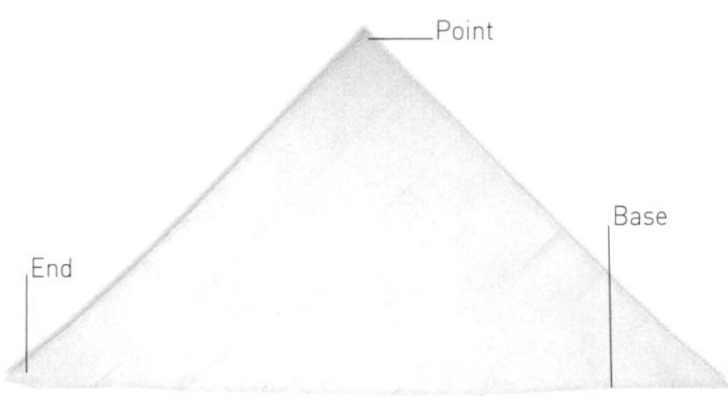

OPEN TRIANGULAR BANDAGE

MAKING A BROAD-FOLD BANDAGE

1 **Open out a triangular bandage and lay it flat on a clean surface. Fold the bandage in half horizontally, so that the point of the triangle touches the centre of the base.**

2 **Fold the bandage in half again in the same direction, so that the first folded edge touches the base. The bandage should now form a broad strip.**

MAKING A NARROW-FOLD BANDAGE

1 **Fold a triangular bandage to make a broad-fold bandage (left).**

2 **Fold the bandage horizontally in half again. It should form a long, narrow, thick strip of material.**

STORING A TRIANGULAR BANDAGE

Keep triangular bandages in their packs so that they remain sterile until you need them. Alternatively, fold them as shown (right) so that they are ready-folded for use as a pad or bandage, or can be shaken open.

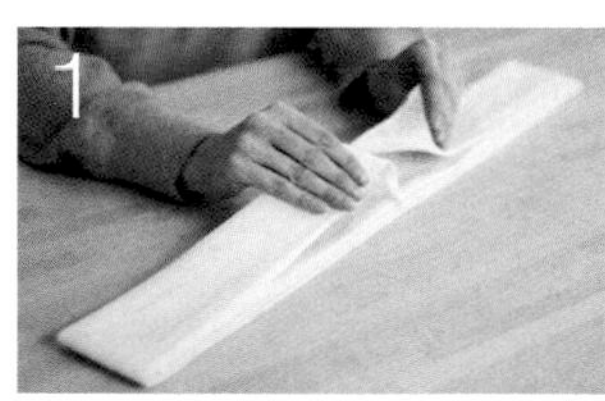

1 **Start by folding the triangle into a narrow-fold bandage (above). Bring the two ends of the bandage into the centre.**

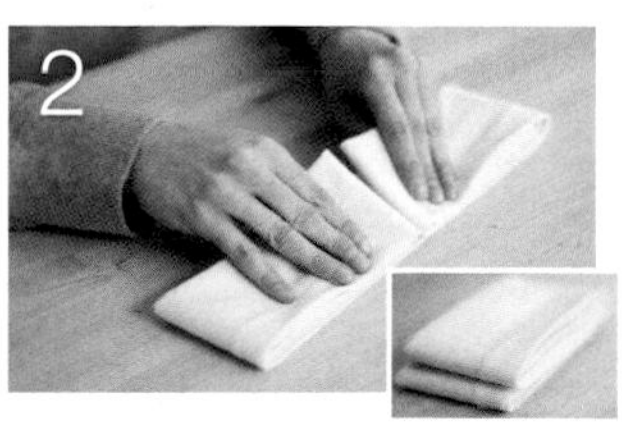

2 **Continue folding the ends into the centre until the bandage is a convenient size for storing. Keep the bandage in a dry place.**

REEF KNOTS

When securing a triangular bandage, always use a reef knot. It is secure and will not slip, it is easy to untie and it lies flat, so it is more comfortable for the casualty. Avoid tying the knot around or directly over the injury, since this may cause discomfort.

TYING AND UNTYING A REEF KNOT

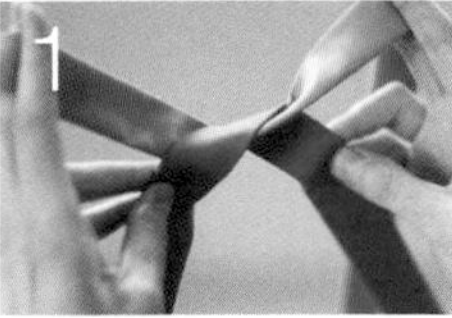

1 Pass the left end of the bandage (dark) over and under the right end (light).

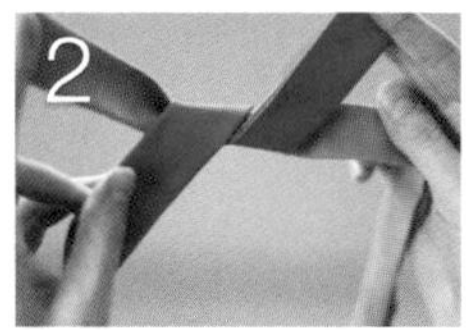

2 Lift both ends of the bandage above the rest of the material.

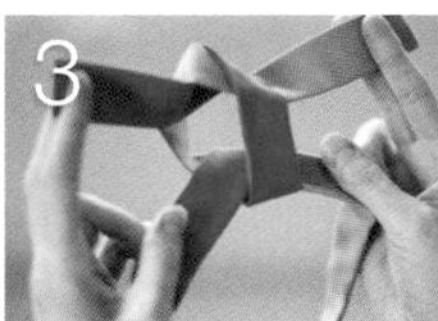

3 Pass the end in your right hand (dark) over and under the left end (light).

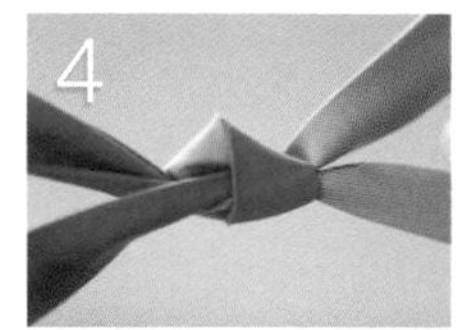

4 Pull the ends to tighten the knot, then tuck them under the bandage.

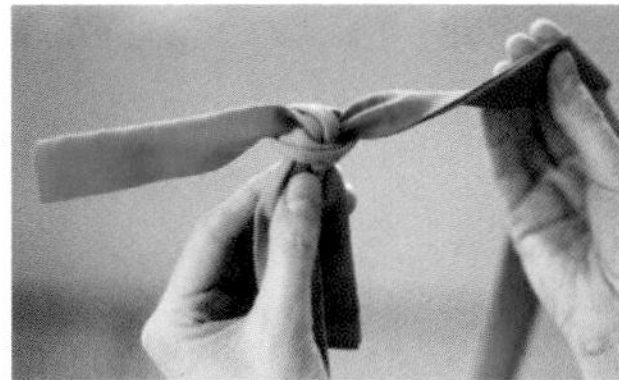

UNTYING A REEF KNOT
Pull one end and one piece of bandage from the same side of the knot firmly so that the piece of bandage straightens. Hold the knot and pull the straightened end through it.

HAND AND FOOT COVER

An open triangular bandage can be used to hold a dressing in place on a hand or foot, but it will not provide enough pressure to control bleeding. The method for covering a hand (right) can also be used for a foot, with the bandage ends tied at the ankle.

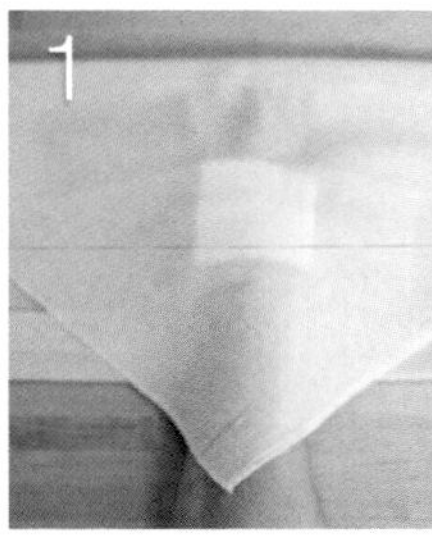

1 Lay the bandage flat. Place the casualty's hand on the bandage, fingers towards the point. Fold the point over the hand.

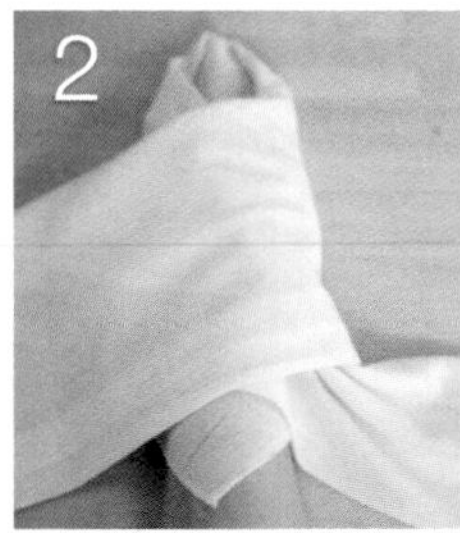

2 Cross the ends over the hand, then pass the ends around the wrist in opposite directions. Tie the ends in a reef knot (above).

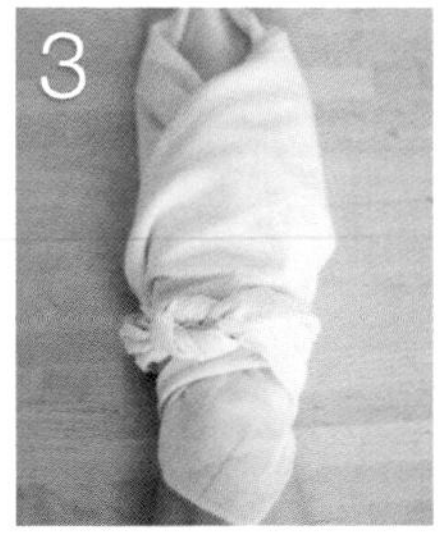

3 Pull the point gently to tighten the bandage. Fold the point up over the knot and tuck it in.

ARM SLING

An arm sling holds the forearm in a slightly raised or horizontal position. It provides support for an injured upper arm, wrist or forearm, on a casualty whose elbow can be bent, or to immobilise the arm for a rib fracture (p.150). An elevation sling (p.252) is used to keep the forearm and hand raised in a higher position.

1 Ensure that the injured arm is supported with the hand slightly higher than the elbow. Fold the base of the bandage under to form a hem. Place the bandage with the base parallel to the casualty's body and level with his little finger nail. Slide the upper end under the injured arm and pull it around the neck to the opposite shoulder.

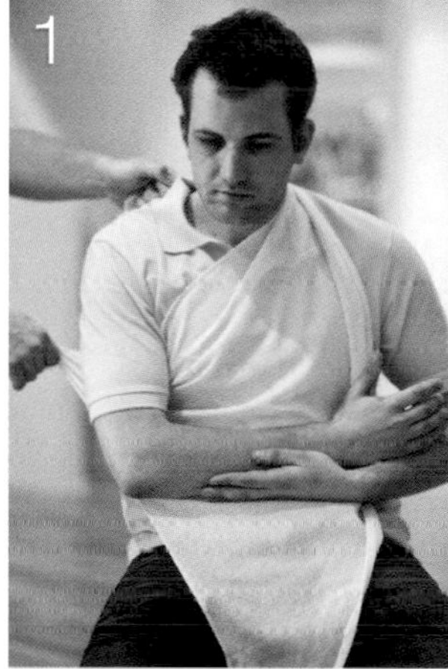

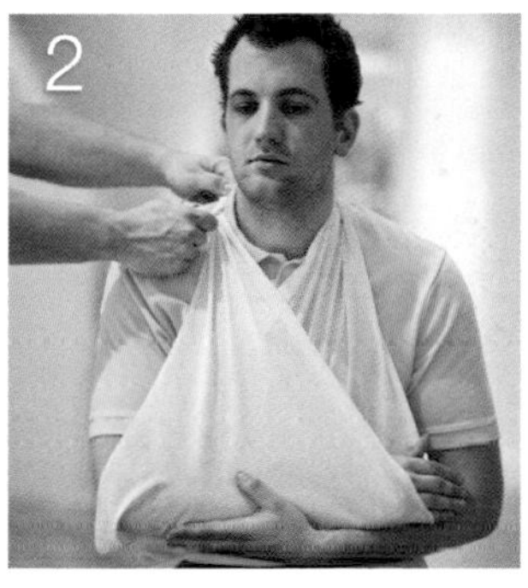

2 Fold the lower end of the bandage up over the forearm and bring it to meet the upper end at the shoulder.

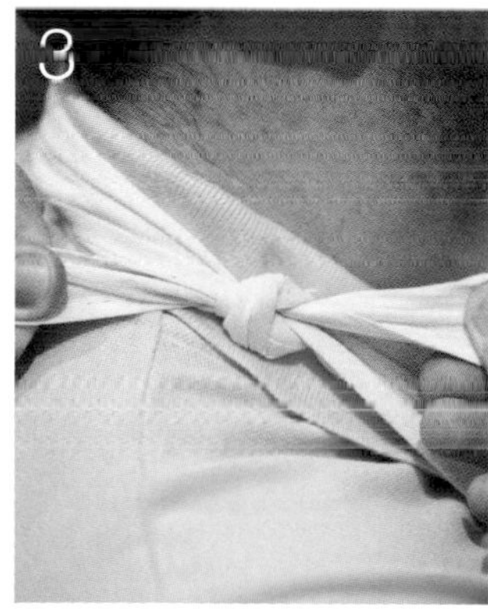

3 Tie a reef knot (opposite) on the injured side, at the hollow above the casualty's collar bone. Tuck both free ends of the bandage under the knot to pad it. Adjust the sling so that the front edge supports the hand – it should extend to the top of the casualty's little finger.

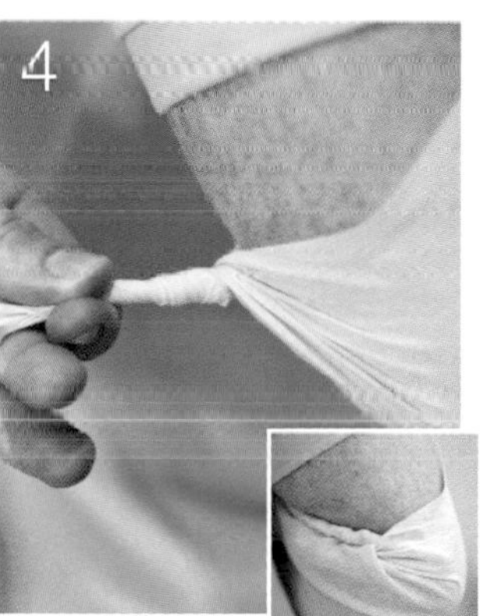

4 Hold the point of the bandage beyond the elbow and twist it until the fabric fits the elbow snugly, then tuck it in. Alternatively, if you have a safety pin, fold the fabric and fasten it to the front.

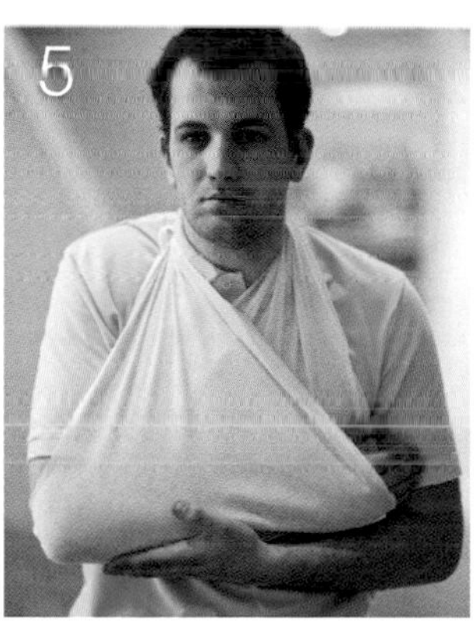

5 As soon as you have finished, check the circulation in the fingers (p.243). Recheck every ten minutes. If necessary, loosen and reapply the bandages and sling.

ELEVATION SLING

This form of sling supports the forearm and hand in a raised position, with the fingertips touching the casualty's shoulder. In this way, an elevation sling helps to control bleeding from wounds in the forearm or hand, to minimise swelling. An elevation sling is also used to support the arm in the case of an injured hand.

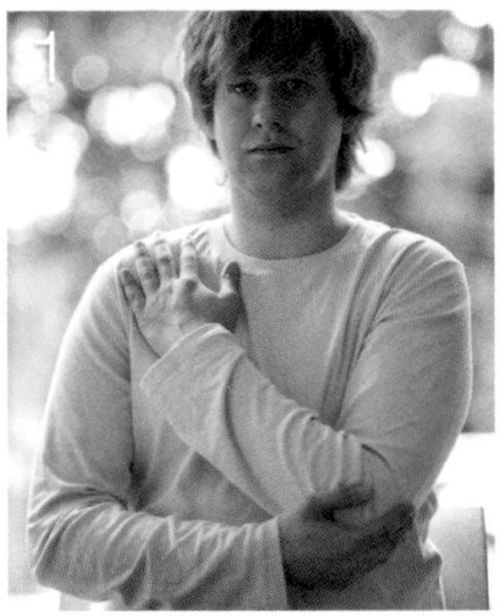

1 Ask the casualty to support his injured arm across his chest, with the fingers resting on the opposite shoulder.

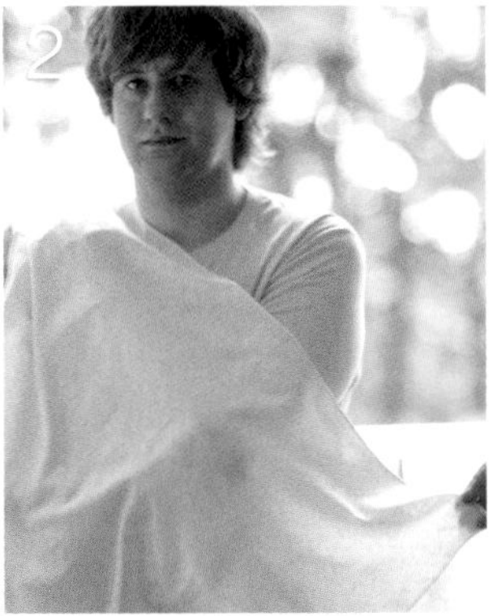

2 Place the bandage over his body, with one end over the shoulder on the uninjured side. Hold the point just beyond his elbow.

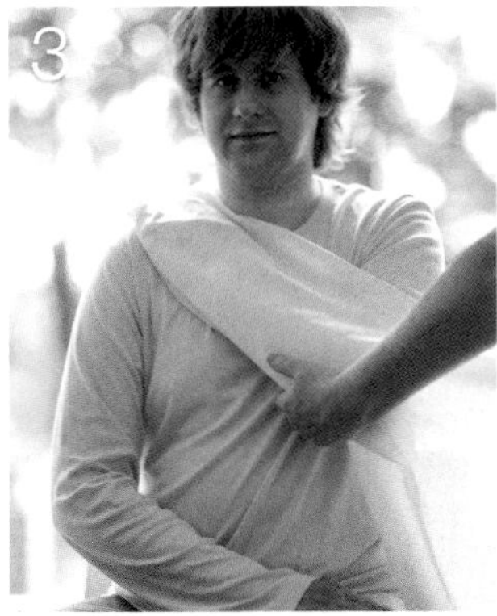

3 Ask the casualty to let go of his injured arm while you tuck the base of the bandage under his hand, forearm and elbow.

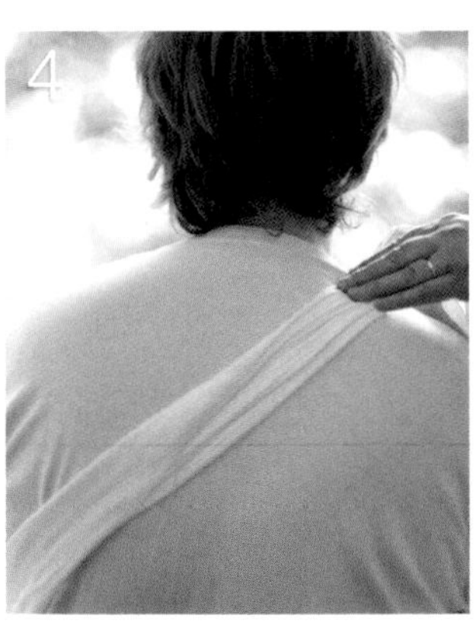

4 Bring the lower end of the bandage up diagonally across his back, to meet the other end at his shoulder.

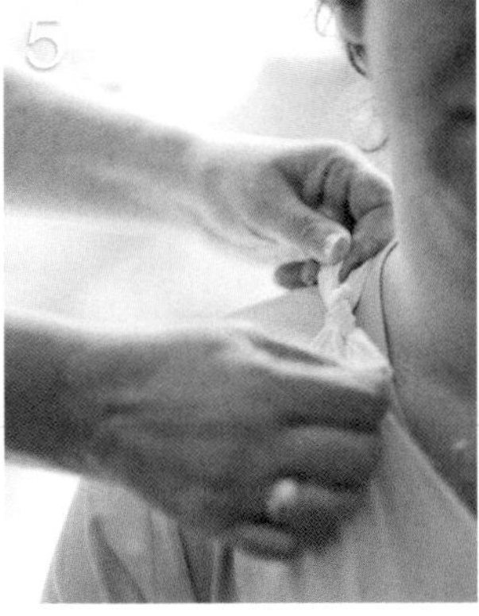

5 Tie the ends in a reef knot (p.250) at the hollow above the casualty's collar bone. Tuck the ends under the knot to pad it.

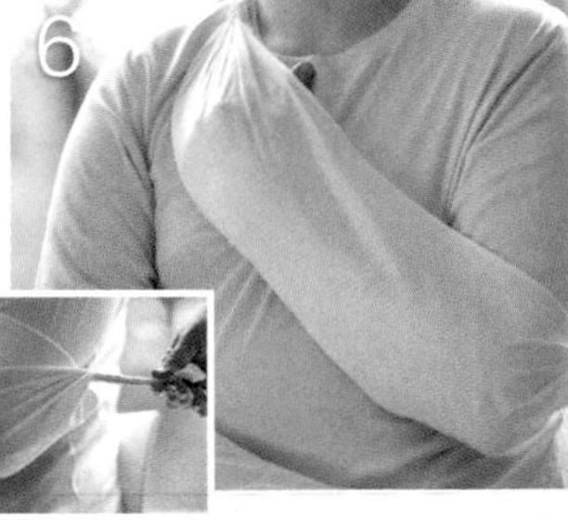

6 Twist the point until the bandage fits closely around the casualty's elbow. Tuck the point in just above his elbow to secure it. If you have a safety pin, fold the fabric over the elbow and fasten the point at the corner. Check the circulation in the thumb every ten minutes (p.243); loosen and reapply if necessary.

IMPROVISED SLINGS

CAUTION

If you suspect that the forearm is broken, use a cloth sling or a jacket corner to provide support. Do not use any other improvised sling: it will not provide enough support.

If you need to support a casualty's injured arm but do not have a triangular bandage available, you can make a sling by using a square metre (just over one square yard) of any strong cloth (p.249). You can also improvise by using an item of the casualty's clothing (below). Check circulation after applying support (p243) and recheck every ten minutes.

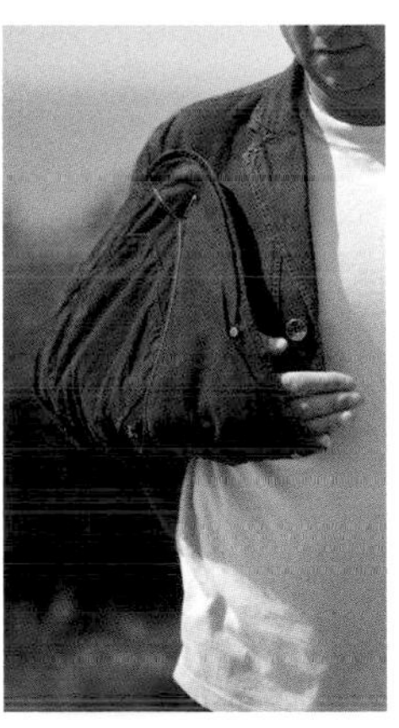

JACKET CORNER

Undo the casualty's jacket. Fold the lower edge on the injured side up over his arm. Secure the corner of the hem to the jacket breast with a large safety pin. Tuck and pin the excess material closely around the elbow.

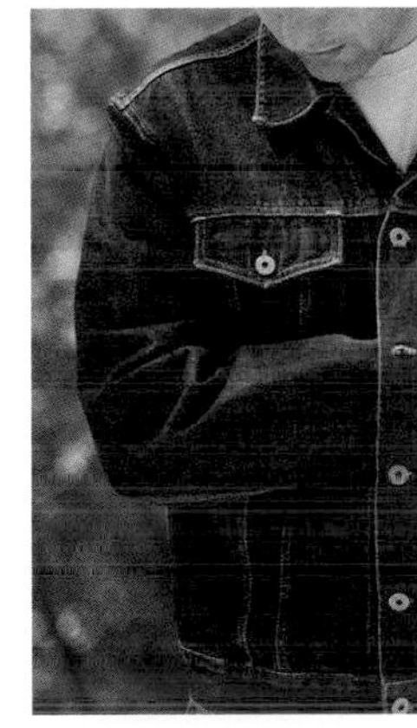

BUTTON-UP JACKET

Undo one button of a jacket or coat (or waistcoat). Place the hand of the injured arm inside the garment at the gap formed by the unfastened button. Advise the casualty to rest his wrist on the button just beneath the gap.

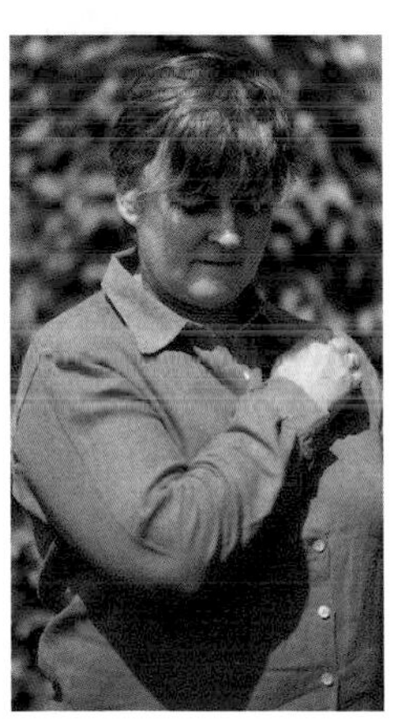

LONG-SLEEVED SHIRT

Lay the injured arm across the casualty's chest. Pin the cuff of the sleeve to the breast of the shirt. To improvise an elevation sling (opposite), pin the sleeve at the casualty's opposite shoulder, to keep her arm raised.

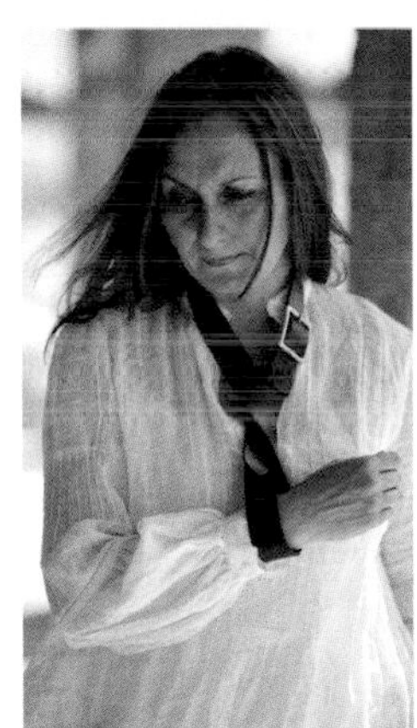

BELT OR THIN GARMENT

Use a belt, a tie or a pair of braces or tights to make a "collar-and-cuff" support. Fasten the item to form a loop. Place it over the casualty's head, then twist it once to form a smaller loop at the front. Place the casualty's hand into the loop.

13

This chapter is designed as a user-friendly quick-reference guide to first aid treatment for casualties with serious illnesses or injuries. It begins with an action plan to help you assess a casualty and identify first aid priorities, using the primary survey (pp.44–45) followed by the secondary survey (pp.46–48) where appropriate.

The chapter goes on to show how to treat unconscious casualties, whose care always takes priority over that of less seriously injured casualties. In addition, there is step-by-step essential first aid for potentially life-threatening illnesses and injuries that benefit from immediate first aid. These include asthma, stroke, severe bleeding, shock, heart attack, burns, broken bones and spinal injuries. Each condition is described in more detail in the main part of the book and cross-referenced here so it can easily be found if you need further advice and background information.

AIMS AND OBJECTIVES

- To protect yourself from danger and make the area safe.
- To assess the situation quickly and calmly and summon appropriate help.
- To assist casualties and provide necessary treatment with the help of bystanders.
- To call 999/112 for emergency help if you suspect a serious illness or injury.
- To be aware of your own needs.

EMERGENCY FIRST AID

ACTION IN AN EMERGENCY

Assess the casualty using the primary survey (pp.44–45). Identify life-threatening conditions and once these are managed carry out a secondary survey (pp.46–48).

START

DANGER
Make sure the area is safe before you approach. *Is anyone in danger?*

YES

NO

RESPONSE
Is the casualty conscious?
Try to get a response by asking questions and gently shaking his shoulders.
Is there a response?

YES

NO

UNCONSCIOUS CASUALTY

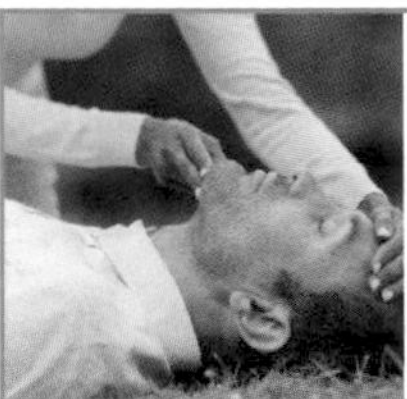

AIRWAY
Is the casualty's airway open and clear?

Open the airway
Tilt the head and lift the chin to open the airway.

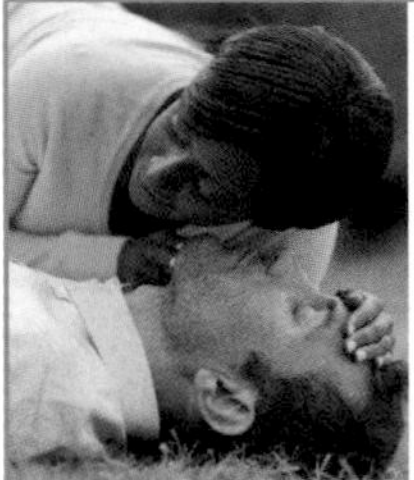

BREATHING
Is the casualty breathing normally?

Check breathing
Look along the chest, and listen and feel for breaths.

NO

Are you on your own?

NO

CPR/CIRCULATION
Ask someone to **call 999/112 for emergency help** and bring an AED if possible. Begin cardiopulmonary resuscitation/CPR (adult p.258, child p.258, infant p.260).

YES

CPR/CIRCULATION
If the casualty is a child or infant, give FIVE initial rescue breaths and cardiopulmonary resuscitation/ CPR for one minute (child p.258, infant p.260). **Call 999/112 for emergency help**, then continue CPR.

If the casualty is an adult, **call 999/112 for emergency help** then begin CPR (p.258).

YES

CIRCULATION
Check for and treat life-threatening conditions, such as severe bleeding.

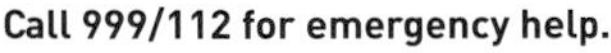

Call 999/112 for emergency help.
Maintain an open airway. Place the casualty on his side in the recovery position.

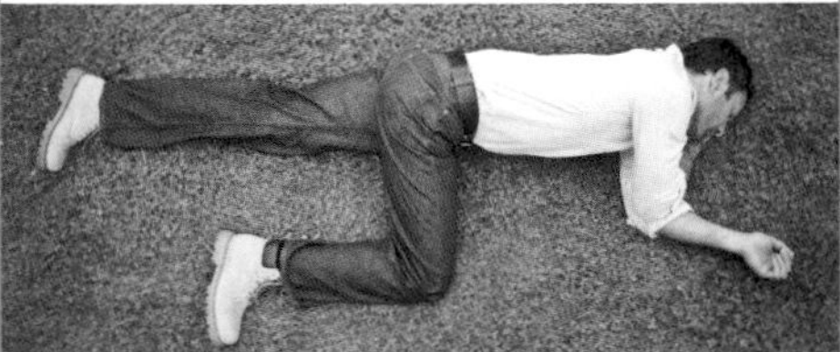

COMPRESSION-ONLY CPR

Give chest compressions only if you have not had formal training in CPR or you are unwilling or unable to give rescue breaths. The ambulance dispatcher will give instructions for chest compression-only CPR.

If it is not safe do not approach.
Call 999/112 for emergency help.

CONSCIOUS CASUALTY

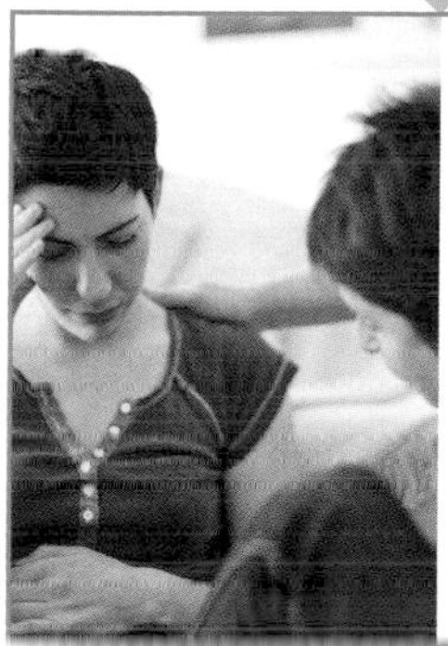

AIRWAY AND BREATHING

If a person is conscious, alert, and responding verbally, it follows that her airway is open and clear and she is breathing.

Breathing may be fast, slow, easy or difficult. Assess and treat any difficulty found.

CIRCULATION

Are there life-threatening conditions, such as severe bleeding or heart attack?

YES

Treat life-threatening injuries or illness.
Call 999/112 for emergency help.
Monitor and record casualty's level of response, breathing and pulse while you wait for help to arrive.

NO

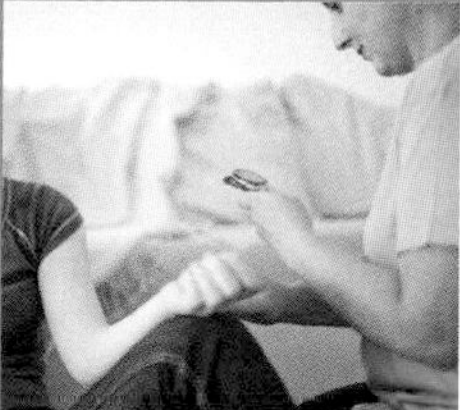

Carry out a secondary survey

Assess the level of consciousness using the AVPU scale (p.52) and carry out a head-to-toe survey to check for signs of illness or injury.

Call for appropriate help. **Call 999/112 for emergency help** if you suspect serious injury or illness. Monitor and record casualty's level of response, breathing and pulse while you wait for help to arrive.

A–Z OF EMERGENCIES

CPR FOR AN ADULT

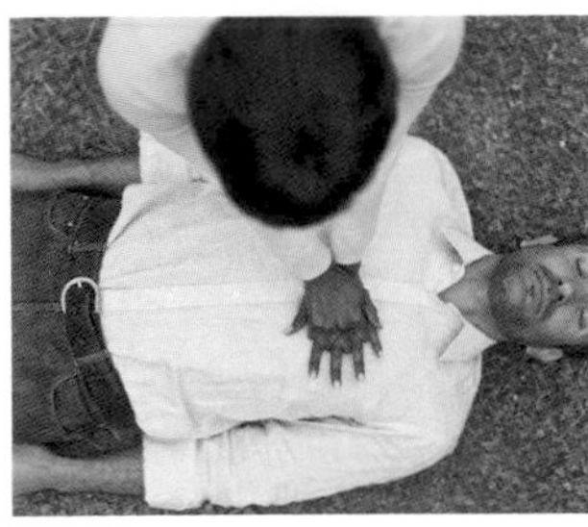

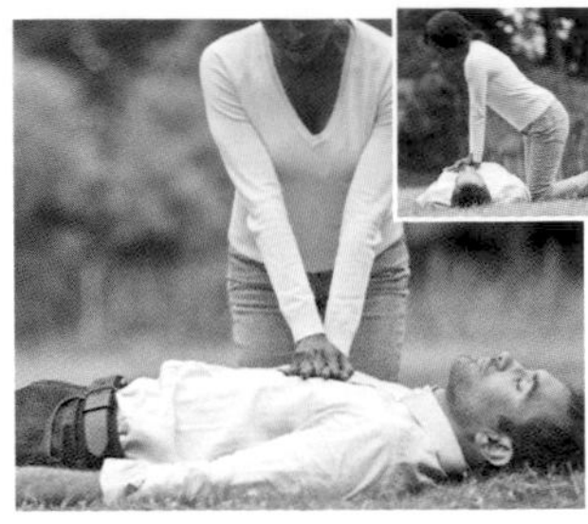

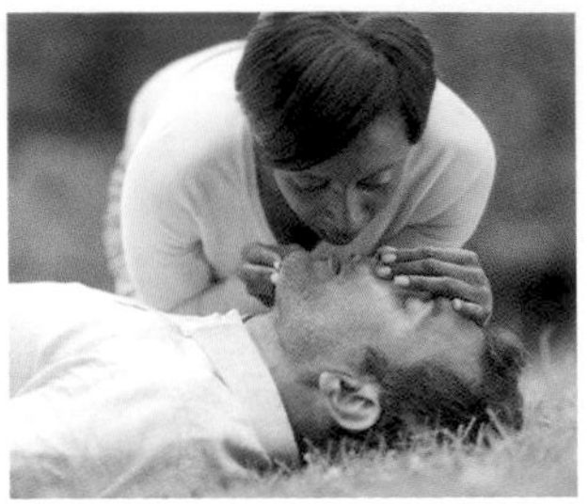

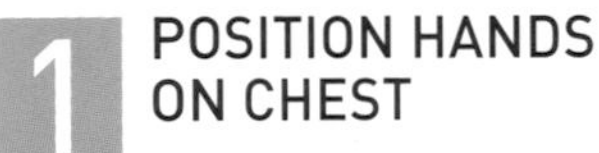

1 POSITION HANDS ON CHEST

Place one hand on the centre of the casualty's chest. Place the heel of your other hand on top of the first and interlock your fingers, but keep your fingers off the casualty's ribs.

2 GIVE 30 CHEST COMPRESSIONS

Lean directly over the casualty's chest and press down vertically about 5–6cm (2–2½in). Release the pressure, but do not remove your hands. Give 30 compressions at a rate of 100–120 per minute.

3 OPEN AIRWAY, BEGIN RESCUE BREATHS

Tilt the casualty's head with one hand and lift the chin with two fingers of your other hand. Pinch the nostrils closed, and allow his mouth to fall open. Take a breath, seal your lips over the casualty's mouth, and blow steadily until the chest rises.

CPR FOR A CHILD (one year to puberty)

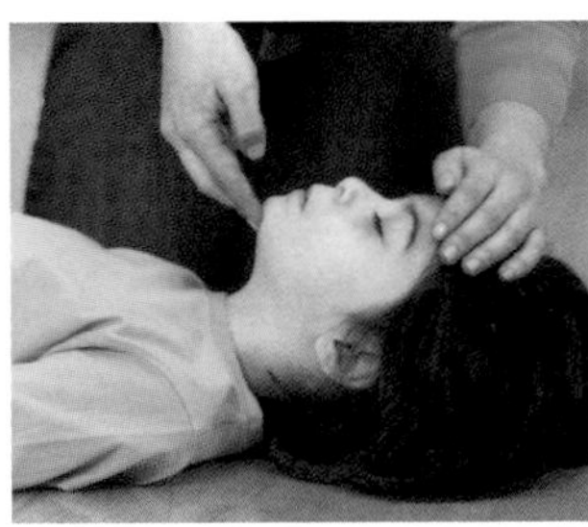

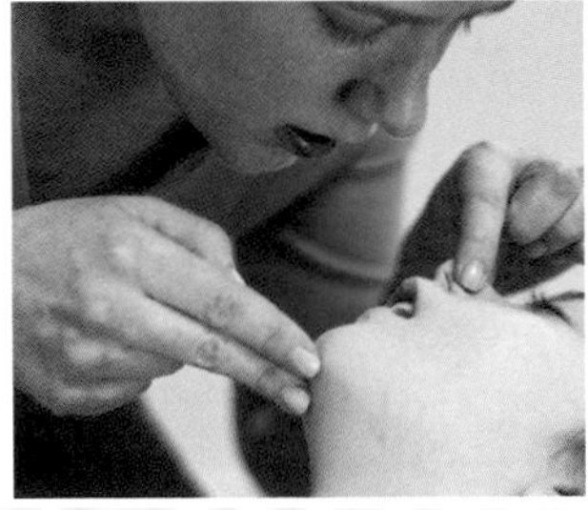

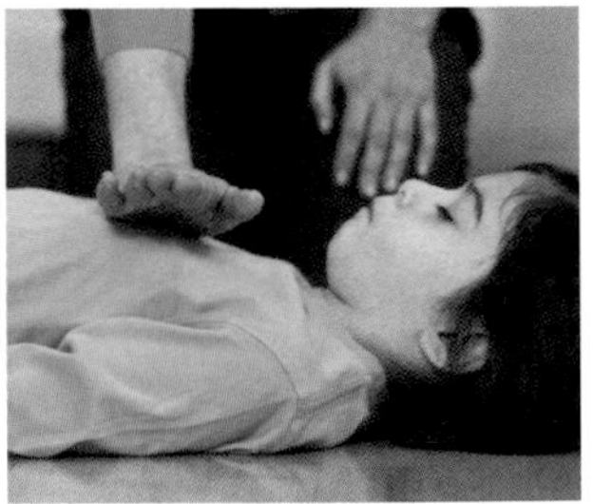

1 CHECK THAT AIRWAY IS OPEN

Tilt the child's head with one hand and lift the chin with two fingers of the other hand to ensure the airway is open.

2 GIVE FIVE INITIAL RESCUE BREATHS

Pinch the nose to close the nostrils. Allow the mouth to fall open. Take a breath and seal your lips over the child's mouth. Blow steadily until the chest rises, then watch it fall; a rescue breath should take one second. Give FIVE rescue breaths.

3 GIVE 30 CHEST COMPRESSIONS

Place the heel of one hand on the centre of the chest. Lean directly over the child's chest and press down to at least one third of its depth, then release the pressure. Give 30 compressions at a rate of 100–120 per minute.

FIND OUT MORE pp.66–67 >>

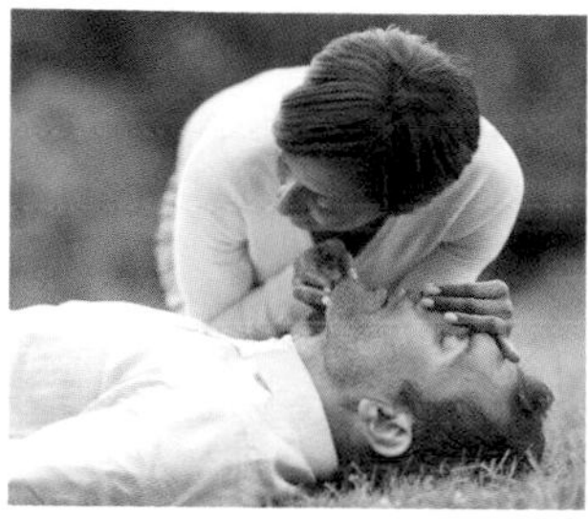

4 WATCH CHEST FALL

Maintaining the open airway, take your mouth away from the casualty's. Look along the chest and watch it fall. Repeat to give TWO rescue breaths; each full breath should take one second. Repeat 30 chest compressions followed by TWO rescue breaths.

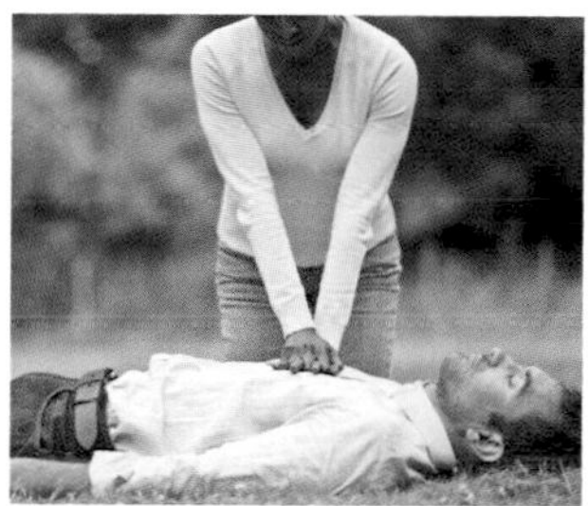

5 CONTINUE CPR

Continue CPR until emergency help arrives, the casualty shows signs of regaining consciousness, such as coughing, opening his eyes, speaking, or moving purposefully, AND starts to breathe normally, or you are too exhausted to continue.

CAUTION

- Give chest compressions only if you have not had formal training in CPR, or you are unwilling or unable to give rescue breaths. The ambulance dispatcher will give instructions for chest compression-only CPR.
- If the casualty vomits during CPR, roll him away from you onto his side, ensuring that his head is turned towards the floor to allow vomit to drain. Clear his mouth, then immediately roll him onto his back again and recommence CPR.
- If there is more than one rescuer, change over every 1–2 minutes, with minimal interruption to chest compressions.

FIND OUT MORE pp.74–75>>

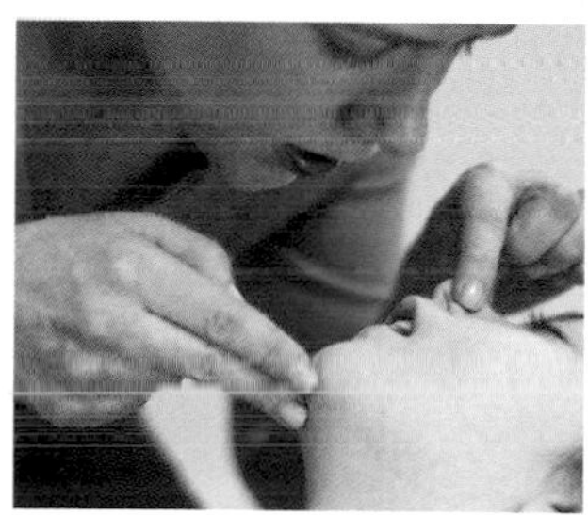

4 GIVE TWO RESCUE BREATHS

Return to the head and give TWO rescue breaths. Repeat 30 chest compressions followed by TWO rescue breaths for one minute. **Call 999/112 for emergency help** if this has not already been done.

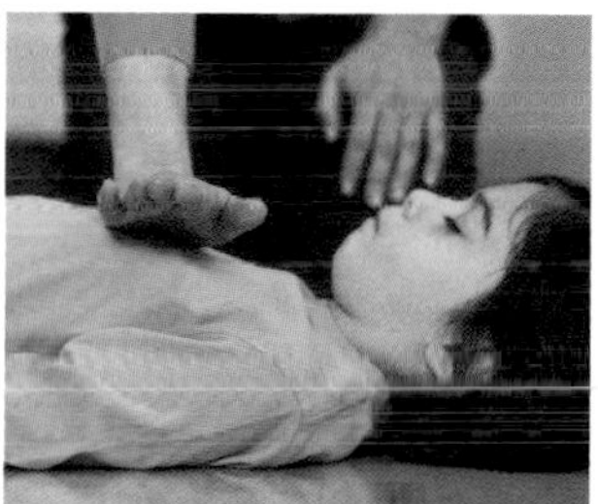

5 CONTINUE CPR

Continue CPR until emergency help arrives, the child shows signs of regaining consciousness, such as coughing, opening her eyes, speaking, or moving purposefully, AND starts to breathe normally, or you are too exhausted to continue.

CAUTION

- Give chest compressions only if you have not had formal training in CPR, or you are unwilling or unable to give rescue breaths. The ambulance dispatcher will give instructions for chest compression-only CPR.
- If the child vomits during CPR, roll her away from you onto her side, ensuring that her head is turned towards the floor to allow vomit to drain. Clear her mouth, then immediately roll her onto her back again and recommence CPR.
- If there is more than one rescuer, change over every 1–2 minutes, with minimal interruption to chest compressions.

CPR FOR AN INFANT (under one year)

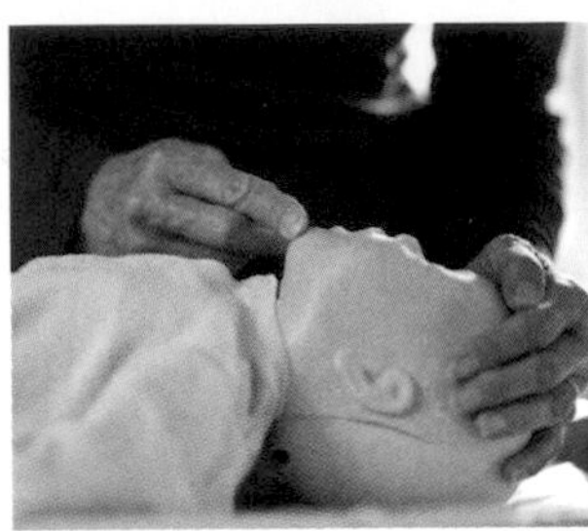

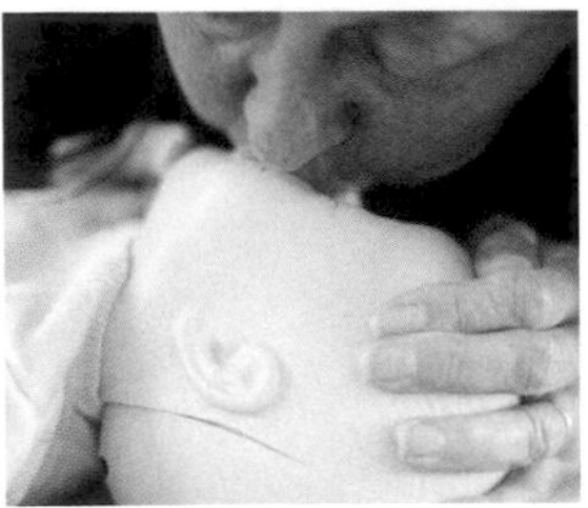

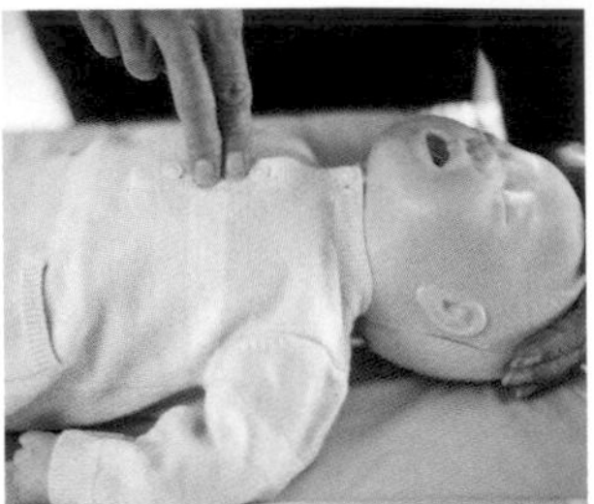

1 CHECK THAT AIRWAY IS OPEN

Place the infant on a firm surface or on the floor. Gently tilt the head with one hand and lift the chin with one finger of the other hand to ensure the airway is open.

2 GIVE FIVE INITIAL RESCUE BREATHS

Take a breath and place your lips over the infant's mouth and nose. Blow steadily into the mouth and nose until the chest rises, then watch it fall. Each full breath should take about one second. Give FIVE rescue breaths.

3 GIVE 30 CHEST COMPRESSIONS

Place the tips of your index and middle finger on the centre of the chest. Lean over the infant's chest and press down vertically to at least one third of its depth. Release the pressure but not your fingers. Give 30 compressions at a rate of 100–120 per minute.

CHOKING ADULT

RECOGNITION

Ask the casualty: "Are you choking?"

Mild obstruction:

- Difficulty in speaking, coughing and breathing.

Severe obstruction:

- Inability to speak, cough or breathe;
- Eventual unconsciousness.

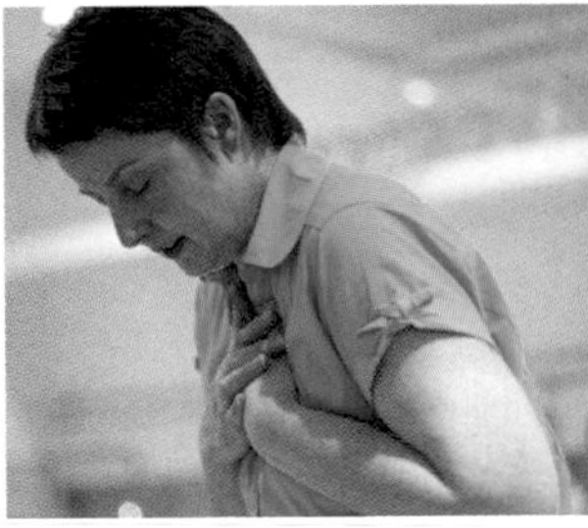

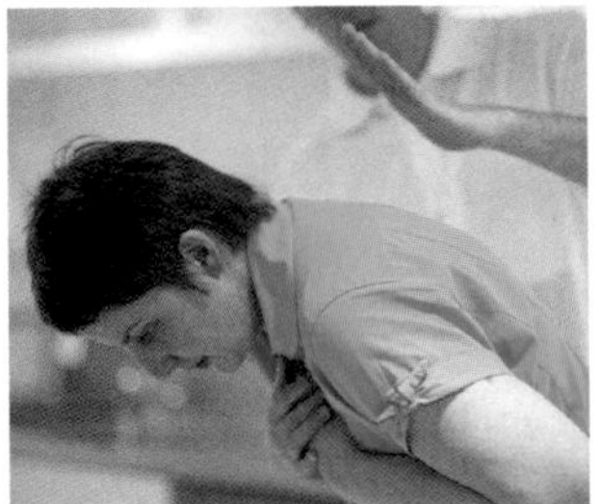

1 ENCOURAGE CASUALTY TO COUGH

If the casualty is breathing, encourage her to cough to try to remove the obstruction herself. If this fails, go to step 2.

2 GIVE UP TO FIVE BACK BLOWS

If the casualty cannot speak, cough or breathe, bend her forward. Give up to five sharp blows between the shoulder blades with the heel of your hand. Check her mouth.
If choking persists, proceed to step 3.

FIND OUT MORE **pp.80–81 >>**

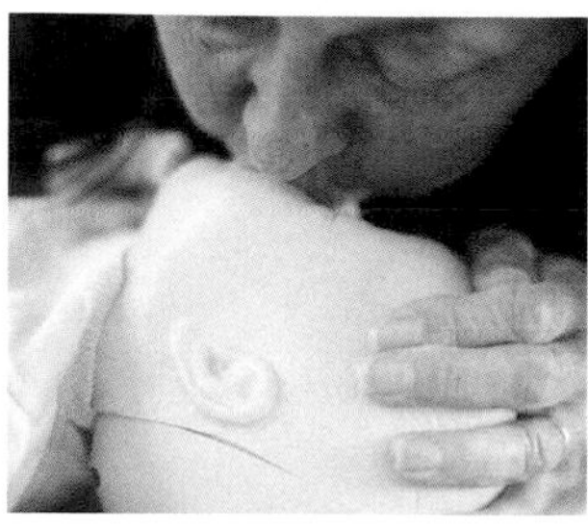

4 GIVE TWO RESCUE BREATHS

Return to the head and give TWO more rescue breaths. Repeat 30 chest compressions followed by TWO rescue breaths for one minute. **Call 999/112 for emergency help** if this has not already been done.

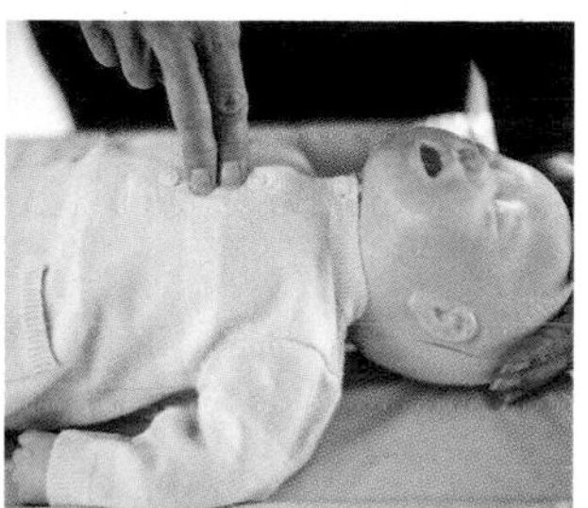

5 CONTINUE CPR

Continue CPR until emergency help arrives, the infant shows signs of regaining consciousness, such as coughing, opening his eyes, speaking, or moving purposefully AND starts to breathe normally or you are too exhausted to continue.

CAUTION

- Give chest compressions only if you have not had formal training in CPR or you are unwilling or unable to give rescue breaths. The ambulance dispatcher will give instructions for chest compression only CPR.
- If the child vomits during CPR, roll her away from you onto her side, ensuring that her head is turned towards the floor to allow vomit to drain. Restart CPR as soon as possible.
- If there is more than one rescuer, change over every 1–2 minutes, with minimal interruption to chest compressions.

FIND OUT MORE **p.91 >>**

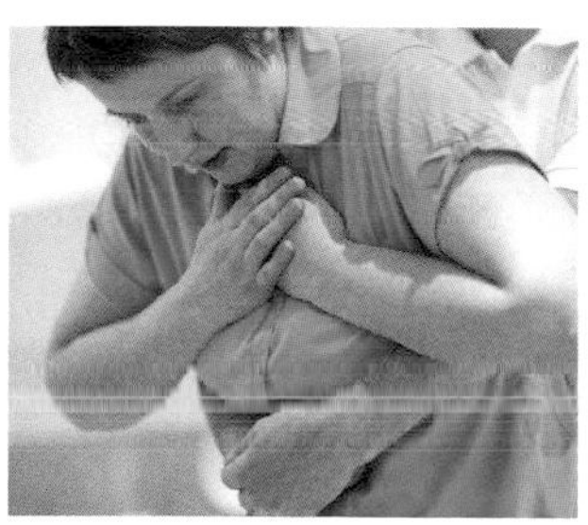

3 GIVE UP TO FIVE ABDOMINAL THRUSTS

Stand behind the casualty. Put both arms around her, and put one fist between her navel and the bottom of her breastbone. Grasp your fist with your other hand, and pull sharply inwards and upwards up to five times. Recheck the mouth.

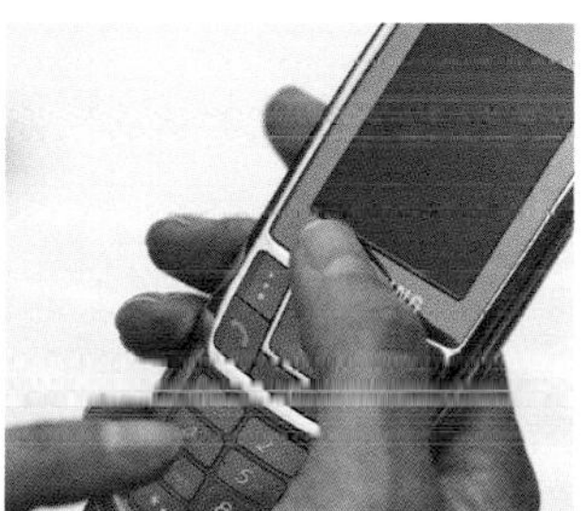

4 CALL FOR EMERGENCY HELP

Repeat steps 2 and 3 until the obstruction clears. If after three cycles it still has not cleared, **call 999/112 for emergency help**. Continue the sequence until help arrives, the obstruction is cleared or the casualty loses consciousness.

CAUTION

- Do not do a finger sweep when checking the mouth.
- If the casualty loses consciousness, open the airway and check breathing (p.256). Be prepared to give CPR (p.258).

CHOKING CHILD (one year to puberty)

RECOGNITION

Ask the child: "Are you choking?"

Mild obstruction:

- Difficulty in speaking, coughing and breathing.

Severe obstruction:

- Inability to speak, cough or breathe;
- Eventual unconsciousness.

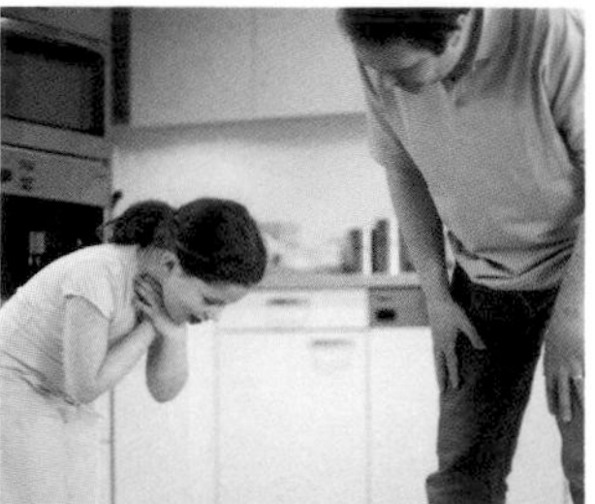

1 ENCOURAGE CHILD TO COUGH

If the child is breathing, encourage her to cough to try to remove the obstruction herself. If this fails, go to step 2.

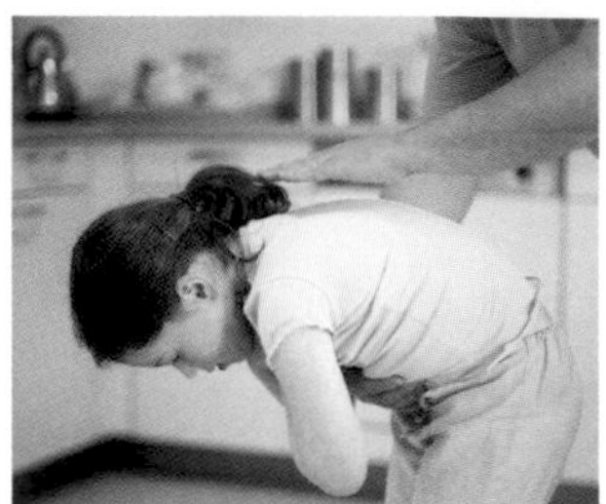

2 GIVE UP TO FIVE BACK BLOWS

If the child cannot speak, cough or breathe, bend her forward. Give up to five sharp blows between the shoulder blades with the heel of your hand. Check her mouth. If choking persists, proceed to step 3.

CHOKING INFANT (under one year)

RECOGNITION

Mild obstruction:

- Able to cough but difficulty in breathing or making any noise.

Severe obstruction:

- Inability to cough, make any noise or breathe;
- Eventual unconsciousness.

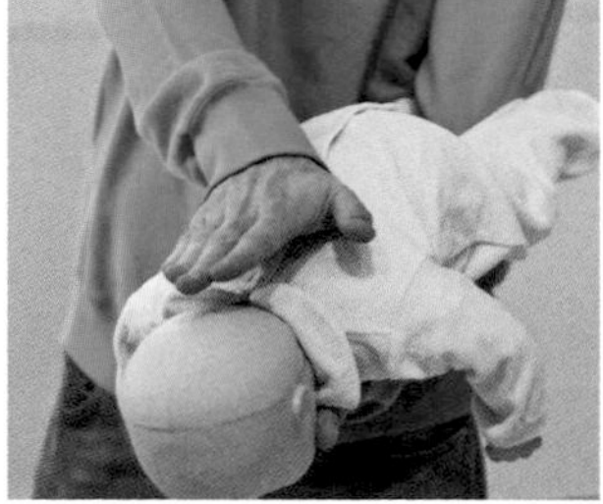

1 GIVE UP TO FIVE BACK BLOWS

If the infant is unable to cough or breathe, lay him face down along your forearm (head low), and support his body and head. Give up to five back blows between the shoulder blades with the heel of your hand.

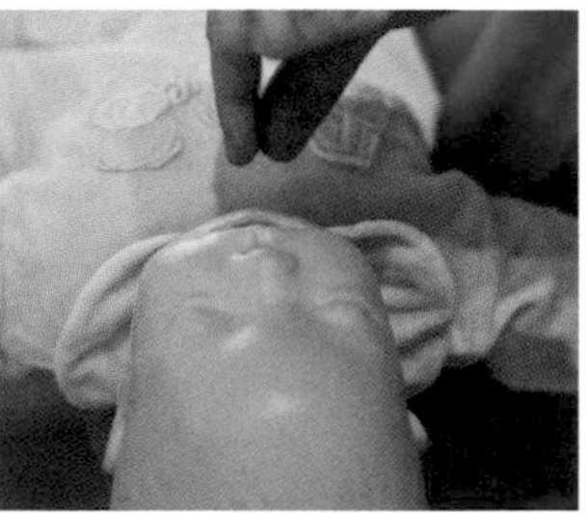

2 CHECK INFANT'S MOUTH

Turn the infant face up along your other forearm, supporting his back and head. Check the mouth. Pick out any obvious obstructions. If choking persists, proceed to step 3.

FIND OUT MORE p.92 >>

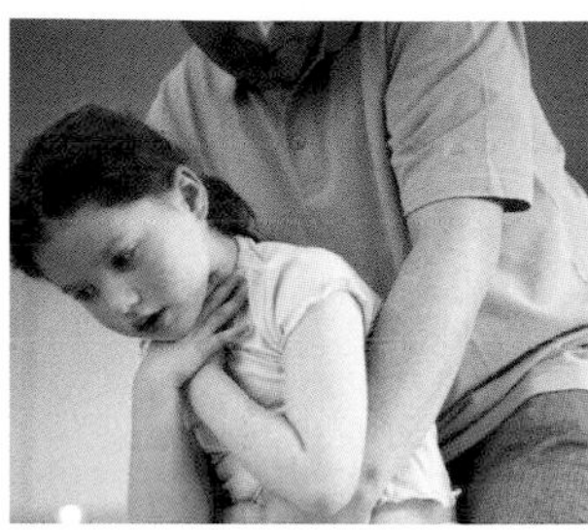

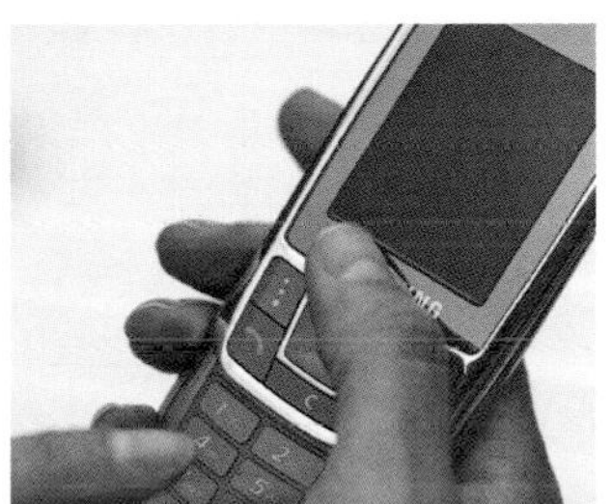

3 GIVE UP TO FIVE ABDOMINAL THRUSTS

Stand behind the child. Put both your arms around her, and put one fist between her navel and the bottom of her breastbone. Grasp your fist with your other hand, and pull sharply inwards and upwards up to five times. Recheck the mouth.

4 CALL FOR EMERGENCY HELP

Repeat steps 2 and 3 until the obstruction clears. If after three cycles it still has not cleared, **call 999/112 for emergency help**. Continue the sequence until help arrives, the obstruction is cleared or the child loses consciousness.

CAUTION

- Do not do a finger sweep when checking the mouth.
- If the child loses consciousness, open the airway and check breathing (p.256). Be prepared to begin CPR (p.258).

FIND OUT MORE p.93 >>

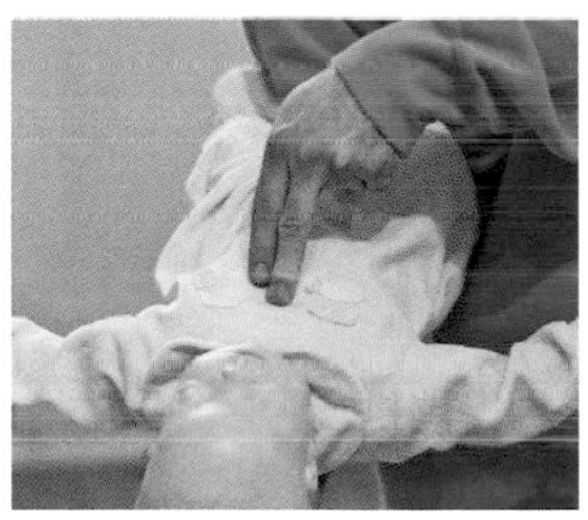

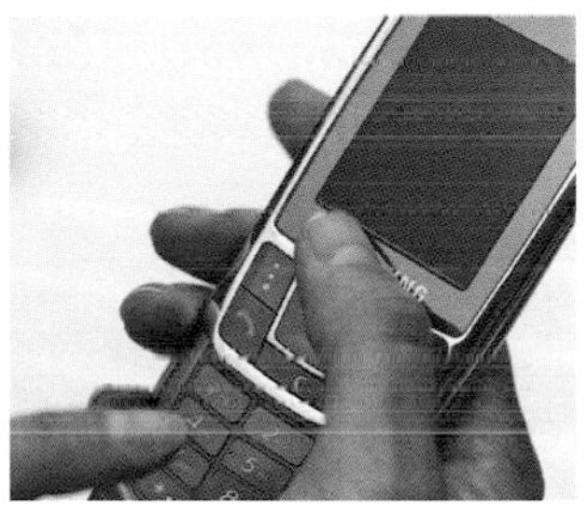

3 GIVE UP TO FIVE CHEST THRUSTS

Place two fingertips on the lower half of the infant's breastbone, a finger's breadth below the nipples. Give up to five sharp thrusts, pushing inwards and towards the head. Recheck the mouth.

4 CALL FOR EMERGENCY HELP

Repeat steps 1 to 3. If after three cycles the obstruction is still not clear, take the infant with you to **call 999/112 for emergency help**. Continue the sequence until help arrives, the obstruction is cleared or the infant loses consciousness.

CAUTION

- Do not do a finger sweep when checking the mouth.
- Do not use abdominal thrusts on an infant.
- If the infant loses consciousness, open the airway and check breathing (p.256). Be prepared to begin CPR (p.260).

ASTHMA

RECOGNITION

Difficulty in breathing, especially breathing out.

There may be:

- Wheezing;
- Difficulty in speaking;
- Grey-blue colouring in skin, lips, earlobes and nailbeds.

In a severe attack:

- Exhaustion and possible loss of consciousness.

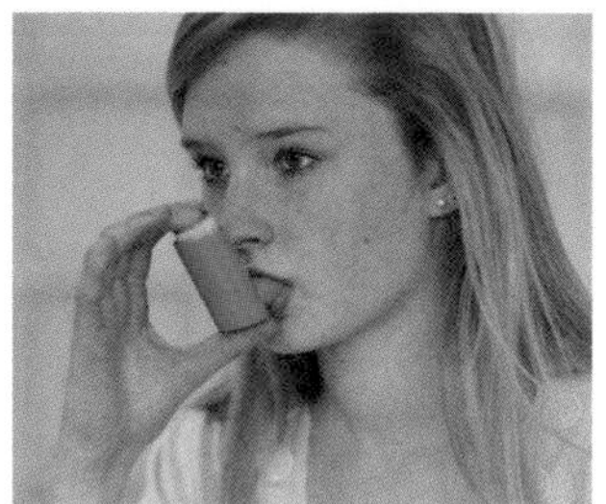

1 HELP CASUALTY USE INHALER

Keep calm and reassure the casualty. Help her to find and use her reliever inhaler (it is usually blue); use a spacer device if she has one. The reliever inhaler should take effect within minutes.

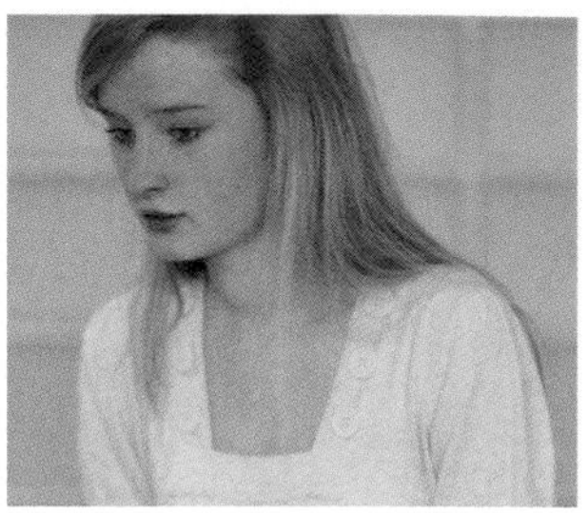

2 ENCOURAGE SLOW BREATHS

Help the casualty into a comfortable breathing position; sitting slightly forwards is best. Tell her to breathe slowly and deeply. A mild attack should ease within a few minutes. If it does not, ask the casualty to take another dose from her inhaler.

HEART ATTACK

RECOGNITION

There may be:

- Vice-like chest pain, spreading to one or both arms;
- Breathlessness;
- Discomfort, like indigestion, in upper abdomen;
- Sudden dizziness or faintness;
- Sudden collapse, with no warning;
- Casualty may have sense of impending doom;
- Ashen skin and blueness of lips;
- Rapid, weak or irregular pulse;
- Profuse sweating;
- Extreme gasping for air (air hunger).

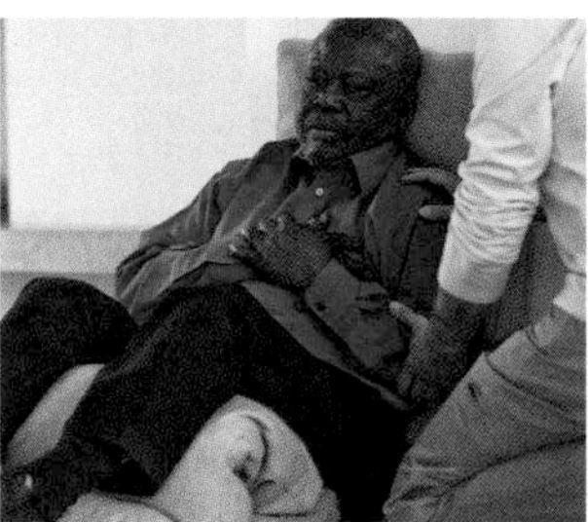

1 MAKE CASUALTY COMFORTABLE

Help the casualty into a half-sitting position. Support his head and shoulders and place cushions under his knees. Reassure the casualty.

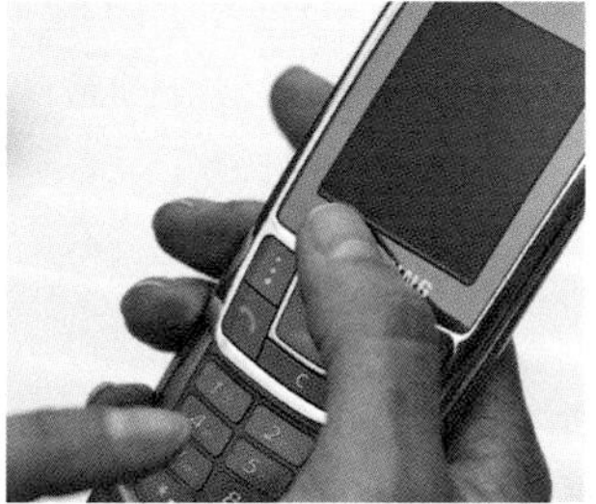

2 CALL FOR EMERGENCY HELP

Call 999/112 for emergency help. Tell ambulance control that you suspect a heart attack. Call the casualty's doctor as well, if he asks you to do so.

FIND OUT MORE p.100 >>

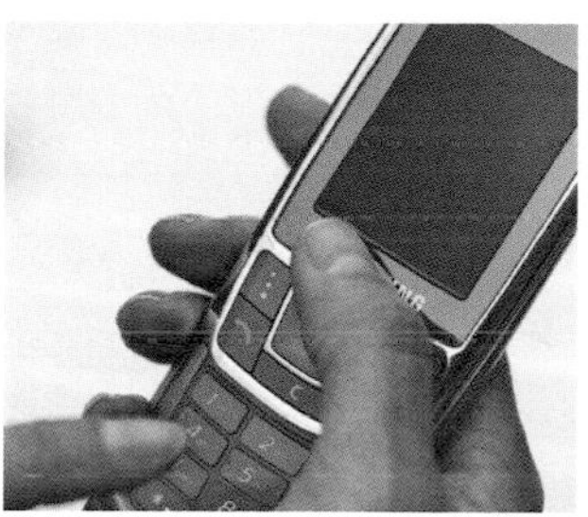

3 CALL FOR EMERGENCY HELP

Call **999/112 for emergency help** if: the inhaler has no effect, breathlessness makes talking difficult or the casualty is becoming exhausted.

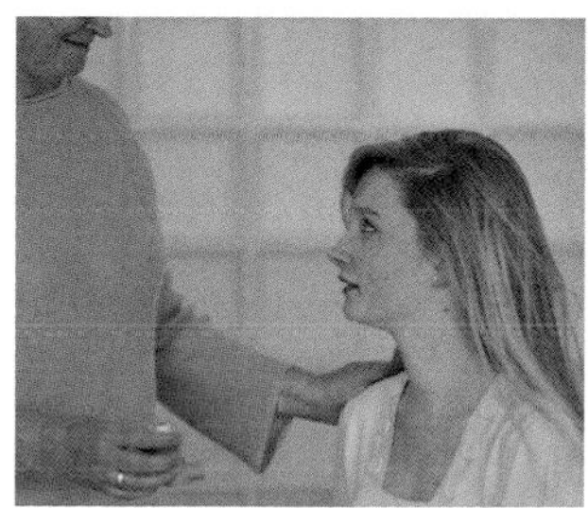

4 MONITOR CASUALTY

Monitor and record the casualty's vital signs – level of response, breathing and pulse – until she recovers or help arrives. Help her to reuse her inhaler as required. Advise the casualty to seek medical advice if she is concerned about the attack.

CAUTION

- Do not let the casualty lie down.
- Do not leave the casualty alone since the attack may quickly worsen.
- If this is a first attack and she has no medication, **call 999/112 for emergency help** immediately.
- If the attack worsens, the casualty may lose consciousness. Open the airway and check breathing (p.256). Be prepared to begin CPR (pp.258–59).

FIND OUT MORE p.110 >>

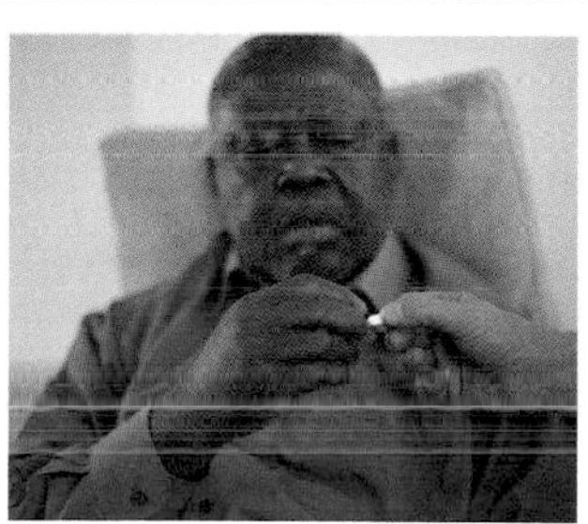

3 GIVE CASUALTY MEDICATION

If the casualty is fully conscious, assist him to take one full dose aspirin tablet (300mg); advise him to chew it slowly. If the casualty has tablets or a puffer for angina, allow him to take it himself. Help him if necessary.

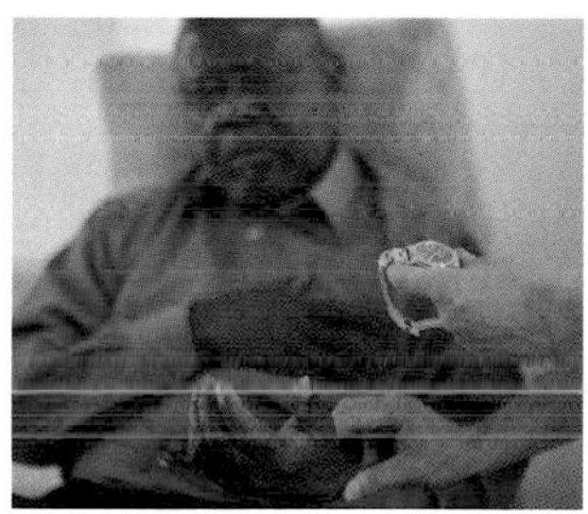

4 MONITOR CASUALTY

Encourage the casualty to rest. Keep any bystanders away. Monitor and record the casualty's vital signs – level of response, breathing and pulse – until emergency help arrives.

CAUTION

- Be aware of the possibility of collapse without warning.
- Do not give the casualty aspirin if you know that he is allergic to it.
- If the casualty loses consciousness, open the airway and check breathing (p.256). Be prepared to begin CPR (pp.258–59).

SEVERE EXTERNAL BLEEDING

CAUTION

- Do not apply a tourniquet.
- If there is an object in the wound, apply pressure on either side of the wound to control bleeding.
- If blood seeps through the bandage, place another pad on top. If blood seeps through the second pad, remove all dressings and apply a fresh one, ensuring that it exerts pressure on the bleeding area.
- Do not give the casualty anything to eat or drink as an anaesthetic may be needed.
- If the casualty loses consciousness, open the airway and check breathing (p.256). Be prepared to begin CPR (pp.258–60).

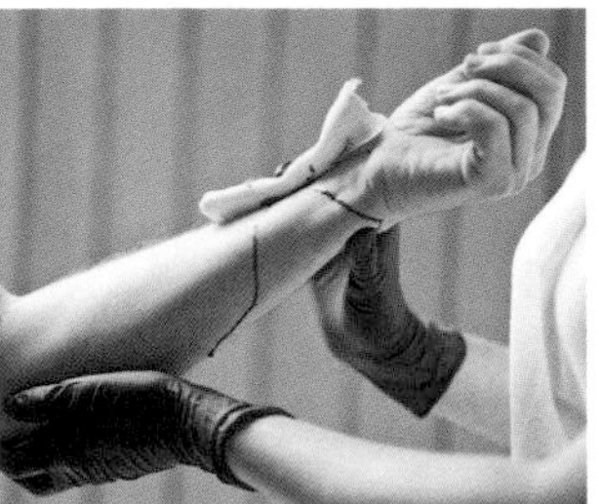

1 APPLY DIRECT PRESSURE TO WOUND

Remove or cut any clothing over the wound if necessary. Place a sterile wound dressing or non-fluffy pad over the wound. Apply firm pressure with your fingers or the palm of your hand.

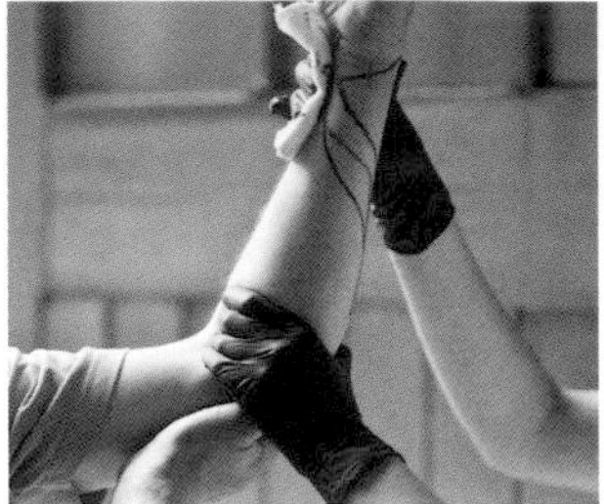

2 RAISE AND SUPPORT INJURED PART

Maintaining pressure on the wound, raise and support the injured part so that it is above the level of the casualty's heart.

SHOCK

RECOGNITION

- Rapid pulse.
- Pale, cold, clammy skin.
- Sweating.

As shock develops:

- Rapid, shallow breathing;
- Weak pulse;
- Grey-blue skin, especially inside lips;
- Weakness and giddiness;
- Nausea and vomiting;
- Thirst.

As the brain's oxygen supply weakens:

- Restlessness;
- Gasping for air;
- Loss of consciousness.

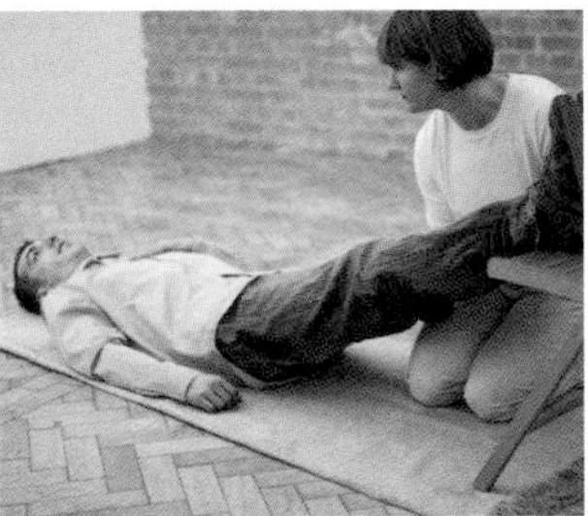

1 HELP CASUALTY TO LIE DOWN

Help the casualty to lie down (ideally on a blanket). Raise and support his legs above the level of his heart. Treat any cause of shock, such as bleeding (above) or burns (p.274).

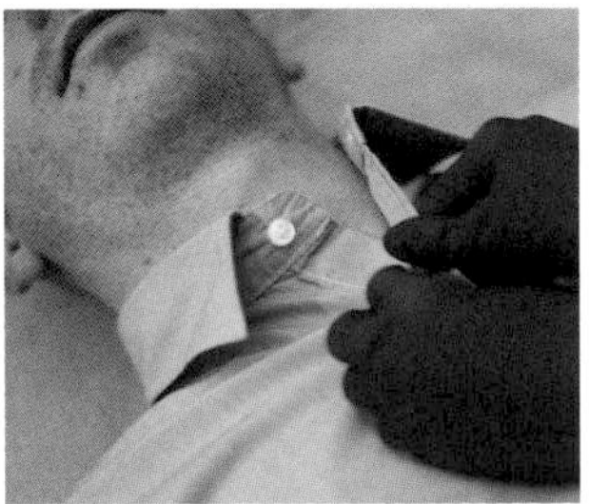

2 LOOSEN TIGHT CLOTHING

Keep the casualty's head low. Loosen any clothing that constricts his neck, chest and waist.

FIND OUT MORE pp.114–15 >>

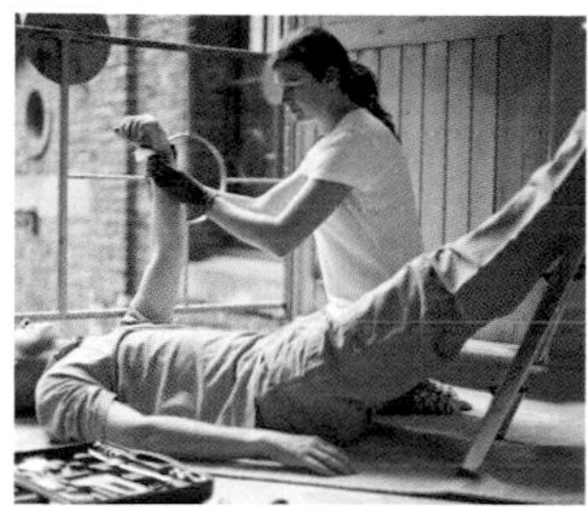

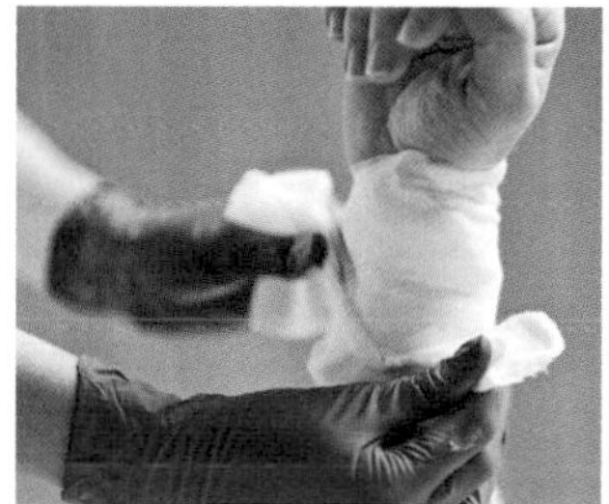

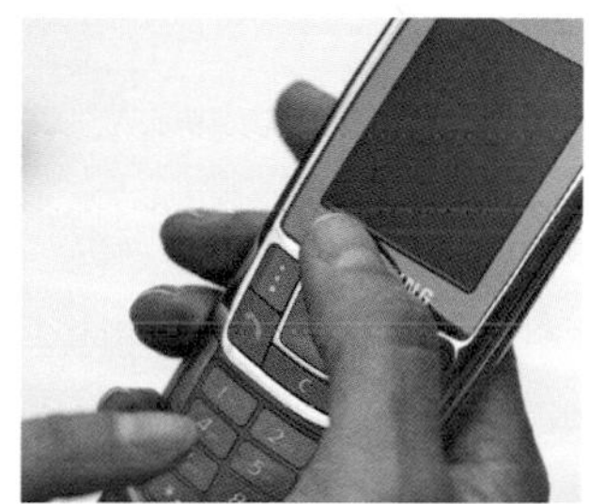

3 LAY CASUALTY DOWN

Keeping the injury high, help the casualty to lie down on a blanket. Raise and support his legs to minimise the risk of shock (below).

4 BANDAGE DRESSING IN PLACE

Secure a pad over the wound with a bandage. Check the circulation beyond the bandage every ten minutes. Loosen and reapply the bandage if necessary.

5 CALL FOR EMERGENCY HELP

Call 999/112 for emergency help. Give details of the site of the injury and the extent of the bleeding when you telephone. Monitor and record vital signs – level of response, breathing and pulse – until emergency help arrives.

FIND OUT MORE pp.116–17 >>

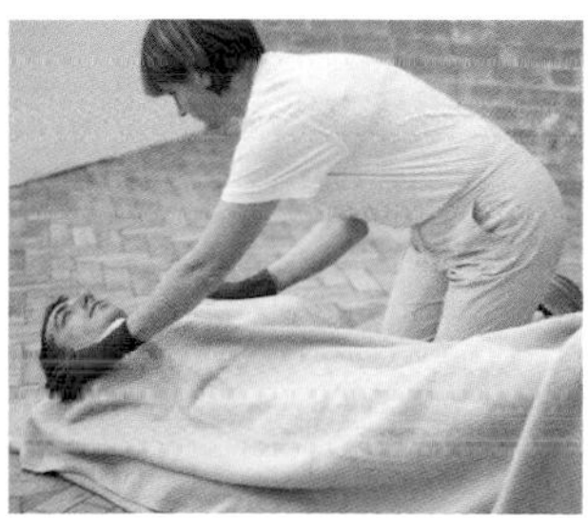

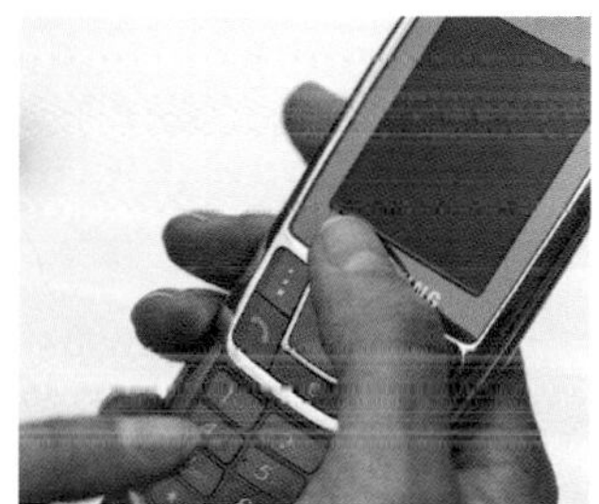

3 KEEP CASUALTY WARM

Cover the casualty with a blanket to keep him warm. Advise the casualty not to move.

4 CALL FOR EMERGENCY HELP

Call 999/112 for emergency help. Give ambulance control details about the cause of shock, if known. Monitor and record vital signs – level of response, breathing and pulse – until help arrives.

CAUTION

- Do not leave the casualty unattended, unless you have to call for emergency help.
- Do not let the casualty move.
- Do not try to warm the casualty with a hot-water bottle or any other form of direct heat.
- Do not give the casualty anything to eat or drink because an anaesthetic may be needed.
- If the casualty loses consciousness, open the airway and check breathing (p.256). Be prepared to begin CPR (pp.258–60).

BROKEN BONES

RECOGNITION

- Distortion, swelling and bruising at the injury site.
- Pain and difficulty in moving the injured part.

There may be:

- Bending, twisting or shortening of a limb;
- A wound, possibly with bone ends protruding.

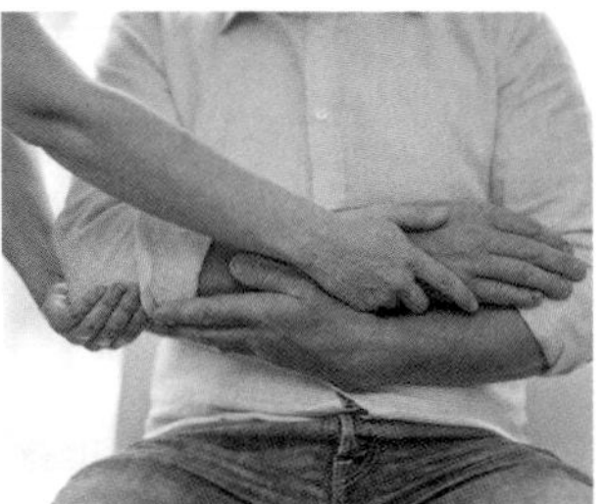

1 SUPPORT INJURED PART

Help the casualty to support the affected part at the joints above and below the injury, in the most comfortable position.

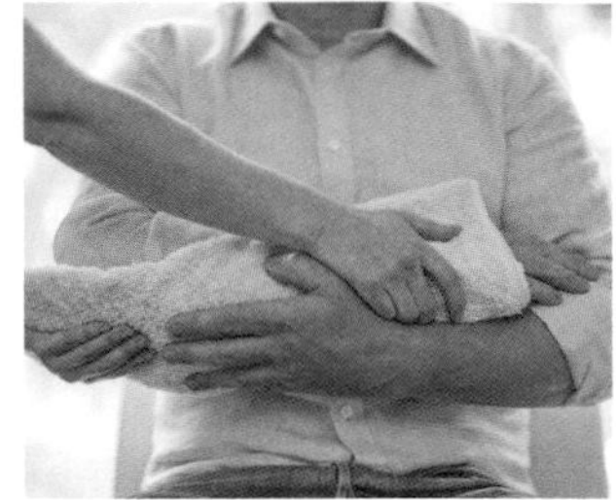

2 PROTECT INJURY WITH PADDING

Place padding, such as towels or cushions, around the affected part, and support it in a comfortable position.

HEAD INJURY

RECOGNITION

There may be:

- A scalp wound;
- Clear fluid or watery blood from the nose or an ear (this indicates a serious underlying head injury).
- Impaired consciousness.

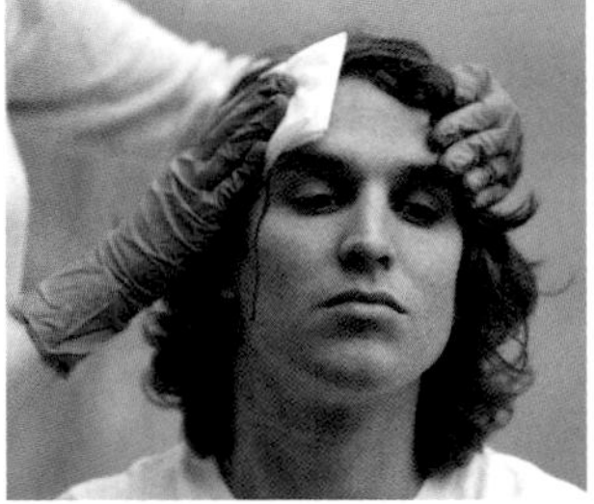

1 APPLY DIRECT PRESSURE TO ANY WOUND

Replace any displaced skin flaps over the wound. Put a sterile dressing or a clean, non-fluffy pad over the wound. Apply firm, direct pressure with your hand to control the bleeding.

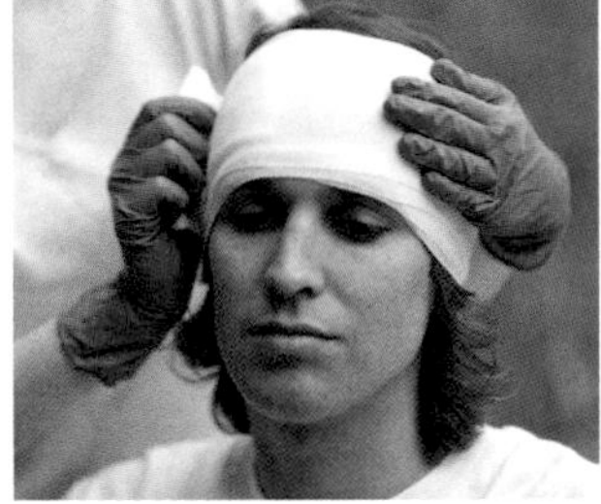

2 SECURE DRESSING WITH BANDAGE

Secure the dressing over the wound with a roller bandage to help maintain direct pressure on the injury.

FIND OUT MORE pp.136–38 ››

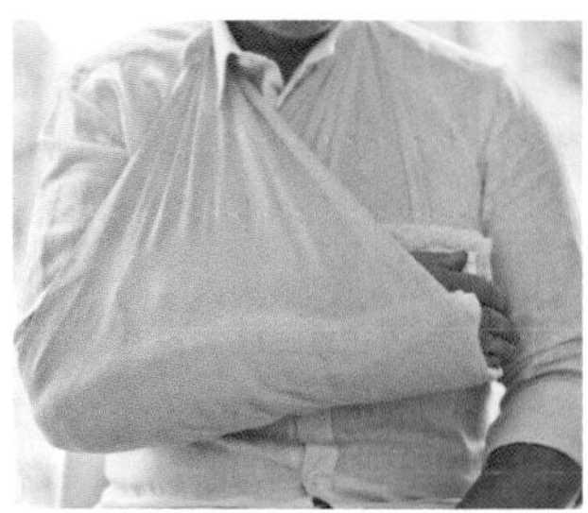

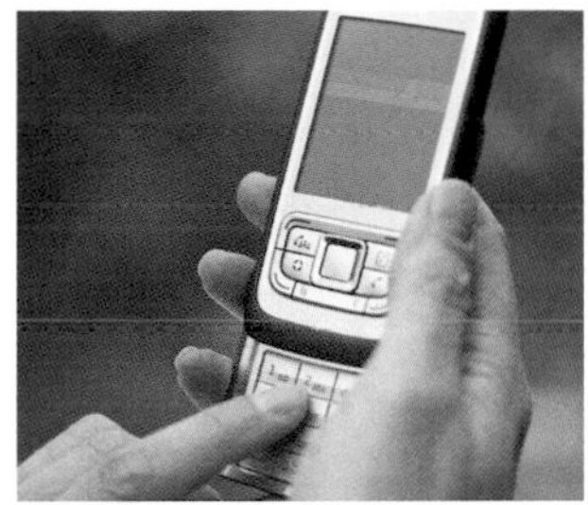

3 SUPPORT WITH SLINGS OR BANDAGES

For extra support or if help is delayed, secure the injured part to an uninjured part of the body. For upper body injuries, use a sling; for lower limb injuries, use broad- and narrow-fold bandages. Tie knots on the uninjured side.

4 TAKE OR SEND CASUALTY TO HOSPITAL

A casualty with an arm injury could be taken by car if not in shock; a leg injury should go by ambulance, so **call 999/112 for emergency help**. Treat for shock. Monitor and record the casualty's level of response, breathing and pulse until help arrives.

CAUTION

- Do not attempt to move an injured limb unnecessarily, or if it causes further pain.
- If there is an open wound, cover it with a sterile dressing or a clean, non-fluffy pad and bandage it in place.
- Do not give the casualty anything to eat or drink as an anaesthetic may be needed.
- Do not raise an injured leg when treating a casualty for shock.

FIND OUT MORE pp.165–67 ››

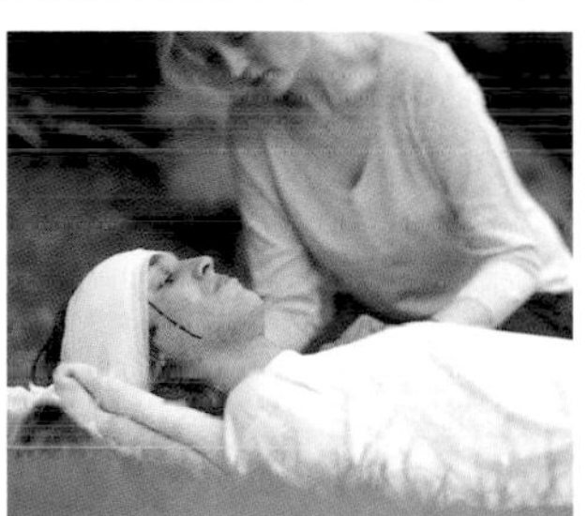

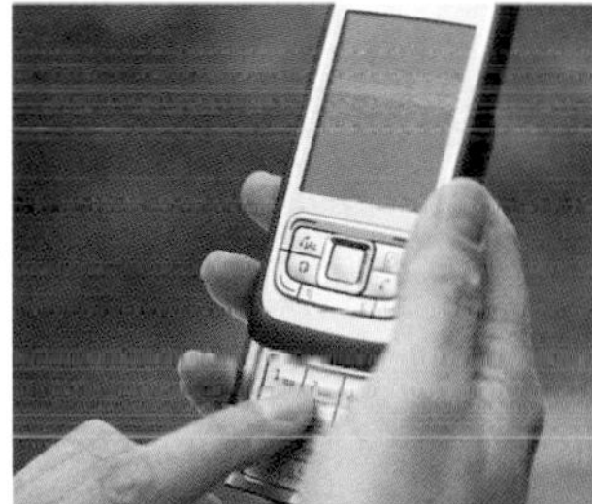

3 HELP CASUALTY TO LIE DOWN

Help the casualty to lie down, ideally on a blanket. Ensure that his head and shoulders are slightly raised. Make him as comfortable as possible.

4 CALL FOR EMERGENCY HELP

Call 999/112 for emergency help. Monitor and record vital signs – level of response, breathing and pulse – until help arrives.

CAUTION

- If blood seeps through the pad, place a second one on top of the first.
- Be aware of the possibility of concussion and compression.
- Monitor a casualty after a head injury. If he recovers initially, but deteriorates hours or days later, **call 999/112 for emergency help** immediately.
- If the casualty loses consciousness, open the airway and check breathing (p.256). Be prepared to begin CPR (pp.258–60).
- Always suspect the possibility of a neck (spinal) injury.

SEIZURES IN ADULTS

RECOGNITION

Seizures often follow a pattern:

- Sudden loss of consciousness, often with a cry;
- Rigidity and arching of the back;
- Breathing may become difficult. The lips may show a grey-blue tinge (cyanosis) and the face and neck may become red and puffy;
- Possible loss of bladder or bowel control;
- Muscles relax;
- After the seizure the casualty may be dazed and unaware of what has happened;
- Casualty falls into a deep sleep.

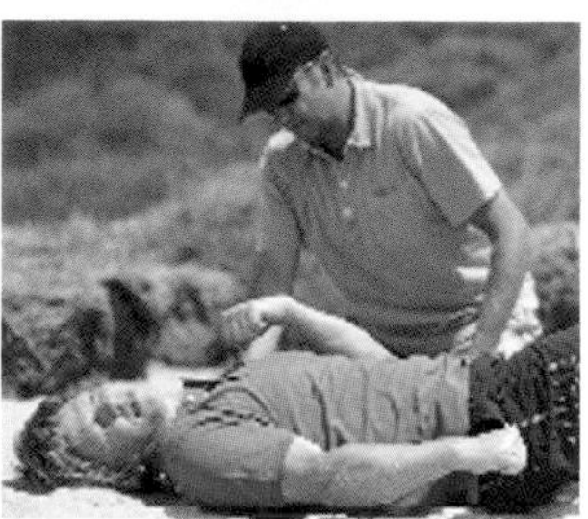

1 PROTECT CASUALTY

Try to ease the casualty's fall. Talk to him calmly and reassuringly. Clear away any potentially dangerous objects to prevent injury to the casualty. Ask bystanders to keep clear. Make a note of when the seizure began.

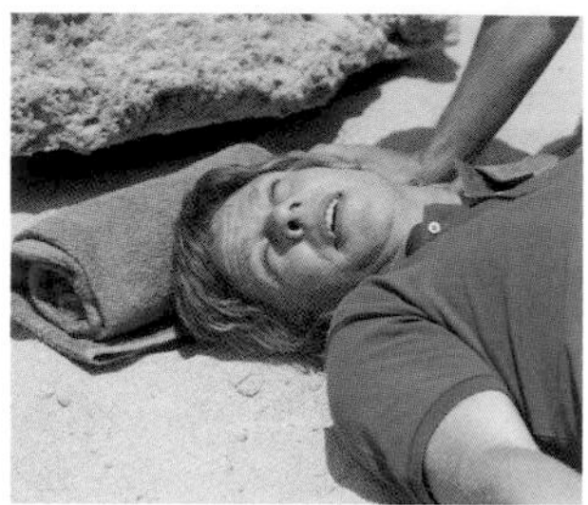

2 PROTECT HEAD AND LOOSEN TIGHT CLOTHING

If possible, cushion the casualty's head with soft material until the seizure ceases. Place padding to protect him from objects that cannot be moved. Loosen any tight clothing around the casualty's neck.

SEIZURES IN CHILDREN

RECOGNITION

- Violent muscle twitching, arched back and clenched fists.
- Signs of fever, such as hot, flushed skin.
- A twitching face and squinting, fixed or upturned eyes.
- Breath-holding, with red, puffy face and neck.
- Drooling at the mouth.
- Loss of, or impaired, consciousness.

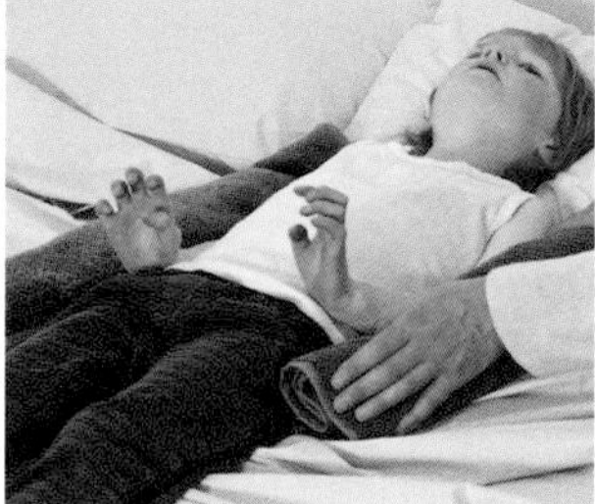

1 PROTECT CHILD FROM INJURY

Clear away any nearby objects and surround the child with soft padding, such as pillows or rolled towels, so that even violent movement will not result in injury.

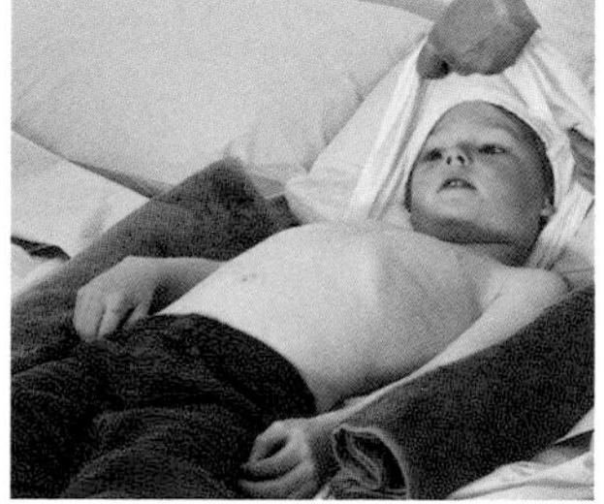

2 HELP THE CHILD COOL DOWN

Remove bedding and clothing, such as a vest or pyjama top; you may have to wait until the seizure stops to do this. Ensure a good supply of cool air, but do not let the child become too cold.

FIND OUT MORE **pp.168–69 ››**

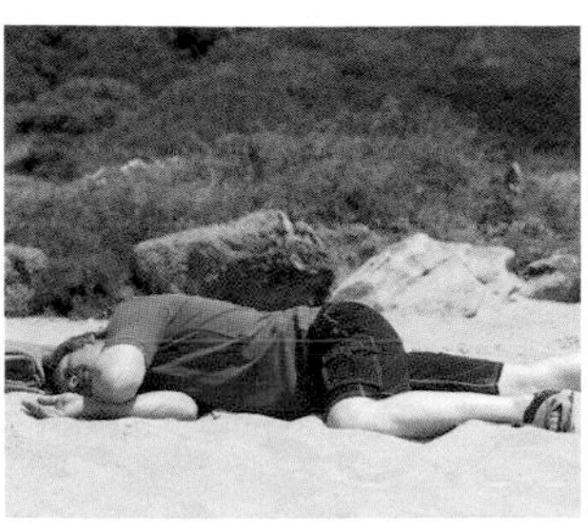

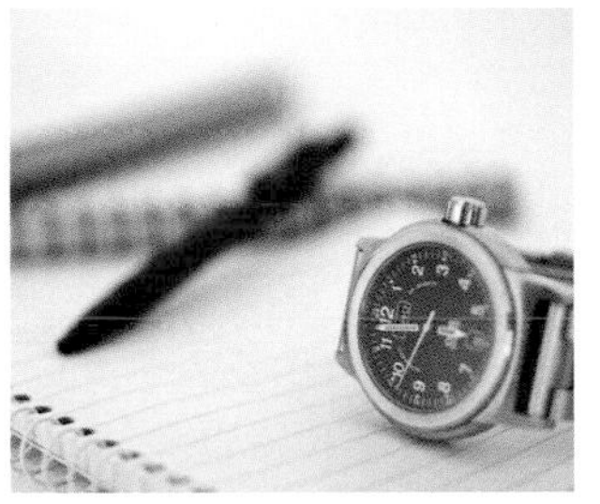

3 PLACE CASUALTY IN RECOVERY POSITION

Once the seizure has stopped the casualty may fall into a deep sleep. Open the airway and check breathing. If he is breathing, place him in the recovery position.

4 MONITOR CASUALTY'S RECOVERY

Monitor and record vital signs – level of response, breathing and pulse – until he recovers. Note the duration of the seizure.

CAUTION

- Do not attempt to restrain the casualty.
- Do not put anything in his mouth during a seizure.
- **Call 999/112 for emergency help** if the casualty is having repeated seizures, a seizure lasts more than five minutes, it is a casualty's first seizure or the casualty remains unconscious for more than ten minutes after the seizure.

FIND OUT MORE **p.170 ››**

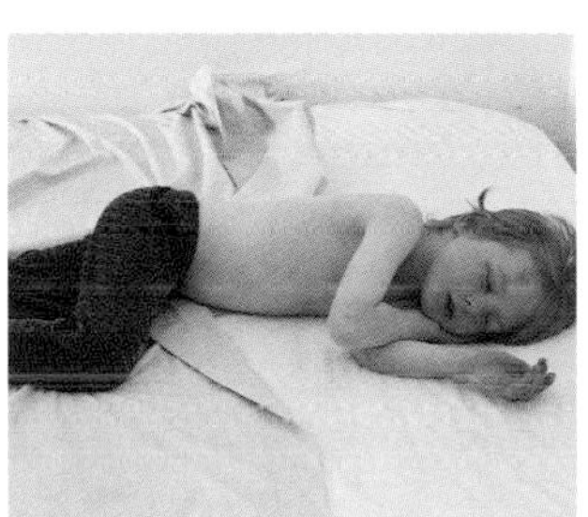

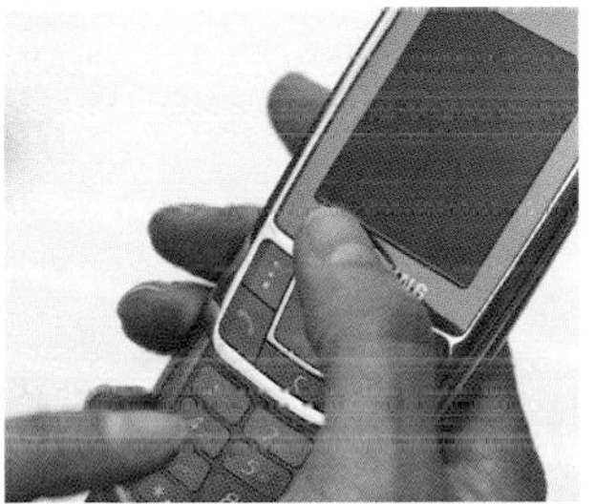

3 PLACE CHILD IN RECOVERY POSITION

Once the seizure has stopped, open the airway and check breathing (p.256). If the child is breathing, place him in the recovery position.

4 CALL FOR EMERGENCY HELP

Call 999/112 for emergency help. Reassure parents or carer, if necessary. Monitor and record the child's vital signs – level of response, breathing, pulse and temperature – until help arrives.

CAUTION

- Do not let the child get too cold.
- If the child loses consciousness, open the airway and check breathing (p.256). Be prepared to begin CPR (pp.258–60).

SPINAL INJURY

RECOGNITION

- Can occur after a fall from a height onto the back, head or feet.

There may be:

- Pain in neck or back;
- Step, irregularity or twist in the normal curve of the spine;
- Tenderness in the skin over the spine.
- Weakness or loss of movement in the limbs;
- Loss of sensation, or abnormal sensation;
- Loss of bladder and/or bowel control;
- Difficulty breathing.

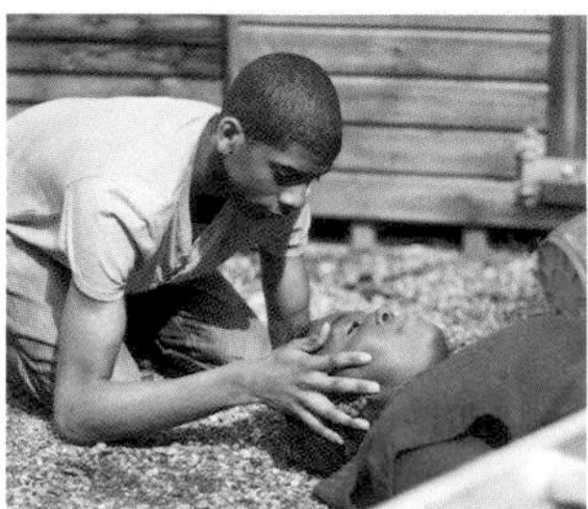

1 STEADY AND SUPPORT HEAD

Tell the casualty not to move. Sit or kneel behind her head and, resting your arms on the ground, grasp either side of the casualty's head and hold it still. Do not cover her ears.

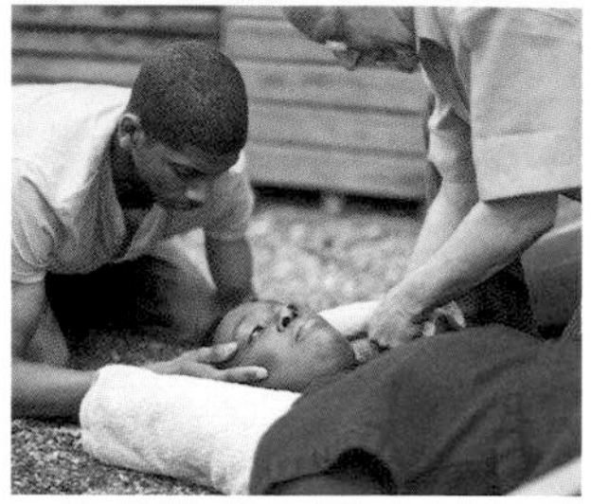

2 PLACE EXTRA SUPPORT AROUND HEAD

Continue to hold her head and ask a helper to place rolled towels, or other padding, around the casualty's neck and shoulders for extra support.

STROKE

RECOGNITION

Use the FAST (Face – Arms – Speech – Time) guide (p.174) to assess the casualty.

- Facial weakness – casualty is unable to smile evenly.
- Arm weakness – casualty may only be able to move his arm on one side of his body.
- Speech problems.

There may also be:

- Weakness or numbness along one side of entire body;
- Sudden blurring or loss of vision;
- Difficulty understanding the spoken word;
- Sudden confusion;
- Dizziness, unsteadiness or a sudden fall.

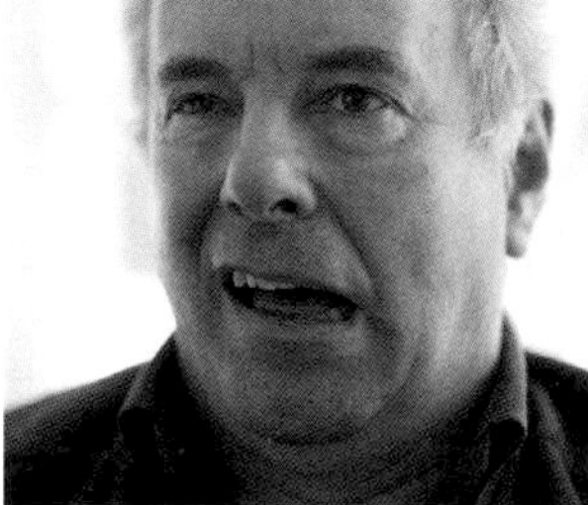

1 CHECK CASUALTY'S FACE

Keep the casualty comfortable. Ask him to smile. If he has had a stroke, he may only be able to smile on one side – the other side of his face may droop.

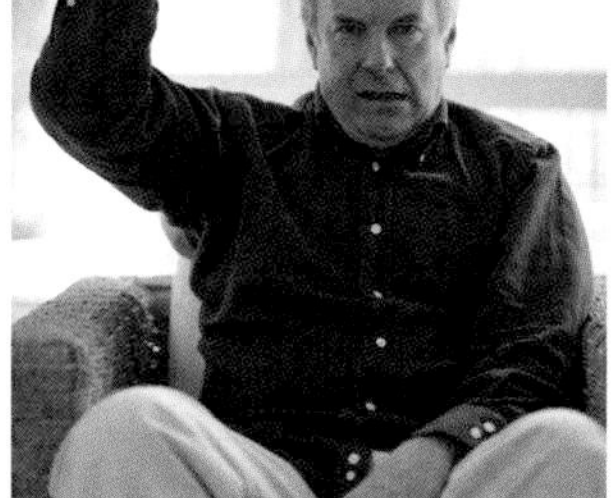

2 CHECK CASUALTY'S ARMS

Ask the casualty to raise his arms. If he has had a stroke, he may only be able to lift one arm.

FIND OUT MORE pp.171–73 ››

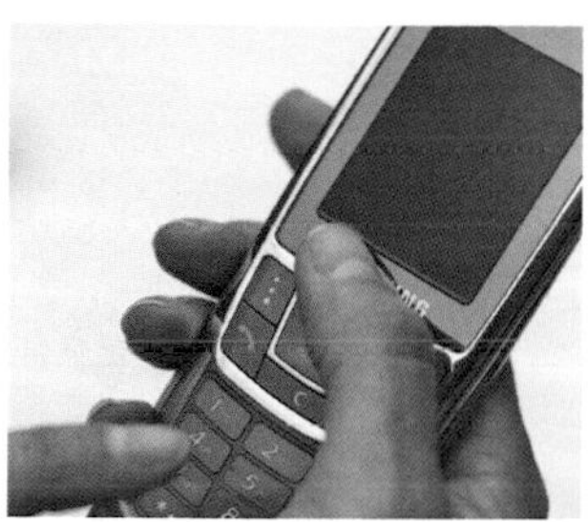

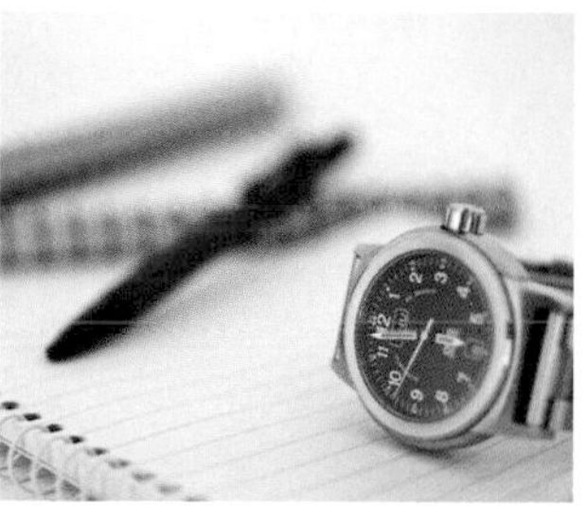

3 CALL FOR EMERGENCY HELP

Call 999/112 for emergency help. If possible, ask a helper to make the call while you support the head and neck. Tell ambulance control that a spinal injury is suspected.

4 MONITOR CASUALTY

Monitor and record the casualty's vital signs – level of response, breathing and pulse – until help arrives.

CAUTION

- Do not move the casualty unless she is in danger.
- If the casualty is unconscious, open the airway by gently lifting the jaw, but do not tilt the head, then check breathing (p.256) Be prepared to begin CPR (pp.258–60).
- If you need to turn the casualty into the recovery position use the log-roll technique.

FIND OUT MORE pp.174–75 ››

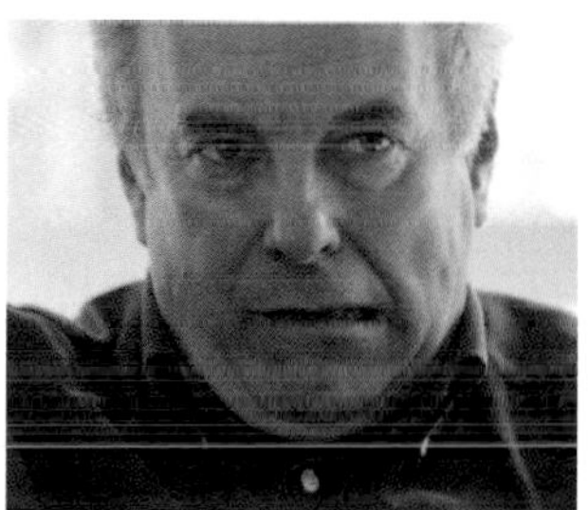

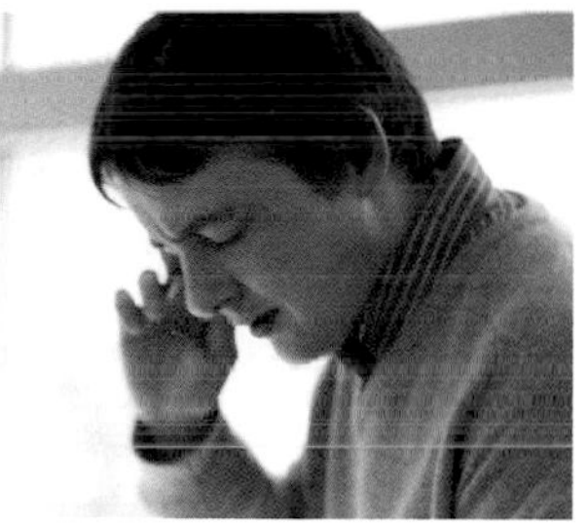

3 CHECK CASUALTY'S SPEECH

Ask the casualty some questions. Can he speak and/or understand what you are saying?

4 CALL FOR EMERGENCY HELP

Call 999/112 for emergency help. Tell ambulance control that you suspect a stroke. Reassure the casualty and monitor and record his vital signs – level of response, breathing and pulse – until help arrives.

CAUTION

- Do not give the casualty anything to eat or drink; he will probably find it difficult to swallow. If the casualty loses consciousness, open the airway and check breathing (p.256). Be prepared to begin CPR (p.258).

BURNS AND SCALDS

RECOGNITION

There may be:

- Possible areas of superficial, partial-thickness and/or full-thickness burns;
- Pain in the area of the burn;
- Breathing difficulties if the airway is affected;
- Swelling and blistering of the skin;
- Signs of shock.

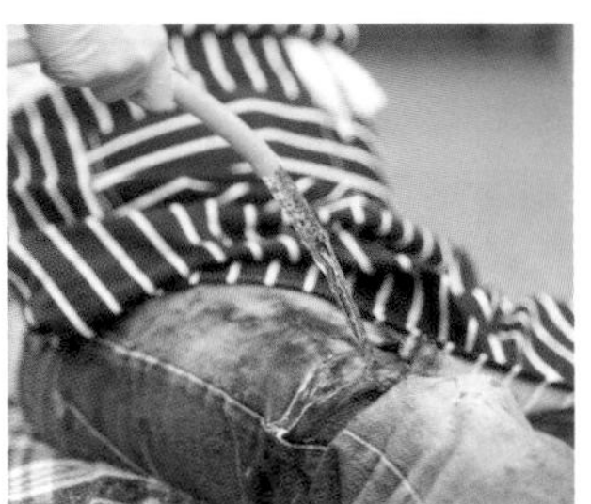

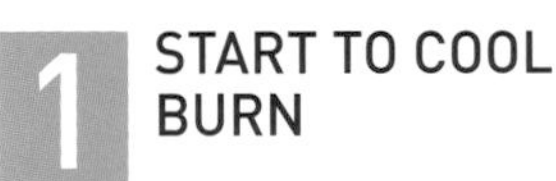

1 START TO COOL BURN

Make the casualty comfortable by helping him to sit or lie down. Flood the injury with cold water; cool for at least ten minutes or until pain is relieved.

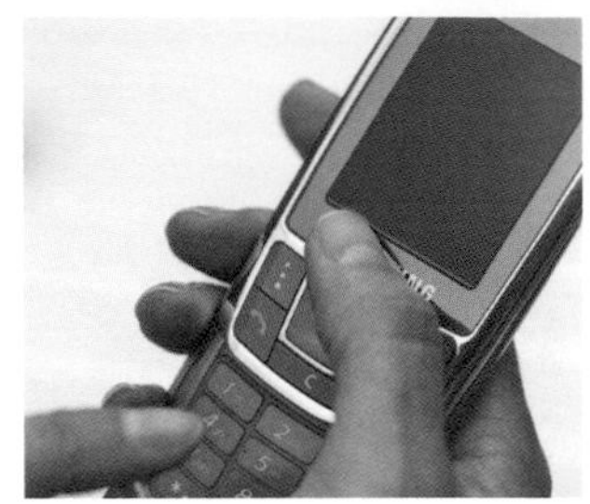

2 CALL FOR EMERGENCY HELP

Call 999/112 for emergency help if necessary. Tell ambulance control that the injury is a burn and explain what caused it, and the estimated size and depth.

HYPOTHERMIA

RECOGNITION

- Shivering, and cold, pale, dry skin.
- Apathy, disorientation or irrational behaviour.
- Lethargy.
- Impaired consciousness.
- Slow and shallow breathing.
- Slow and weakening pulse. In extreme cases, the heart may stop altogether.

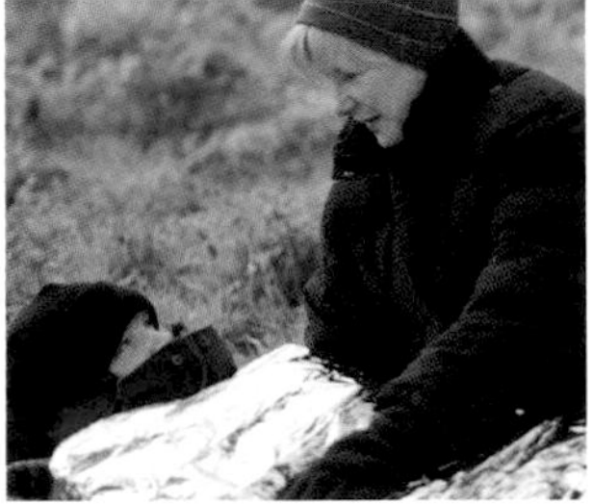

1 RE-WARM CASUALTY GRADUALLY

Shelter the casualty. Lay him on a layer of dry insulating material. Put him in a sleeping bag and/or wrap him in a survival blanket. Do not heat the casualty too rapidly. Warm him with your body too.

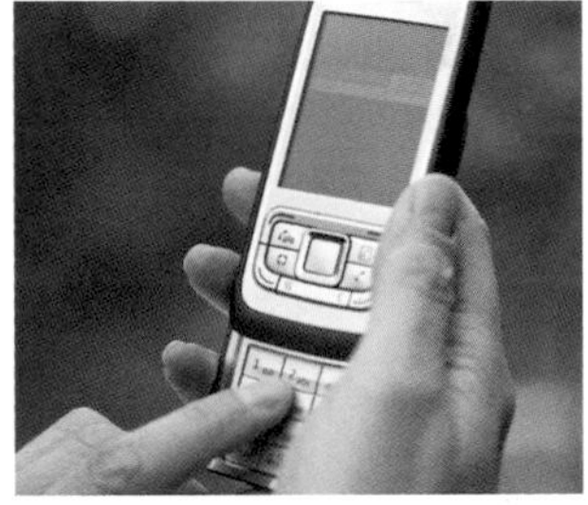

2 CALL FOR EMERGENCY HELP

Call 999/112 for emergency help. Ideally, two people should go for help if you are in a remote area, staying together at all times. Someone must remain with the casualty.

FIND OUT MORE **pp.182–87>>**

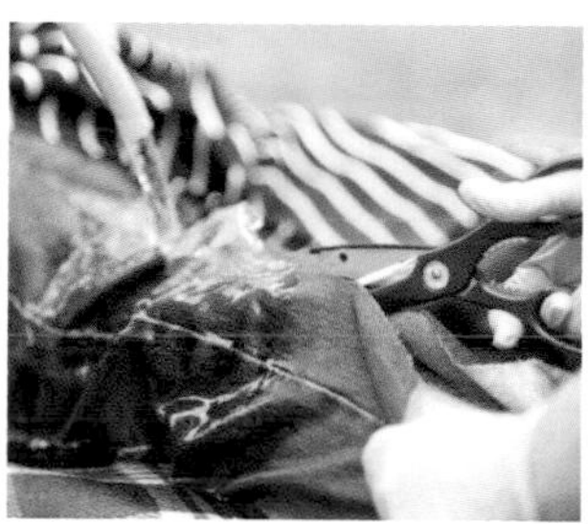

3 REMOVE ANY CONSTRICTIONS

While you are cooling the burn, carefully remove any clothing or jewellery from the area before it starts to swell; a helper can do this for you. Do not remove anything that is sticking to the burn.

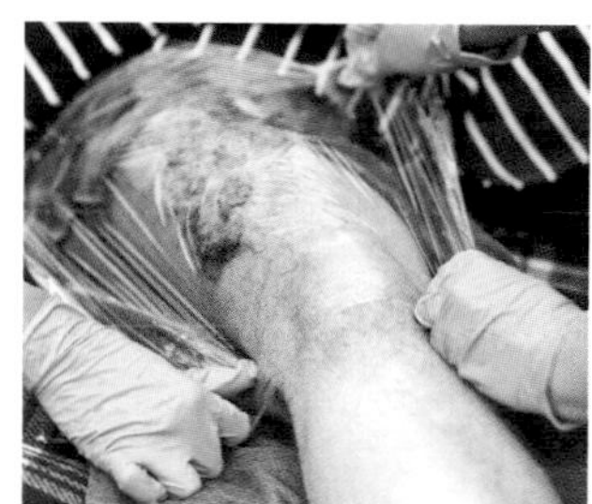

4 COVER BURN

Cover the burn with kitchen film placed lengthways over the injury, or use a plastic bag. Alternatively, use a sterile dressing or clean, non-fluffy pad. Monitor and record the casualty's level of response, breathing and pulse while waiting for help.

CAUTIONS

- Do not apply lotions, ointment or fat to a burn; specialised dressings are also not recommended.
- Do not use adhesive dressings.
- Do not touch the burn or burst any blisters.
- If the burn is severe, treat the casualty for shock (p.266).
- If the burn is on the face, do not cover it. Keep cooling with water until help arrives.
- If the burn is caused by contact with chemicals, wear protective gloves and cool for at least 20 minutes.
- Watch the casualty for signs of smoke inhalation, such as difficulty breathing.

FIND OUT MORE **pp.194–96 >>**

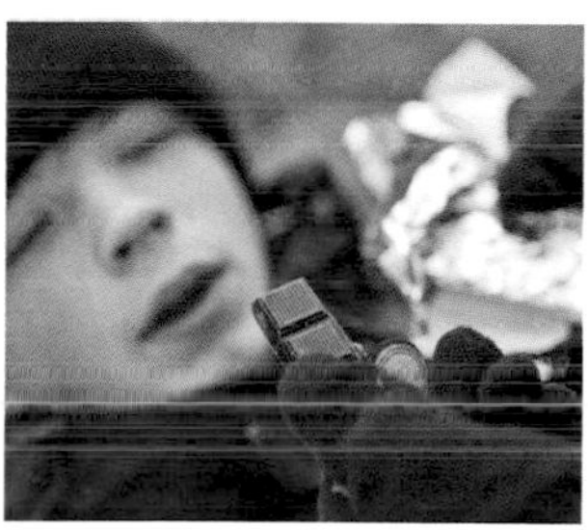

3 GIVE CASUALTY HIGH-ENERGY FOODS

Give the casualty high-energy foods – chocolate and/or a warm drink such as soup – to help re-warm him.

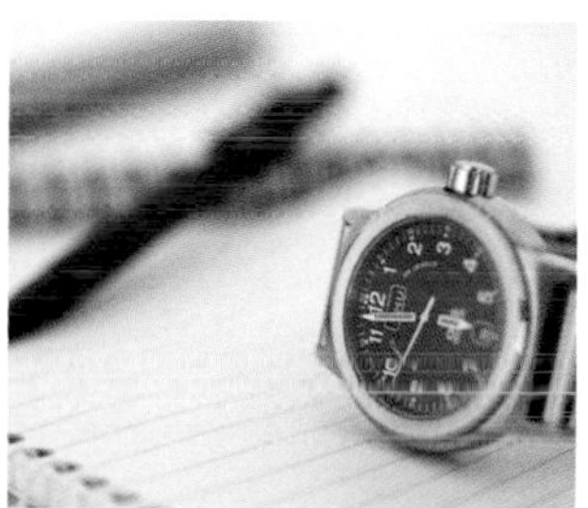

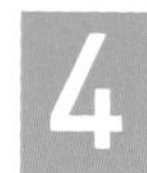

4 MONITOR CASUALTY

Monitor and record vital signs – level of response, breathing, pulse and temperature – until emergency help arrives. The casualty needs to be taken to hospital on a stretcher.

CAUTION

- Hypothermia in an elderly person may disguise the symptoms of a heart attack, stroke or an underactive thyroid gland.
- Do not place a heat source such as a hot water bottle or fire next to a casualty. It can mobilise blood too rapidly and divert it suddenly from the heart and brain to the skin. It could also burn the casualty.
- Do not give the casualty alcohol because this will worsen the hypothermia.
- Make sure you keep warm.
- Re-warm an elderly casualty indoors by wrapping him in blankets. Put a hat on his head for extra warmth.

SWALLOWED POISONS

RECOGNITION

- A history of ingestion/ exposure to poison; evidence of poison nearby.

Depending on what the casualty has taken, there may be:

- Vomit that may be bloodstained;
- Diarrhoea;
- Cramping abdominal pains;
- Pain or burning sensation;
- Impaired consciousness.

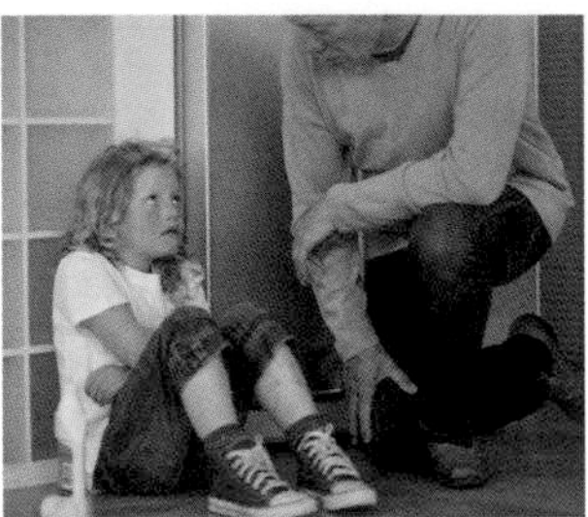

1 IDENTIFY THE POISON

Reassure the casualty. If she is conscious, ask her what she has swallowed. Look for clues such as poisonous leaves or berries, containers or pill bottles.

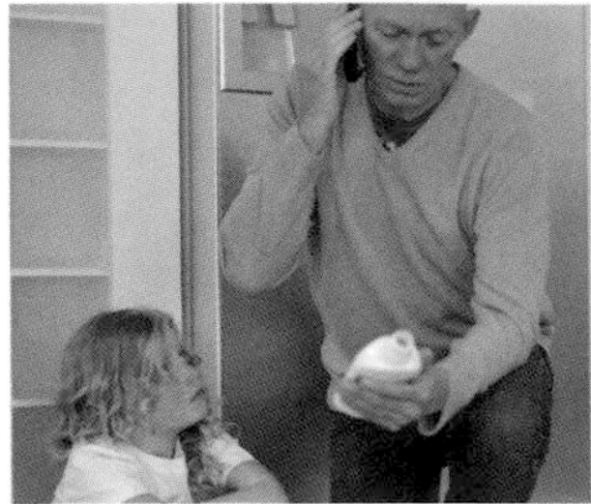

2 CALL FOR EMERGENCY HELP

Call 999/112 for emergency help. Give ambulance control as much information as possible. Find out what she took, how much and when. This helps doctors to give the casualty the correct treatment.

HYPOGLYCAEMIA

RECOGNITION

There may be:

- A history of diabetes – the casualty may recognise the onset of a hypo (low blood sugar) attack;
- Weakness, faintness or hunger;
- Confusion and irrational behaviour;
- Sweating with cold, clammy skin;
- Palpitations and muscle tremors;
- A deteriorating level of response;
- A medical alert tag or bracelet, glucose gel, medication or insulin syringe/pen in his possessions.

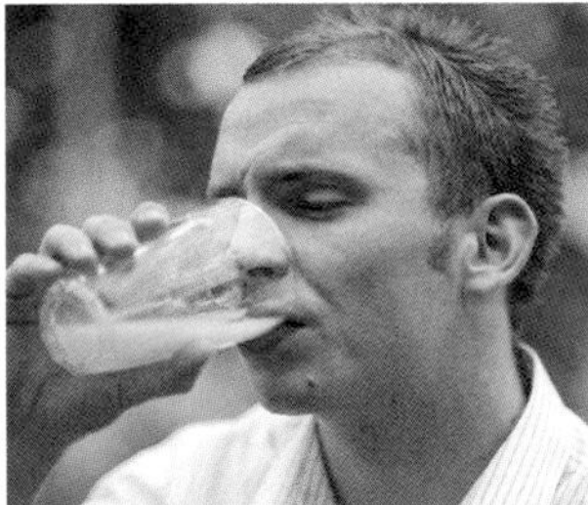

1 GIVE CASUALTY SUGAR

Help the casualty to sit down. Give him a sugary drink.

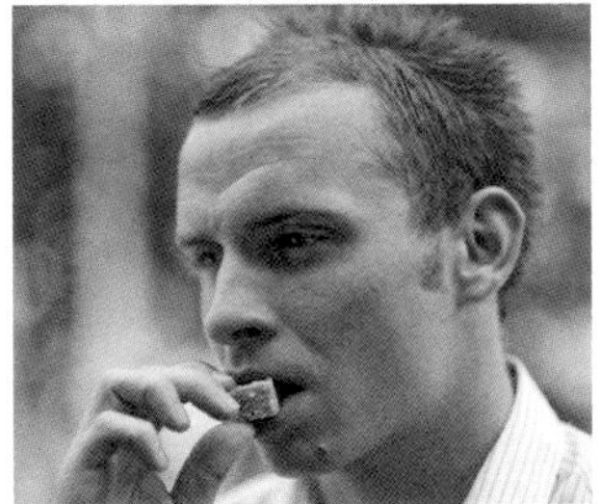

2 GIVE SOME SUGARY FOOD

If the casualty responds to the drink, give him more sugar in the form of sugar lumps or sweet food. If he has glucose gel help him take it. Help him to find his glucose testing kit so that he can check his glucose levels.

FIND OUT MORE pp.207–10 ››

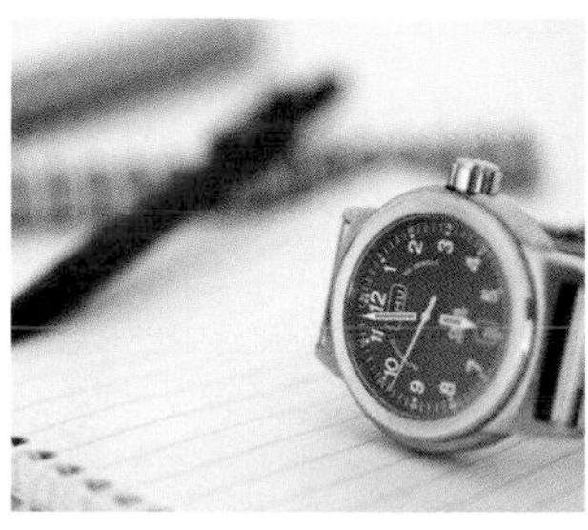

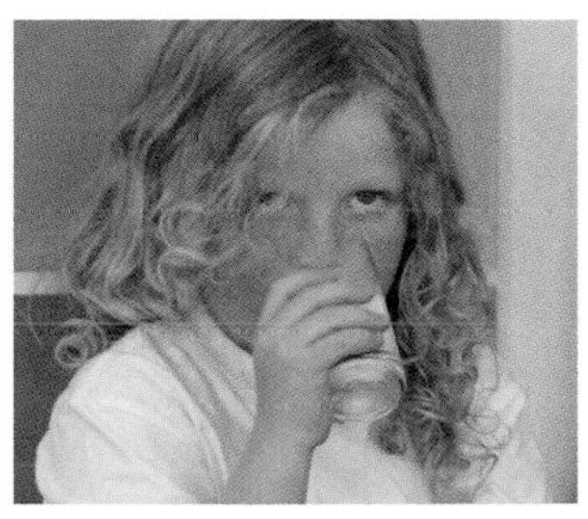

3 MONITOR CASUALTY

Monitor and record the casualty's vital signs – level of response, breathing and pulse – until help arrives.

4 IF CASUALTY'S LIPS ARE BURNT

If the casualty has swallowed a substance that has burnt her lips, give her frequent sips of cool milk or water.

CAUTION

- Do not attempt to induce vomiting.
- If the casualty is contaminated with chemicals, wear protective equipment such as disposable gloves, a mask and goggles if you have them.
- If the casualty loses consciousness, make sure that there is no vomit or other matter in the mouth. Open the airway and check breathing (p.256). Be prepared to begin CPR (pp.258–60).
- If there are chemicals on the casualty's mouth, protect yourself by using a face shield or pocket mask when giving rescue breaths.

FIND OUT MORE p.219››

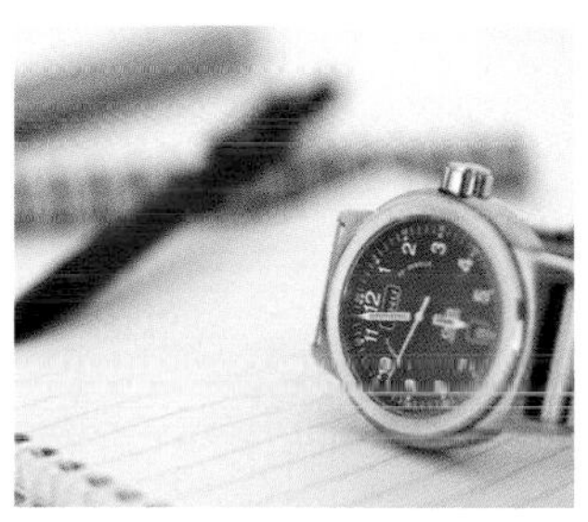

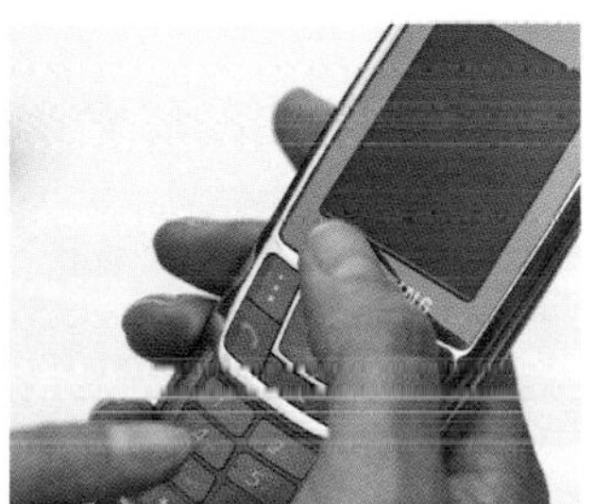

3 MONITOR CASUALTY

Monitor and record the casualty's vital signs – level of response, breathing and pulse – until he is fully recovered.

4 CALL FOR EMERGENCY HELP

If the casualty's condition does not improve, look for other causes of his condition. **Call 999/112 for emergency help.** Continue to monitor his vital signs until help arrives.

CAUTION

- If consciousness is impaired, do not give the casualty anything to eat or drink.
- If the casualty loses consciousness, open the airway and check breathing (p.256). Be prepared to begin CPR (pp.258–59).

ANAPHYLACTIC SHOCK

RECOGNITION

There may be:

- Anxiety;
- Red, blotchy skin, itchy rash and red, itchy, watery eyes;
- Swelling of hands, feet and face;
- Puffiness around the eyes;
- Abdominal pain, vomiting and diarrhoea;
- Difficulty breathing, ranging from tight chest to severe difficulty, which causes wheezing and gasping for air;
- Swelling of tongue and throat;
- A feeling of terror;
- Confusion and agitation;
- Signs of shock (p.266) leading to unconsciousness.

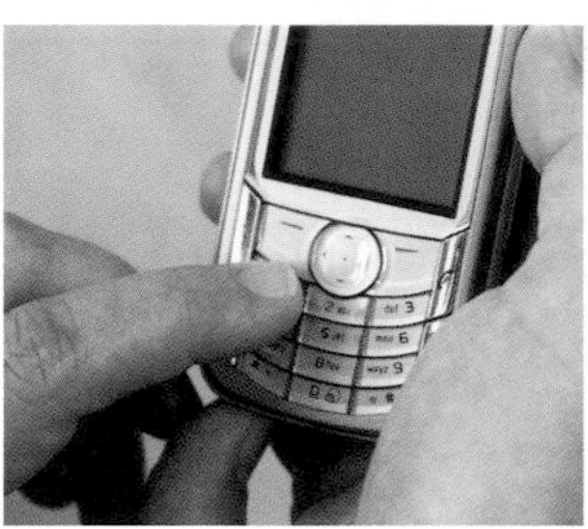

1 CALL FOR EMERGENCY HELP

Call 999/112 for emergency help. Ideally, ask someone to make the call while you treat the casualty. Tell ambulance control that you suspect anaphylaxis and let them know the possible cause.

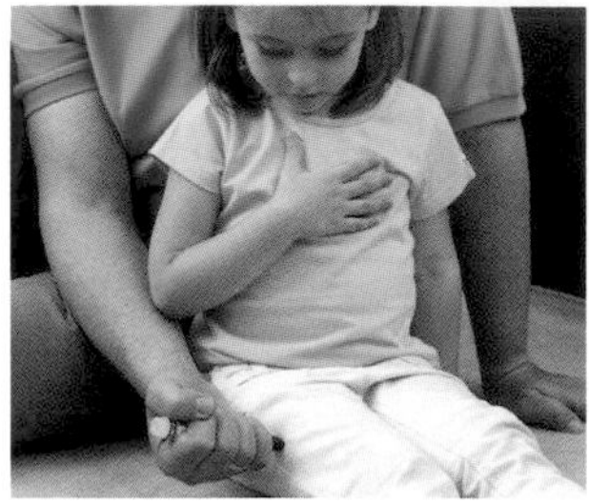

2 HELP CASUALTY WITH MEDICATION

Check whether the casualty has a syringe or an auto-injector of adrenaline (epinephrine). If trained, help her use it. Hold it in your fist, pull off the safety cap and place the tip firmly against the casualty's thigh (through clothing if necessary).

MENINGITIS

RECOGNITION

Some, but not all, of these symptoms may be present:

- Flu-like illness with a high temperature;
- Cold hands and feet;
- Joint and/or limb pain;
- Mottled or very pale skin.

As infection develops:

- Neck stiffness;
- Eyes become sensitive to light;
- Drowsiness;
- A distinctive rash of red or purple spots that look like bruises and do not fade when pressed;
- In infants, a high-pitched moaning or whimpering cry, floppiness and a tense or bulging fontanelle (soft part of the skull).

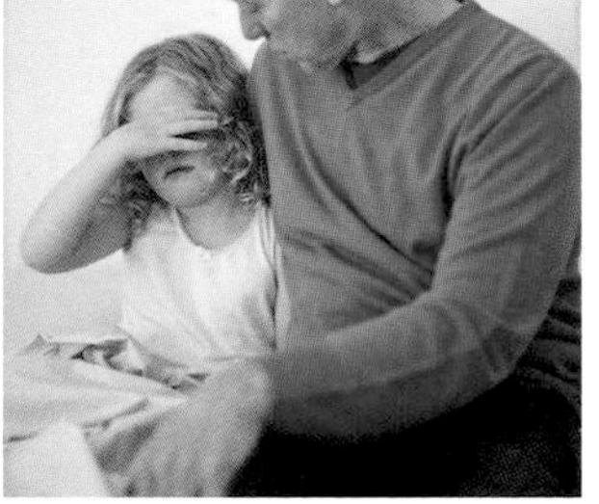

1 SEEK MEDICAL ADVICE

If you notice any signs of meningitis, such as the casualty shielding her eyes from light or a stiff neck, seek urgent medical advice.

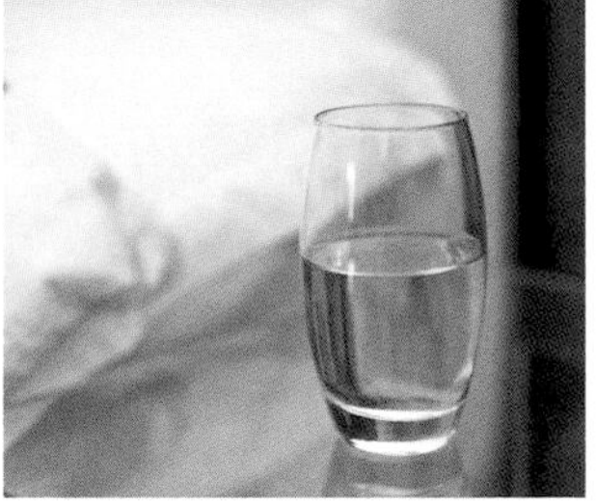

2 TREAT FEVER

Keep the casualty cool and give plenty of water to replace fluids lost through sweating. An adult may take the recommended dose of paracetamol tablets; a child may have the recommended dose of paracetamol syrup.

FIND OUT MORE p.221>>

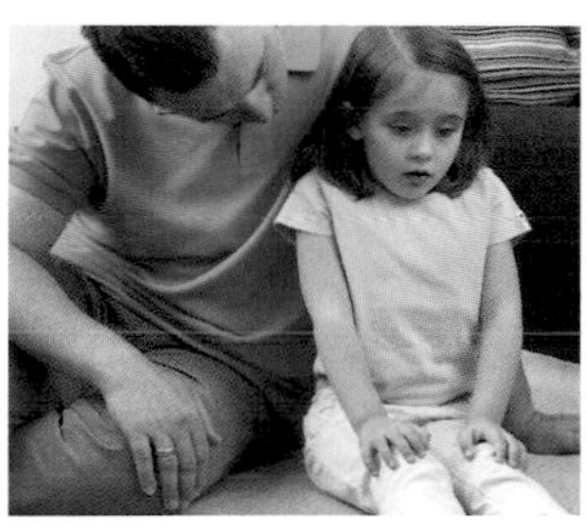

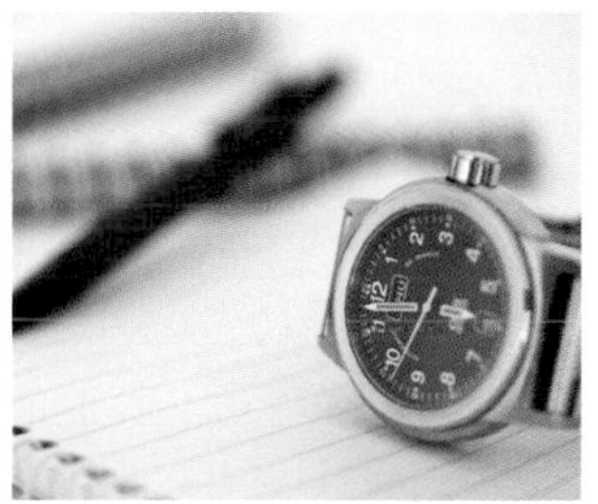

3 MAKE CASUALTY COMFORTABLE

Reassure the casualty and help her to sit in a position that eases any breathing difficulties. If she becomes very pale with a weak pulse, lay her down with legs raised as for shock.

4 MONITOR CASUALTY

Monitor and record vital signs – level of response, breathing and pulse – until help arrives. Repeat the adrenaline (epinephrine) dose every five minutes if there is no improvement or the casualty's symptoms return.

CAUTION

- If the casualty loses consciousness, open the airway and check breathing (p.256). Be prepared to begin CPR (pp.258–60).

FIND OUT MORE p.223 >>

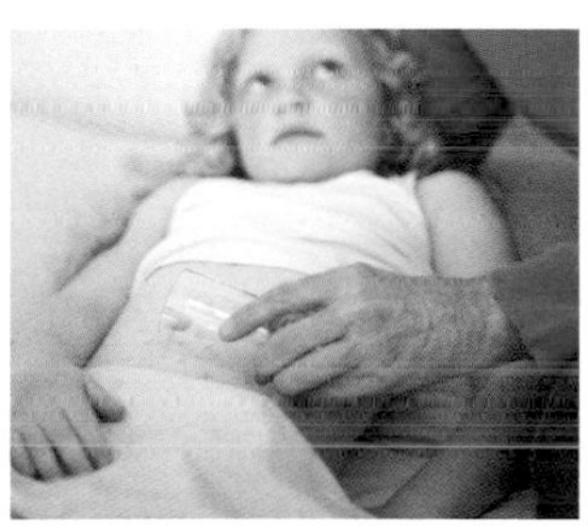

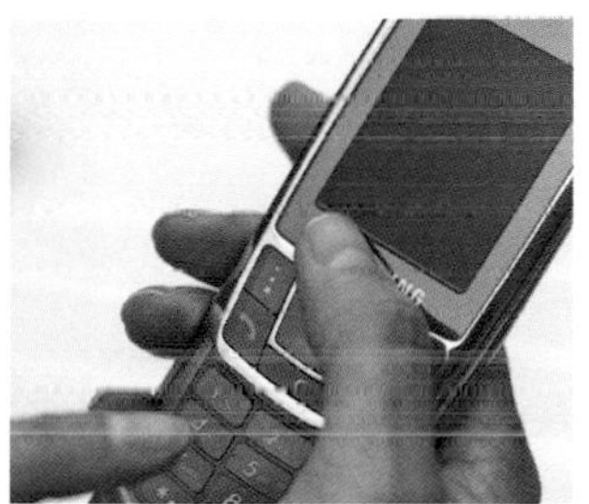

3 CHECK FOR SIGNS OF RASH

Check the casualty for signs of the meningitis rash: press against the rash with the side of a glass. Most rashes will fade when pressed; if you can still see the rash through the glass, it is probably meningitis.

4 CALL FOR EMERGENCY HELP

Call 999/112 for emergency help if you see signs of the rash, or if medical help is delayed. Reassure the casualty. Keep her cool and monitor and record level of response, breathing and pulse until help arrives.

CAUTION

- If the casualty loses consciousness, open the airway and check breathing (p.256). Be prepared to begin CPR (pp.258–60).

FIRST AID REGULATIONS

First aid may be practised in any situation where injuries or illnesses occur. In many cases, the first person on the scene is a volunteer who wants to help, rather than someone who is medically trained. However, in certain circumstances the provision of first aid, and first aid responsibilities, is defined by statutes. In the UK, these regulations apply to incidents occurring in the workplace and to mass gatherings.

FIRST AID AT WORK

The Health and Safety (First Aid) Regulations of 1981 place a general duty on employers to make first aid provision for employees in case of injury or illness in the workplace. The practical aspects of this statutory duty for employers and for self-employed persons are set out in the Approved Code of Practice (ACOP), which is revised periodically to ensure that the appropriate standards are maintained. Regular occupational first aiders should make sure they are familiar with the ACOP and Guidance Notes.

The current ACOP stresses the aims of the first aid provision and encourages all employers to assess their organisation's ability to meet those aims. The number of specific first aiders required in a specific workplace is dependent on the needs assessment, which should be carried out by the Health and Safety Representative in the workplace. There is a checklist (opposite) to help determine the personnel required: depending on the workplace, this ranges from an appointed person, to those trained in emergency first aid at work (EFAW) or first aid at work (FAW). The ACOP also contains guidance on first aid materials, equipment and facilities.

Comprehensive advice can also be found at www.hse.gov.uk/firstaid/.

ACCIDENT BOOK

An employer has the overall responsibility for an accident book, but it is the responsibility of the first aider or appointed person to look after and note details of incidents in the book.

If an employee is involved in an incident in the workplace, the following details should be recorded in the accident book.

- **Date, time and place** of incident;
- **Name and job** of the injured or ill person.
- **Details of the injury/illness** and what first aid was given.
- **What happened** to the person immediately afterwards (for example, went home or taken to hospital).
- **Name and signature** of the first aider or person dealing with the incident.

REPORTING OF INJURIES, DISEASES AND DANGEROUS OCCURRENCES

In the event of injury or ill health at work, an employer has a legal obligation to report the incident. The Reporting of Injuries, Diseases and Dangerous Occurrences Regulations 1995 (RIDDOR) requires an employer to report the following:

- **Deaths.**
- **Major injuries.**
- **Injuries lasting more than three days** – where an employee or self-employed person is away from work or unable to perform their normal work duties for more than three consecutive days;
- **Injuries to members of the public** or people not at work, where they are taken from the scene of an accident to hospital;
- **Some work-related diseases.**
- **Some dangerous occurrences** such as a near miss, where something happens that could have resulted in an injury, although it did not.

CHECKLIST FOR ASSESSMENT OF FIRST AID NEEDS	
FACTORS TO CONSIDER	
Is your workplace low risk (for example, shops, offices and libraries)?	**The minimum provision is:** ■ An appointed person to take charge of first aid arrangements ■ A suitably stocked first aid box. As there is a possibility of an accident or sudden illness consider providing a qualified first aider. **First aider requirements:** ■ For fewer than 25 employees, one appointed person; for 25–50 employees, at least one first aider trained in EFAW; for over 50 employees, one FAW trained first aider for every 100 employees (or part thereof). **Where there are large numbers of employees consider:** ■ Additional first aid equipment ■ A first aid room.
Is your workplace higher risk (for example light engineering and assembly work, food processing, warehousing, extensive work with dangerous machinery or sharp instruments, construction or chemical manufacture). Do your work activities involve special hazards, such as hydrofluoric acid or confined spaces?	**The minimum provision is:** ■ An appointed person to take charge of first aid arrangements ■ A suitably stocked first aid box. **First aider requirements:** ■ For fewer than five employees, one appointed person; for 5–50 employees, at least one first aider trained in EFAW or FAW dependng on the type of injuries that could occur; for over 50 employees, at least one FAW trained first aider for every 50 employees (or part thereof). **Consider:** ■ Additional training for first aiders to deal with injuries resulting from special hazards ■ Additional first aid equipment ■ Precise siting of first aid equipment ■ Providing a first aid room ■ Informing the emergency services if there are chemicals on site.
Are there inexperienced workers on site, or employees with disabilities or special health problems?	**Consider:** ■ Additional training for first aiders ■ Additional first aid equipment ■ Local siting of first-aid equipment. Your first aid provision should cover any work experience trainees.
What is your record of accidents and ill health? What injuries and illness have occurred and where?	Ensure your first aid provision caters for the type of injury and illness that might occur in your workplace. Monitor accidents and ill health and review your first aid provision as appropriate.
Do you have employees who travel a lot, work remotely or work alone?	**Consider:** ■ Personal first aid kits ■ Personal communicators or mobile phones for remote or lone workers.
Do any of your employees work shifts or work out of hours?	Ensure there is adequate first aid provision at all times while people are at work.
Are the premises spread out; for example, are there several buildings on the site or multi-floor buildings?	**Consider:** ■ First aid provision in each building or on each floor.
Is your workplace remote from emergency medical services?	**Consider:** ■ Special arrangements with the emergency services ■ Informing the emergency services of your location
Do any of your employees work at sites occupied by other employers?	Make arrangements with other site occupiers to ensure adequate provision of first aid. A written agreement between employers is strongly recommended.
Do you have sufficient provision to cover absences of first aiders or appointed persons?	**Consider what cover is needed for:** ■ Annual leave and other planned absences ■ Unplanned and exceptional absences.
Do members of the public visit your premises (for example, schools, places of entertainment, fairgrounds, shops)?	Under the regulations, there is no legal obligation to provide first aid for non-employees, but the Health and Safety Executive (HSE), strongly recommends that you consider the members of the public when planning your first aid provision.

INDEX

ACKNOWLEDGMENTS

AUTHORS OF 9TH EDITION (REVISED)

ST JOHN AMBULANCE
Dr Margaret Austin LRCPI LRSCI LM
Deputy Chief Medical Officer

ST ANDREW'S FIRST AID
Mr Rudy Crawford MBE BSc (Hons) MB ChB FRCS (Glasg) FCEM
Chairman of the Board

BRITISH RED CROSS
Dr Vivien J. Armstrong MBBS DRCOG FRCA PGCE (FE)
Chief Medical Adviser

CO-AUTHORS OF 9TH EDITION
Dr Meng AwYong BSc MBBS DFMS Medical Adviser, St John Ambulance; **John Newman** Head of Emergency Operations, St John Ambulance; **Joe Mulligan** Head of First Aid Education, British Red Cross; **Dr Sarah Davidson** MBE BSc (Hons) Clin PsyD CPsychol Psychosocial Adviser, British Red Cross

TRIPARTITE COMMERCIAL COMMITTEE

ST JOHN AMBULANCE
Richard Evens
Director of Training
Richard Fernandez
Head of Communications
Andrew New
Commercial Project Manager

ST ANDREW'S FIRST AID
Carla Mackay
Communications Manager
Jim Dorman
Training Manager
John Roche
Supplies Manager

BRITISH RED CROSS
Katrina Thornton
Head of Purchasing and Supply
Nadine Gower
First Aid Education Marketing Manager

AUTHORS' ACKNOWLEDGMENTS
The authors would like to extend special thanks to: Alison Stevens, Marketing Information Manager, St John Ambulance; Jim Dorman, Training Manager, St Andrew's First Aid; Stewart Simpson, Training Adviser, St Andrew's First Aid; Joslyn Kofi Opata, Administrator British Red Cross; Dr Peter Beaumont; Steven Hines.

PUBLISHERS' ACKNOWLEDGMENTS
Dorling Kindersley would like to thank: Cardiac Science for the loan of the AED, Frith Manor Riding Stables, Simon Tuite for editorial assistance, Steve Woosnam-Savage for design assistance, Steve Willis for colour retouching, Caroline Hunt and Diana Vowles for proofreading the text and Dorothy Frame for the index.

Dorling Kindersley would also like to thank the following people who appear as models:
Lyndon Allen, Gillian Andrews, Kayko Andrieux, Mags Ashcroft, Nicholas Austin, Neil Bamford, Jay Benedict, Joseph Bevan, Bob Bridle, Gerard Brown, Helen Brown, Jennifer Brown, Val Brown, Michelle Burke, Tamlyn Calitz, Tyler Chambers, Evie Clark, Tim Clark, Junior Cole, Sue Cooper, Linda Dare, Julia Davies, Simon Davis, Tom Defrates, Louise Dick, Jemima Dunne, Maria Elia, Phil Fitzgerald, Alex Gayer, John Goldsmid, Stephen Hines, Nicola Hodgson, Clare Joyce, Jennifer Irving, Dan James, Megan Jones, Dallas Kidman, Carol King, Andrea Kofi-Opata, Andrews Kofi-Opata, Edna Kofi-Opata, Joslyn Kofi-Opata, Tim Lane, Libby Lawson, Wren Lawson-Foley, Daniel Lee, Crispin Lord, Danny Lord, Harriet Lord, Phil Lord, Gareth Lowe, Mulkina Mackay, Ethan Mackay-Wardle, Ben Marcus, Catherine McCormick, Fiona McDonald, Alfie McMeeking, Cath McMeeking, Archie Midgley, David Midgley, Gary Moore, Sandra Newman, Matt Robbins, Dean Morris, Eva Mulligan, Priscilla Nelson-Cole, Emma Noppers, Phil Ormerod, Julie Oughton, Andrew Roff, Ian Rowland, Phil Sergeant, Vicky Short, Gregory Small, Andrew Smith, Emily Smith, Sophie Smith, Bev Speight, Silke Spingies, David Swinson, Hannah Swinson, Laura Swinson, Becky Tennant, Laura Tester, Pip Tinsley, Daniel Toorie, Adam Walker, Jonathan Ward, David Wardle, Dion Wardle, Angela Wilkes, Liz Wheeler, Jenny Woodcock, Nigel Wright, Nan Zhang.

Picture credits Dorling Kindersley would like to thank the following for their kind permission to reproduce their photographs: Getty Images: Andrew Boyd 176–77.